Human Metapneumovirus

Advances in Research and Clinical Applications

nova
Medicine & Health
New York

Pulmonary and Respiratory Diseases and Disorders Series

Pulmonary Hypertension and Lung Transplantation
Roberto G. Carbone, MD, FCCP, Francesco Puppo, MD and Deborah Jo Levine, MD
ISBN: 979-8-89530-598-0
eBook ISBN: 979-8-89530-704-5

Respiratory Care in Heliox Therapy Physiology and Technology
Antonio M. Esquinas, MD, PhD, FCCP, FAARC
ISBN: 979-8-89530-385-6
eBook ISBN: 979-8-89530-519-5

Bronchopneumonia: Pathogenesis, Clinical Insights and Therapeutic Approaches
Salim Surani, MD, MPH, MSHM, FACP, FAASM, FCCP, FCCM and Nitesh K. Jain, MD
ISBN: 979-8-89530-341-2
eBook ISBN: 979-8-89530-477-8

High-Frequency Chest Wall Oscillation Therapy in Critically Ill Patients: A Rational Approach
Antonio M. Esquinas, MD, PhD, FCCP, FAARC
ISBN: 979-8-89530-264-4
eBook ISBN: 979-8-89530-403-7

Pulmonary Emergencies
Aysegül Bayýr
ISBN: 979-8-89113-658-8
eBook ISBN: 979-8-89113-755-4

Understanding and Treating Acute Pulmonary Embolism
James K. Edwards (Editor)
ISBN: 979-8-88697-149-1
eBook ISBN: 979-8-88697-398-3

More information about this series can be found at
https://novapublishers.com/product-category/series/pulmonary-and-respiratory-diseases-and-disorders/

Anjali Sharma
Vishnu Mittal
Devkant Sharma
Himani Bajaj
Editors

Human Metapneumovirus

Advances in Research and Clinical Applications

nova
Medicine & Health
New York

DOI: https://doi.org/10.52305/AYXB0445

Additional color graphics may be available in the e-book version of this book.

Library of Congress Cataloging-in-Publication Data
Library of Congress Control Number: 2025950034
ISBN: 979-8-90134-063-9 (Hardcover)
ISBN: 979-8-90134-146-9 (eBook)

Published by Nova Science Publishers, Inc. † New York

Contents

Preface

Human Metapneumovirus (HMPV) has rapidly gained global recognition as a significant respiratory pathogen, particularly impacting vulnerable populations such as infants, elderly individuals, and immunocompromised patients. Since its identification in 2001, HMPV has been associated with a broad spectrum of respiratory tract infections, ranging from mild upper respiratory illnesses to severe lower respiratory complications, including bronchiolitis and pneumonia. Despite its clinical relevance, HMPV remains underrecognized and underreported, mainly due to limitations in diagnostic capacity and the overlapping symptomatology it shares with other respiratory viruses. With the increasing emergence of respiratory infections and the growing awareness of viral pandemics, the need for a comprehensive, up-to-date resource on HMPV has become more critical than ever.

This book, *Human Metapneumovirus: Advances in Research and Clinical Applications*, is a timely and extensive compilation of the latest scientific, clinical, and technological developments concerning HMPV. It is designed to serve as a vital academic and practical reference for researchers, virologists, epidemiologists, clinicians, healthcare professionals, policymakers, and graduate students engaged in the prevention, diagnosis, treatment, and surveillance of respiratory viruses.

The book opens with foundational chapters that provide a clear understanding of the virus itself, beginning with an Introduction to Human Metapneumovirus (HMPV) and followed by its Epidemiology: Global Trends and Insights, and Molecular Virology, which detail the virus's structure, replication, and transmission mechanisms. The subsequent chapters delve into Pathogenesis and Clinical Manifestations, focusing on the diverse presentations of HMPV, particularly in high-risk groups. Special attention is given to Pediatric Populations, where HMPV accounts for a significant disease burden worldwide.

A significant strength of this book lies in its critical evaluation of Diagnostic Approaches and Therapeutic Strategies, covering both conventional and advanced methodologies. Readers will gain insights into the role of molecular diagnostics, including RT-PCR, LAMP, and CRISPR-based platforms, as well as updates on antiviral interventions and supportive therapies. Another essential component addresses Vaccine Development, an area of increasing interest given the virus's global impact and the absence of licensed vaccines to date.

Expanding beyond the clinical sphere, chapters on Environmental and Ecological Factors, Genotypic Variations, and Emerging Technologies offer a multidisciplinary perspective on HMPV spread, evolution, and surveillance. The book also highlights Global Initiatives and collaborative efforts to control HMPV outbreaks, with particular emphasis on implementation in Low-Resource Settings, where diagnostic and therapeutic disparities often persist.

Innovative themes such as Artificial Intelligence and Machine Learning in HMPV research are introduced to showcase the potential of digital technologies in diagnostics, outbreak prediction, and personalized treatment planning. The book concludes with a forward-looking chapter on Future Directions, exploring the integration of genomics, AI, immunology, and public health for developing next-generation vaccines and therapeutics.

Ultimately, this book aims to provide a cohesive narrative that bridges laboratory research, clinical practice, and public health strategy. We hope that this collective work will empower the scientific and medical communities to address the global challenge posed by HMPV more effectively, while also contributing to the broader field of respiratory virus management.

Editors:
Dr. Anjali Sharma
Mr. Vishnu Mittal
Dr. Devkant Sharma
Dr. Himani Bajaj

Chapter 1

Introduction to Human Metapneumovirus (HMPV)

**Shefali Mehla*
and Yunes M. M. A. Alsayadi**
University Institute of Pharma Sciences, Chandigarh University, Chandigarh, India

Abstract

A widespread respiratory pathogen, Human Metapneumovirus, or HMPV, is the cause of acute respiratory tract infections, particularly in immunocompromised individuals, geriatric, and newborns. First identified within the Netherlands back in 2001, analyses suggest that it circulated among humans for decades before. HMPV relates genetically as well as clinically to respiratory Syncytial virus (RSV). It also belongs to the family of Pneumoviridae. Its genome is made up of negative-sense RNA (single strand). It encodes surface proteins that, such as the fusion (F) and glycoprotein (G) proteins, which have roles in pathogenesis and immune evasion. HMPV is common epidemiologically, and seasonal peaks are typically observed during early spring and late winter, though regional variations exist. Mostly, children are infected before age five. Reoccurrence chances are there in a person's life due to partial or incomplete immunity. In clinical practice, HMPV causes varied respiratory diseases, varying from moderate upper respiratory problems to severe pneumonia and bronchiolitis, which commonly look just like other viral respiratory illnesses. Diagnosis depends greatly upon molecular techniques such as reverse transcription-polymerase chain reaction (RT-PCR) since antigen-based methods have some limits. At present, no one treats HMPV specifically with antiviral drugs or approves

* Corresponding Author's Email: shefalimehla19@gmail.com

In: Human Metapneumovirus
Editors: Anjali Sharma, Vishnu Mittal, Devkant Sharma et al.
ISBN: 979-8-90134-063-9

a vaccine; management supports it. However, research continues, and it also explores vaccine candidates as well as antiviral agents. Since the virus puts a burden so prominent upon healthcare systems, it underscores a need for improved surveillance and diagnostic capabilities with more focused actions. The epidemiology, virology, clinical features, and public health impact of HMPV are reviewed in this paper, so continued research plus public health preparedness should reduce global health effects.

Keywords: metapneumovirus, glycoprotein, RT-PCR, bronchiolitis, respiratory infection

List of Abbreviations

HMPV	Human Metapneumovirus
RSV	Respiratory Syncytial Virus
RNA	Ribonucleic Acid
F Protein	Fusion Protein
G Protein	Glycoprotein
RT-PCR	Reverse Transcription Polymerase Chain Reaction
ARIs	Acute Respiratory Infections
ARTIs	Acute Respiratory Tract Infections
SARS-CoV-2	Severe Acute Respiratory Syndrome Coronavirus 2
AMPV	Avian Metapneumovirus
URTI	Upper Respiratory Tract Infection
LRTI	Lower Respiratory Tract Infection
ARDS	Acute Respiratory Distress Syndrome
COPD	Chronic Obstructive Pulmonary Disease
IgM	Immunoglobulin M
IgG	Immunoglobulin G.

Introduction

Across the entire world, children, along with older adults and people who have weak immune systems, are still affected by respiratory tract infections (RTIs), a large cause of illness and also of death. RTIs are caused by a wide variety of viruses that exist within humans. These include influenza viruses, respiratory Syncytial virus (RSV), rhinoviruses, adenoviruses, and also coronaviruses

(Mistry et al., 2025). These pathogens explain a large percentage of acute respiratory illnesses, also they cause great healthcare use and economic strain worldwide (Mazzoncini Jr et al., 2010). Certain viruses, such as the severe acute respiratory syndrome coronavirus virus2 (SARS-CoV-2), can impact respiration. It is indeed important to have vigilant surveillance, and also very rapid response mechanisms (Waghmode et al., 2021). Continuous monitoring along with research is needed for promptly identifying then novel respiratory pathogens because viral evolution's nature evolves rapidly, as well as zoonotic spillover events' potential (Adedokun et al., 2025).

Metapneumovirus shares a close relationship with Respiratory Syncytial Virus (RSV) because it is a member of the Pneumovirus genus within the same subfamily. Across age groups, viruses are the leading causes for acute respiratory tract infections (ARTIs), and they possess enveloped, non-segmented, negative-sense RNA genomes. HMPV clinically overlaps feature RSV infections present. The symptoms represent hypoxia plus wheezing along with a cough. However, these distinctions actually do exist; RSV patients manifest less fever, and are younger than HMPV patients. HMPV infections will commonly link to asthma exacerbations as well as pneumonia, while RSV associates itself more frequently with bronchiolitis (Ng, 2024).

Breakthrough

The first detection of Human metapneumovirus (HMPV) occurred in 2001 when Dutch scientists isolated the virus from young children's nasopharyngeal aspirates with existing respiratory tract infections (Mistry et al., 2025). Serological evidence from 1958 indicated HMPV circulated within the human population a minimum of 50 years prior to discovery. Phylogenetic investigations propose HMPV separated from avian metapneumovirus around 200 years ago. This suggests HMPV existed within humans throughout antiquity (Mistry et al., 2025). HMPV detection filled in some blanks regarding respiratory infection origins, most notably when common pathogens remained unobserved. Pneumoviridae constitutes the virus family, as the genetic structure and clinical manifestations are shared with RSV (Swagatika Panda et al., 2014). Since its unveiling, HMPV has considerably contributed to respiratory system maladies among all demographics. It notably correlates with bronchiolitis plus pneumonia among young children, and it may gravely result in respiratory disease among the elderly and immunocompromised people. Within epidemiological studies, about 5-10% pediatric for acute respiratory infections are caused by HMPV (Swagatika Panda et al., 2014).

HMPV infection frequently manifests clinically indistinguishably from other respiratory viruses. This identical manifestation confounds the manner in which clinicians diagnose and manage it. Leadership stays largely encouraging, and additionally, there exist now no definite antiviral therapies or sanctioned inoculations for HMPV. Given that targeted therapies are absent, we require heightened awareness, improved diagnostic capabilities, coupled with the development of effective preventive measures. Recent surges in HMPV cases have underscored the virus's potential for important outbreaks. Susceptible demographics are especially endangered, as evidenced by accounts originating from China around late 2024. These events highlight continued monitoring as well as investigation because understanding HMPV's transmission characteristics, pathogenesis, and influence upon community wellness is important (Porwal et al., 2025).

Molecular Structure and Virology

Categorization

Human metapneumovirus (HMPV) exists within the genus Metapneumovirus in Pneumoviridae as an enveloped RNA virus having a negative-sense, non-segmented single-stranded form. This grouping also includes the Respiratory Syncytial Virus (RSV). Important genetic similarities exist between HMPV and RSV. HMPV relates in an intimate manner to avian metapneumovirus (AMPV) in phylogenetic analyses because it indicates a genealogical source shared by them both (Chittiprol et al., 2025; Mackie, 2003).

Genomic Characterization

The HMPV genome comes to about 13.3 kilobases in length and codes for eight genes, making nine proteins. That is 3′-N-P-M-F-M2-SH-G-L-5′ regarding that genetic. The RNA genome of the virus is enveloped by nucleoprotein. In consequence, the nucleocapsid is generated (Biacchesi et al., 2003). Phosphoprotein (P) acts as a cofactor with the polymerase. It participates in RNA creation as well. Matrix protein (M): Budding, along with virus assembly, contributes to the functions it performs. Glycoprotein of fusion (F) eases coalescence of the viral casing. It acts thusly upon the host cell membrane. M2-1 and M2-2 proteins: Participate in transcriptional modulation and RNA production. Small hydrophobic protein (SH): Although its precise function remains incompletely elucidated, scientists hypothesise a role in virus-host interactions. Adhesion glycoprotein (G): Eases viral adhesion to host cells. Large polymerase protein (L): It operates as RNA-dependent RNA polymerase(Wei et al., 2023). Figure 1 illustrates the structure of human metapneumovirus (Soto, 2018). HMPV mostly replicates in the cytoplasm of infected cells, affecting the respiratory tract's epithelial cells. The virus binds to host cells using the G glycoprotein. Membrane fusion for entrance is then facilitated by the F protein (Liu, 2008).

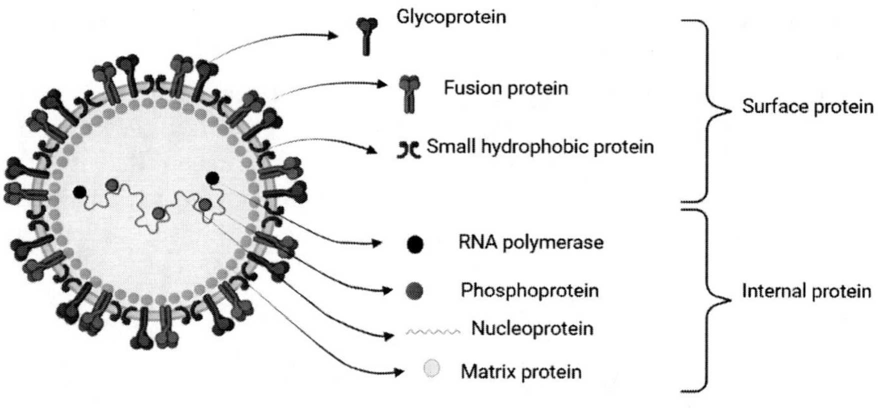

Figure 1. Molecular structure of human metapneumovirus.

Subgroups and Genetic Diversity

HMPV is sorted within two main genetic lineages, A and B, which are further divided into subgroups A1, A2, B1, and B2. Subgroup A2 has been further divided into A2a coupled with A2b, with recent studies proposing additional subline ages such as A2c, A2b1, coupled with A2b2 (Krüger et al., 2025; Nao et al., 2020). The basic idea studies suggested is that there is genetic variation across these subgroups in the genes that encode surface glycoproteins, particularly in the G and F proteins. The antigenic properties of the virus may be impacted by these changes. When combined with advancements in vaccines, the immunological response can also have consequences (Márquez-Escobar, 2017).

Epidemiology

Seasonality and Worldwide Distribution

HMPV possesses a global prevalence exhibiting documented infections spanning every continent. HMPV displays a clear seasonal trend within temperate regions. The frequency culminates throughout the late winter and near the beginning of spring months. Incidents frequently transpire during January until March within the Northern Hemisphere, for instance, while maxima are generally perceived during June until July within the Southern Hemisphere. This seasonality is in close alignment with the actions of other respiratory viruses, including influenza and Respiratory Syncytial Virus (RSV) (Panda et al., 2014). HMPV circulates worldwide, showing its worthiness as a respiratory pathogen. Observed trends denote that HMPV decidedly constitutes a large portion of the affliction of acute respiratory infections throughout the globe because it has an impact on varied demographics regardless of the terrestrial position (Kulkarni et al., 2025).

Age-Related Prevalence and Seroprevalence

Seroprevalence investigations have indicated that HMPV does infect almost all children at an early stage. Around age 5, roughly 90–100% of children show HMPV infection. They exhibit serological evidence regarding it. Children less than 2 years of age are mainly vulnerable to HMPV-caused severe lower respiratory tract infections, exhibit the highest occurrence rates (Heikkinen et al., 2008). Reoccurrence of infections is possible across a lifespan, though initial infection occurs mainly in young children. Even though frequently milder than initial infections in young children, adults, especially elderly as well as immunocompromised people, remain at risk for HMPV-linked respiratory illnesses(Williams et al., 2010).

Recent Trends and Post-Corona Surveillance

The pandemic of COVID-19 has largely impacted the study of respiratory viruses since it includes HMPV. Several respiratory pathogens circulated less due to public health protocols like mask wearing, social isolation, and lockdowns. Aberrant trends surfaced when these regulations were loosened. Remarkably, people have indicated off-season HMPV proliferations, and this alters the duration and strengthens seasonal maxima (García-García et al., 2023). Following COVID-19, improved monitoring endeavours. Following COVID-19, improved monitoring efforts have increased HMPV case identification. Instances of HMPV are now reported with greater frequency. A large escalation of HMPV occurrences within China, as an instance, came into observation near the end of 2024, subsequent to augmented dispatches throughout countries such as Pakistan, India, and the USA. These inclinations underscore the call for sustained observation as well as inquiry. Grasping HMPV's shifting epidemiology amid evolving public health factors necessitates this (Adedokun et al., 2025).

Clinical Manifestations

Indications and Symptoms

The respiratory symptoms of Human metapneumovirus (HMPV) comprise minor upper respiratory tract infections (URTIs) as well as severe lower respiratory tract infections (LRTIs). Common symptoms and manifestations include rhinorrhea, nasal blockage, and tussis, along with fever and sore throat. In more severe cases, particularly in vulnerable populations, Human metapneumovirus can cause acute respiratory distress syndrome, or ARDS, bronchiolitis, and pneumonia (Kahn, 2006).

Categories at High Risk

Some groups are more vulnerable to serious disease linked to HMPV: including infants and young children under age five, geriatric groups due to less effective immune system, and immunocompromised patients who are receiving chemotherapies and have had organ transplant surgeries are more prone. Additionally, HMPV infection may worsen symptoms for people who already have underlying chronic diseases such as asthma or chronic obstructive pulmonary disease (Anderson et al., 2012; Papenburg et al., 2012).

Recurrence and Immunity

Recurrence of HMPV is common across all age groups; also, this indicates the virus does not confer long-lasting immunity upon infection. People may be re-infected with HMPV repeatedly during their existence. The investigations have depicted that the intensity of the recurrence may fluctuate. Sustained investigation of impactful prophylactic strategies is required for durable immunity deficits that present obstacles regarding vaccine origination (González et al., 2017; Walsh et al., 2008).

Diagnosis of Human Metapneumovirus (HMPV)

Laboratory Methods

The precise identification of HMPV is important because it mirrors other respiratory pathogens symptomatically. When it comes to respiratory specimens, the reverse transcription-polymerase chain reaction (RT-PCR) is deemed the quintessential benchmark for ascertaining HMPV RNA. This molecular technique offers high sensitivity as well as specificity; therefore, it identifies low viral loads and eases early diagnosis. Quantitative RT-PCR may also elucidate the viral burden. The intensity of that burden can correspond to an ailment (Mohammadi et al., 2025).

Multiplex RT-PCR assays were created to simultaneously reveal HMPV coupled with influenza and respiratory Syncytial virus (RSV). Expeditious detection of such a causative agent is vital to proper management when co-infections are typical within clinical settings, using these assays (Dayakar et al., 2016). Alternative diagnostic routes include serological assays for the recognition of HMPV-specific IgM and IgG antibodies, with antigen detection tactics that aim at viral proteins. Nonetheless, these techniques prove typically less perceptive. These modalities are not typically employed for rapid diagnosis (Mohammadi et al., 2025).

Challenges in Diagnosis

HMPV diagnosis presents a number of difficulties, like clinical overlap: The symptoms of an HMPV infection, which include fever, coughing, obstruction of the nose, and dyspnea, are widespread and closely resemble those of other respiratory viruses, such as influenza, rhinoviruses, and RSV. Ignoring HMPV-specific testing can result in overlap and inaccurate diagnosis. Limited awareness regarding HMPV is still underrated in the field of medicine. This is true even though it is widespread throughout the world. HMPV may not always be taken into consideration by many medical practitioners when diagnosing respiratory conditions. Resource limitations for diagnosis are another challenge. RT-PCR is a sophisticated molecular diagnostic technologies that require specialized equipment and experienced personnel, and they might not always be immediately available in all healthcare settings, especially in low-resource areas. In light of these challenges, healthcare professionals should become more aware, should provide diagnostic tools, and individuals should develop affordable, quick diagnostic procedures to facilitate the prompt and precise detection of HMPV infections (Costa-Filho et al., 2025; Roy et al., 2025).

Treatment and Prevention of Human Metapneumovirus (HMPV)

Existing Management

To date, no sanctioned specific antiviral agents address HMPV infections. Leadership mainly furnishes assistance since it reduces manifestations and sustains sufficient oxygenation along with hydration. Acute instances can involve treatments such as oxygen support. Respiratory assistance might also prove necessary, notably among immunodeficient people (Verma et al., 2025). Certain investigations have scrutinised the employment of ribavirin for the management of HMPV infections. Ribavirin represents an antiviral pharmaceutical. Nevertheless, Ribavirin's effectiveness remains unproven, so it is not regularly advised. Further investigation toward strong antiviral therapies for HMPV is required, given the absence of targeted treatments (Yin et al., 2009).

Vaccine Progress

Currently, HMPV lacks a licensed vaccine at present. Nevertheless, vaccine research has demonstrated substantial advancement. Numerous vaccine candidates are being examined because they include subunit vaccines, live attenuated vaccines, and virus-like particle (VLP) vaccines. Recently, two mRNA vaccines, along with VLP vaccine aspirants, have commenced Phase 1 clinical investigations (NCT05664334 and NCT05743881) (Guo et al., 2023; Topalidou et al., 2023).

Preventive Strategies

Preventive strategies are essential for halting the spread of HMPV in the absence of targeted antiviral therapies and vaccinations. Important tactics include- Hand hygiene: Using alcohol-based hand sanitisers or washing your hands often with soap and water will help prevent the spread of the disease. Respiratory Etiquette: To stop respiratory droplets from spreading, cover your mouth and nose when you cough or sneeze. Isolation of Infected Individuals: Transmission can be reduced by keeping infected people apart from susceptible groups, such as young children and the elderly. Personal Protective Equipment (PPE) Use: Masks, gloves, and gowns are examples of PPE that can be used in healthcare settings to safeguard patients and healthcare personnel. To protect high-risk groups from serious HMPV infections, it is crucial to put these preventative measures into place during times when respiratory viruses are most prevalent (Satapathy et al., 2025).

Impact on Public Healthcare System

Healthcare Weigh Down

HMPV constitutes a major cause of disease for young children, especially in acute respiratory infections (ARIs). According to a global analysis, HMPV caused about 14.2 million acute lower respiratory infections (ALRI) cases in children under five in 2018. This also led to approximately 643,000 hospital admissions as well as 16,100 deaths all over the world. HMPV constitutes a large fraction of hospitalisations that occur because of respiratory ailments among children within the United States. This frequently mandates critical care and extended hospitalisation (Wang et al., 2021). The virus also presents hazards to other susceptible demographics, including senior citizens and immunocompromised people, engendering heightened sickness and healthcare consumption. Occurrences within extended residential establishments stress the possibility of swift contagion alongside grave consequences there (Spires et al., 2017).

Economic Variables

HMPV's financial consequence is substantial. This impact includes both direct and indirect costs. Direct medical outlays include hospitalisation, supportive treatments, and diagnostic testing. One study conveyed that the hospitals expended a median of $5,513 for each pediatric patient when HMPV infected those patients, and they observed elevated costs in patients showing underlying chronic conditions. Investigators approximated that the yearly economic burden for HMPV hospitalisations within Japan's older population exceeds $50 million(Davis et al., 2016). The economic encumbrance is additionally strengthened by indirect expenditures like diminished productivity as well as caregiver absenteeism. Consequently, efficacious prophylactic strategies are requisite. Furthermore, focused treatments must be created for diminishing HMPV's burden upon healthcare systems and the resultant fiscal effects (Twumasi et al., 2025).

Necessity of Surveillance

Improved monitoring identifies and governs HMPV outbreaks promptly and decisively. Since HMPV's clinical manifestations correspond to other respiratory viruses, laboratory validation is important for precise diagnosis. Genomics are surveyed by real-time monitors for helping identify emerging strains, including helping understand transmission dynamics (Adedokun et al., 2025). The World Health Organization (WHO) stresses fortifying monitoring infrastructure under the International Health Regulations (IHR) construct. It is vital to discern early onsets of respiratory viruses, which include HMPV. Strong monitoring approaches may influence public health initiatives, direct resource distribution, and finally lessen the HMPV impact on global health (Gnanasekaran et al., 2025).

Future Perspective

Understanding HMPV pathophysiology, immunological responses, and the long-term consequences of infection is essential to expand our knowledge. Contemporary investigations have accentuated the capability of the virus to circumvent the immune system of the host. Such circumvention gives rise to repeated maladies plus difficulties in engendering durable invulnerability. Investigating HMPV infection's molecular mechanisms is important for discerning possible therapeutic targets and for understanding viral protein roles, plus host factors. To completely grasp the virus's influence on public health, an investigation into the lasting respiratory aftereffects of HMPV infection is necessary, especially in children and immunocompromised people. The absence of specific antiviral treatments for HMPV accentuates the fact that researchers must cultivate specialised therapeutics. Contemporary investigations probe assorted antiviral compounds that include fusion inhibitors with monoclonal antibodies.

The HMPV fusion (F) protein remains vital to viral entry into host cells; therefore, later agents should target it into host cells. These endeavours principally target efficacious treatment modalities, notably for immunocompromised patients, the elderly, and infants. An additional meaningful subject for concentration involves vaccine origin. Many vaccine prospects, including live-attenuated vaccines, subunit vaccines, and virus-like particle (VLP) vaccines, are under investigation. Due to modern progress, Phase 1 clinical trials commenced regarding mRNA and VLP-based vaccines. This commencement signifies a large advancement in this sphere. The worldwide character of HMPV transmission calls for public health tactics and, furthermore, international collaboration in investigation. Entities such as the World Health Organization (WHO) are vital toward encouraging such alliances. They also guarantee a cohesive strategy as they confront HMPV and diminish its repercussions on global health.

Conclusion

Around the world, Human metapneumovirus, or HMPV, has emerged as a significant respiratory infection, greatly impacting immunocompromised people, the elderly, and young children. Since its discovery in 2001, HMPV has been acknowledged to cause many respiratory illnesses. These maladies range from more benign upper airway infections to more critical lower airway diseases such as bronchiolitis and pneumonia. Across the world, current epidemiological data show a return of HMPV cases, along with outbreaks within long-term care homes and marked increases in child hospital intakes. The virus is able to co-circulate along with the other respiratory pathogens, which include Respiratory Syncytial Virus (RSV) and influenza, thereby complicating diagnosis and management. This highlights the necessity for improved monitoring with more heightened diagnostic capacities. HMPV represents a significant healthcare system burden since hospitalizations increased and therapeutics residence grew. Expenses related to caregiver absence, coupled with reduced production, further strengthen the economic impact since they stress the need for strong preventative strategies through therapeutic interventions. In consideration of each of these issues, a detailed tactic is required. Sustained investigation into the virus pathogenesis, immune responses, and sequelae is required now for cultivating bespoke therapies and vaccines. Investigators and also health officials, in addition to political leaders, must cooperate at an international level so as to institute efficacious monitoring frameworks. They should likewise share data and synchronize reactions to outbreaks. Ultimately, it is in that HMPV affects communal well-being that investigators, monitors, and global entities must pledge without ceasing. We can reduce viral effects by prioritising these efforts as we prepare for respiratory pathogen outbreaks.

References

Adedokun, K. A., Adekola, S. A., Tajudeen, A., Bello-Ibiyemi, A. A., Babandina, M. M., Magwe, E. A., & Bello, A. (2025). Rising global threat of Human metapneumovirus (hMPV in 2024/2025): pathogenesis, immune dynamics, vulnerabilities in immunocompromised individuals, and lessons from past pandemics. *Journal of Rare Diseases, 4*(1), 1–20.

Anderson, E. J., Simões, E. A., Buttery, J. P., Dennehy, P. H., Domachowske, J. B., Jensen, K., Yogev, R. (2012). Prevalence and characteristics of Human metapneumovirus infection among hospitalised children at high risk for severe lower respiratory tract infection. *Journal of the Pediatric Infectious Diseases Society, 1*(3), 212–222.

Biacchesi, S., Skiadopoulos, M. H., Boivin, G., Hanson, C. T., Murphy, B. R., Collins, P. L., & Buchholz, U. J. (2003). Genetic diversity between Human metapneumovirus subgroups. *Virology, 315*(1), 1-9.

Chittiprol, N., Kandi, V., Pinnelli, V. B. K., Suvvari, T. K., Madamsetti, N., CA, J., Challa Jr, S. T. (2025). The Re-emergence of Human Metapneumovirus: Virus Classification,

Characteristics, Mechanisms of Infection, Clinical Features, Diagnosis, Epidemiology, Prevention, and Treatment. *Cureus, 17*(6).

Costa-Filho, R. C., Saddy, F., Costa, J. L. F., Tavares, L. R., & Castro Faria Neto, H. C. (2025). The silent threat of Human metapneumovirus: clinical challenges and diagnostic insights from a severe pneumonia case. *Microorganisms, 13*(1), 73.

Davis, C. R., Stockmann, C., Pavia, A. T., Byington, C. L., Blaschke, A. J., Hersh, A. L., Ampofo, K. (2016). Incidence, morbidity, and costs of Human metapneumovirus infection in hospitalised children. *Journal of the Pediatric Infectious Diseases Society, 5*(3), 303–311.

Dayakar, S., Pillai, H. R., Thulasi, V. P., & Nair, R. R. (2016). Development of a multiplex RT-PCR for simultaneous diagnosis of Human metapneumovirus (HMPV) and human respiratory syncytial virus (HRSV) from clinical specimens. *Virusdisease, 27*, 375–381.

García-García, M. L., Pérez-Arenas, E., Pérez-Hernández, P., Falces-Romero, I., Ruiz, S., Pozo, F., Calvo, C. (2023). Human metapneumovirus infections during the COVID-19 pandemic, Spain. *Emerging infectious diseases, 29*(4), 850.

Gnanasekaran, S., Bashar, M. A., Rajan, A. K., & Prabhat, P. (2025). Emerging threat of Human metapneumovirus (HMPV) and strategies for its containment and control. *Infection, Genetics and Evolution*, 105758.

González, A. E., Lay, M. K., Jara, E. L., Espinoza, J. A., Gómez, R. S., Soto, J., Riedel, C. A. (2017). Aberrant T cell immunity triggered by human Respiratory Syncytial Virus and Human metapneumovirus infection. *Virulence, 8*(6), 685–704.

Guo, L., Li, L., Liu, L., Zhang, T., & Sun, M. (2023). Neutralising antibodies against Human metapneumovirus. *The Lancet Microbe, 4*(9), e732-e744.

Heikkinen, T., Österback, R., Peltola, V., Jartti, T., & Vainionpää, R. (2008). Human metapneumovirus infections in children. *Emerging infectious diseases, 14*(1), 101.

Kahn, J. S. (2006). Epidemiology of Human Metapneumovirus. *Clinical microbiology reviews, 19*(3), 546–557.

Krüger, N., Laufer, S. A., & Pillaiyar, T. (2025). An overview of progress in Human metapneumovirus (hMPV) research: Structure, function, and therapeutic opportunities. *Drug Discovery Today*, 104364.

Kulkarni, D., Cong, B., Ranjini, M. J. K., Balchandani, G., Chen, S., Liang, J., Li, Y. (2025). The global burden of Human metapneumovirus-associated acute respiratory infections in older adults: a systematic review and meta-analysis. *The Lancet Healthy Longevity*.

Liu, L. (2008). Molecular biology of Human metapneumovirus (HMPV) attachment protein.

Mackie, P. (2003). The classification of viruses infecting the respiratory tract. *Paediatric respiratory reviews, 4*(2), 84-90.

Márquez-Escobar, V. A. (2017). Current developments and prospects on Human metapneumovirus vaccines. *Expert review of vaccines, 16*(5), 419-431.

Mazzoncini Jr, J. P., Crowell, C. B., & Kang, C. S. (2010). Human metapneumovirus: an emerging respiratory pathogen. *The Journal of Emergency Medicine, 38*(4), 456-459.

Mistry, L. N., Agarwal, S., Jaiswal, H., Kondkari, S., Mulla, S. A., & Bhandarkar, S. D. (2025). Human metapneumovirus: Emergence, Impact, and Public Health Significance. *Cureus, 17*(3).

Mohammadi, K., Faramarzi, S., Yaribash, S., Valizadeh, Z., Rajabi, E., Ghavam, M., Seifi, A. (2025). Human metapneumovirus (hMPV) in 2025: emerging trends and insights from community and hospital-based respiratory panel analyses—a comprehensive review. *Virology Journal, 22*(1), 1-21.

Nao, N., Saikusa, M., Sato, K., Sekizuka, T., Usuku, S., Tanaka, N., Takeda, M. (2020). Recent molecular evolution of Human metapneumovirus (HMPV): subdivision of HMPV A2b strains. *Microorganisms, 8*(9), 1280.

Ng, D. C. E., Liew, C. H., Tan, K. K., Awang, E. H. B., Nazri, F. N. B. A., Maran, A. K. T., & Khoo, E. J. (2024). Clinical comparison of HMPV and RSV infections in hospitalised Malaysian children: A propensity score matched study. *The clinical respiratory journal, 18*(3).

Panda, S., Mohakud, N. K., Pena, L., & Kumar, S. (2014). Human metapneumovirus: review of an important respiratory pathogen. *International journal of infectious diseases, 25*, 45-52.

Papenburg, J., Hamelin, M.-È., Ouhoummane, N., Carbonneau, J., Ouakki, M., Raymond, F., Frenette, L. (2012). Comparison of risk factors for Human metapneumovirus and respiratory syncytial virus disease severity in young children. *The Journal of Infectious Diseases, 206*(2), 178-189.

Porwal, S., Malviya, R., Sridhar, S. B., Shareef, J., & Wadhwa, T. (2025). Global impact of hMPV virus: Transmission, pathogenesis, diagnosis and treatment. *Diagnostic Microbiology and Infectious Disease*, 116809.

Roy, A., Singh, P. K., Dutt, K. R., Yadav, M. K., Singh, A., Mahto, I. K., Kashyap, S. (2025). The Hidden Menace: Human metapneumovirus Infection (hMPV): A Review of Clinical Manifestations, Diagnosis, and Management Strategies. *International Journal of Scientific Research and Technology*.

Satapathy, T., Satapathy, A., Satapathy, A., Yadav, N., Chandrakar, M., & Chandrakar, K. (2025). Recent outbreaks of Human metapneumovirus (HMPV): Prevention, Diagnosis and Therapeutic insights. *Journal of Drug Delivery & Therapeutics, 15*(2).

Soto, J. A., Gálvez, N. M., Benavente, F. M., Pizarro-Ortega, M. S., Lay, M. K., Riedel, C.,& Kalergis, A. M. (2018). Human metapneumovirus: mechanisms and molecular targets used by the virus to avoid the immune system. *Frontiers in immunology, 9*, 2466.

Spires, S. S., Talbot, H. K., Pope, C. A., & Talbot, T. R. (2017). Paramyxovirus outbreak in a long-term care facility: the challenges of implementing infection control practices in a congregate setting. *infection control & hospital epidemiology, 38*(4), 399-404.

Swagatika Panda, S. P., Mohakud, N., Lindomar Pena, L. P., & Subrat Kumar, S. K. (2014). Human metapneumovirus: review of an important respiratory pathogen.

Topalidou, X., Kalergis, A. M., & Papazisis, G. (2023). Respiratory syncytial virus vaccines: a review of the candidates and the approved vaccines. *Pathogens, 12*(10), 1259.

Twumasi, S., Ansah, R. O., Ayirebi, A. A., Antonio, D. N. M., Asafoakaa, Y. A., Tawiah, E., & Opoku, A. (2025). Human metapneumovirus: A Review of Its Epidemiology,

Clinical Features, Public Health Implications and Treatment Options. *Reviews in Medical Virology, 35*(4), e70043.

Verma, M., Kumar, A., Kumar, S., Mehta, R., Sah, R., & Verma, A. (2025). Human metapneumovirus–A Clickbait clickbait or a real pandemic Threat? *Clinical Infection in Practice*, 100410.

Waghmode, R., Jadhav, S., & Nema, V. (2021). The burden of respiratory viruses and their prevalence in different geographical regions of India: 1970–2020. *Frontiers in Microbiology, 12*, 723850.

Walsh, E. E., Peterson, D. R., & Falsey, A. R. (2008). Human metapneumovirus infections in adults: another piece of the puzzle. *Archives of internal medicine, 168*(22), 2489–2496.

Wang, X., Li, Y., Deloria-Knoll, M., Madhi, S. A., Cohen, C., Ali, A., Chittaganpitch, M. (2021). Global burden of acute lower respiratory infection associated with Human metapneumovirus in children under 5 years in 2018: a systematic review and modelling study. *The Lancet Global Health, 9*(1), e33-e43.

Wei, T., Wang, C., Ma, F., Guo, J., Chen, A., Huang, Y., Zheng, L. (2023). Whole genome sequencing and evolution analyses of Human metapneumovirus. *Virus genes, 59*(4), 524–531.

Williams, J. V., Edwards, K. M., Weinberg, G. A., Griffin, M. R., Hall, C. B., Zhu, Y., Silva, D. (2010). Population-based incidence of Human metapneumovirus infection among hospitalised children. *The Journal of Infectious Diseases, 201*(12), 1890-1898.

Yin, M. T., Brust, J. C., Tieu, H. V., & Hammer, S. M. (2009). Antiherpesvirus, Anti-Hepatitis Virus, and Anti-Respiratory Virus Agents. *Clinical virology*, 217–264.

Chapter 2

Epidemiology of Human Metapneumovirus (HMPV): Global Trends and Insights

Shivani Sharma[1,*]
Muskan Shingari[2]
Neha Saini[1]
Anu Chaudhary[1]
and Ashwani Kumar Dhingra[1]
[1]Global Research Institute of Pharmacy, Nachraun, Radaur, Haryana, India
[2]Guru Gobind Singh College of Pharmacy, Yamunanagar, Haryana, India

Abstract

The Human Metapneumovirus (HMPV) is a significant cause of respiratory illnesses. The human respiratory syncytial virus (HRSV) is not like this. A member of its closely related family, no specific vaccine or antiviral medication has been developed since the virus was identified in 2001. The signs of HMPV, which can range from mild cold symptoms to pneumonia, can resemble those of other respiratory viruses, like COVID-19 and RSV, making early detection and treatment more difficult. The reemerging respiratory disease known as human metapneumovirus (HMPV) is a cause of illness and mortality, particularly in the elderly, small children, and those with compromised immune systems. During the winter months, HMPV was the sixth common virus, primarily affecting small children. 70% of HMPV isolates, such as influenza A and B viruses, adenoviruses, and parainfluenza, were responsible for 26% of HMPV infections in samples

* Corresponding Author's Email: shivanisharma1524@gmail.com

In: Human Metapneumovirus
Editors: Anjali Sharma, Vishnu Mittal, Devkant Sharma et al.
ISBN: 979-8-90134-063-9

having clinical manifestation data during the respiratory season in the previous few years. Compared to those who had HRSV, those who had these infections had reduced respiratory tract symptoms. As with other respiratory virus infections, upper respiratory tract symptoms or illness were associated with about 13% of HMPV infections. This chapter highlights the most recent developments in diagnosis, treatment, and preventive techniques while examining the seasonal patterns, epidemiological trends, and worldwide impact of HMPV. Polymerase chain reaction (PCR) and other molecular diagnostic methods have increased detection rates. Because the symptoms can be confused with those of other respiratory illnesses, there are still problems. Since there is no specific antiviral medication available at the moment and care is primarily supportive, successful vaccine research is crucial. New antiviral treatments and recent vaccination research initiatives provide promise for lowering the burden of illness. Comprehending these patterns is essential for formulating effective public health regulations, refining monitoring systems, and preventing future outbreaks through enhanced preventive and control strategies.

Keywords: HMPV, clinical manifestation, pneumonia, vaccine, clinical characteristics

List of Abbreviations

HMPV	Human Metapneumovirus
RSV	Respiratory Syncytial Virus
RNA	Ribonucleic Acid
RT-PCR	Reverse Transcription Polymerase Chain Reaction
PCR	Polymerase Chain Reaction
ARIs	Acute Respiratory Infections
LRTIs	Lower Respiratory Tract Infections
COPD	Chronic Obstructive Pulmonary Disease
mAbs	Monoclonal Antibodies
ELISA	Enzyme-Linked Immunosorbent Assay
APV	Avian Pneumovirus
RGD	Arginine-Glycine-Aspartic Acid (motif in F protein)
tMK	Tertiary Monkey Kidney (cells).

Introduction

First discovered in 2001 in children displaying symptoms resembling those of respiratory syncytial virus, human metapneumovirus (HMPV) is a major respiratory virus that affects people all over the world (Van den Hoogen et al., 2001). Numerous investigations have now confirmed the importance of HMPV, typically establishing it as the leading cause of acute respiratory tract infection in young children. People of all ages, including infants and young toddlers, are susceptible to severe sickness from HMPV, which is more likely to impact those with weakened immune systems and underlying cardiac disorders (Papenburg and Boivin et al., 2010).

Most people have been exposed to this virus by the time they are five years old, according to Seroprevalence surveys. Reinfections are frequent (Van den Hoogen et al., 2001). A AHMPV infection can be lethal and cause a variety of symptoms, including feverish seizures, pneumonia, bronchiolitis, and moderate cold symptoms (Kahn et al., 2006; Papenburg et al., 2010). The structure of HMPV is demonstrated in Figure 1.

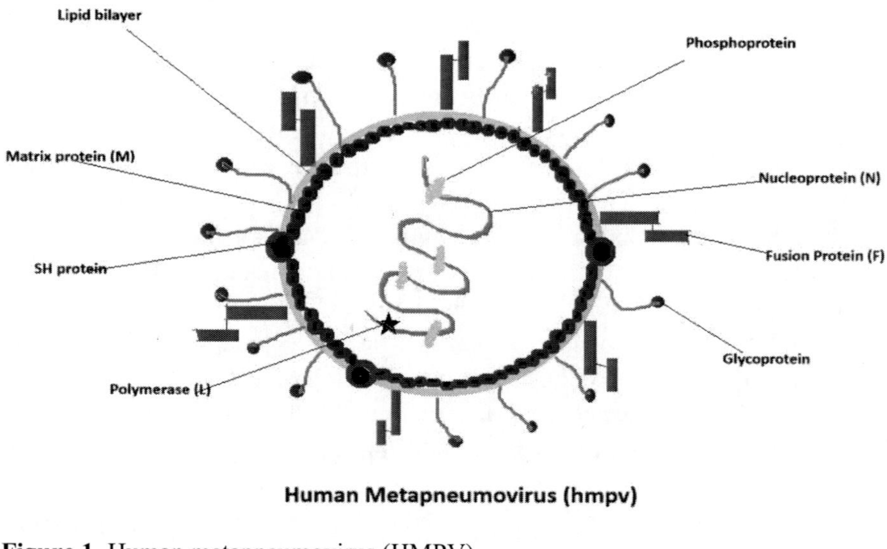

Figure 1. Human metapneumovirus (HMPV).

Although they aid in the battle against viral infections, Cytokine-induced inflammatory immune responses also cause persistent lung issues and severe bronchiolitis, which mostly affect adults, children, and those with compromised immune systems. Of younger children with HMPV, 5.3% to

9.0% had a major respiratory pathogen (Zhao et al., 2022). A seasonal pattern of HMPV migration was noted in arid regions, with a peak incidence of HMPV activity during winter. There have been cases in North America and Europe, and in some Asian nations, there may be a peak during the wet seasons (Du et al., 2022; Lim et al., 2020). However, according to a recent study, weather patterns may influence the seasonal occurrence of HMPV. Additionally, the fight is now, medical care is supportive, and there are no known treatments or vaccines.

Statistics and Clinical Characteristics

Global epidemiological research shows that the majority of children under five will already have an HMPV infection. HMPV will account for 10% of all respiratory infections that necessitate hospital treatment, followed by hRSV at 40% and adenoviruses at 5% (Freymuth et al., 2004; Kahn et al, 2006). In adults, 4%to 5% of severe acute respiratory illnesses are caused by HMPV. Similar to hRSV, HMPV has the following epidemiologic characteristics: (i) it is found on every continent; (ii) it is seasonal, with the majority of cases in the winter season; and (iii) it is spread mainly by airborne respiratory droplets. Additionally, chimpanzees have been discovered to be infected with HMPV (61% Seroprevalence in caged animals in one investigation), which may result in human-to-gorilla transmission cases (Skiadopoulos et al, 2004; Palacios et al., 2021).

The ciliated epithelial cells of the human respiratory tract are the main target of HMPV. The virus takes four to six days to incubate, and it takes two to five weeks for it to be excreted. In children, HMPV often causes 5–15% of hospital treatment for lower respiratory tract infections, or the clinical symptoms frequently mimic those of bronchiolitis (Louie et al., 2007). Young individuals who are infected typically exhibit flu-like symptoms; however, elderly or immunocompromised patients may experience a more severe illness. There have been reports of significant HMPV infection case fatality rates close to 10% (Boivin et al., 2007). Notably, it has also been discovered that older mice have significantly greater clinical severity (Darniot et al., 2009). Although HMPV is diagnosed more frequently in childhood, recurrences are more common in the elderly. This would imply that unfinished protective immune responses or infection by a distinct virus might be the cause of HMPV re-infection in adulthood. On the other hand, it has also been proposed that the inadequate immunological response results from increased G protein glycosylation (Van den Hoogen et al., 2001).

Diagnosis

These characteristics might account for the virus's recent identification. Nevertheless, cell culture methods have low sensitivity for diagnosing HMPV in respiratory tract secretions. Notable outbreaks of HMPV are in Table 1. Currently, the most widely used technique for detecting HMPV is RT-PCR. Several HMPV genes have been identified as targets for primers used in genomic amplification. Primers that bind to portions of the N and L genes have a high sensitivity for both HMPV strain genotypes (Côté et al., 2003). Detecting HMPV or other respiratory viruses can also be accomplished with real-time reverse transcription (PCR). For real-time experiments, a number of genes have been targeted, and viruses from both genotype groups can be identified using particular primers (Kuypers et al., 2005; Mackay et al., 2004; Maertzdorf et al., 2004; Scheltinga et al., 2005). A common method in diagnostic labs for quickly identifying respiratory viruses is immuno-fluorescence, which uses antibodies unique to the virus. Although RT-PCR may be more sensitive for detecting HMPV, immunofluorescence approaches have been developed using HMPV-specific antibodies (Ebihara et al., 2005; Landry et al., 2005; Percivalle et al., 2005). Commercial vendors provide fluorescent antibodies specific to HMPV.

HPMV Classification's Virological Features

On the basis of its gene configuration and sequence identity with avian pneumovirus 9 (APV), HMPV is believed to be the first virus belonging to genus metapneumovirus, subfamily Pneumoviridae (Fouchier et al., 2003). In the subfamily Pneumoviridae, the RSV is the other member of the Pneumovirus genus. According to Ling et al., (1992) and Yu et al., (1992), the primary feature that distinguishes the two genera is the gene constellation variation. The amino acid sequences of HMPV and APV are highly similar (56–87%) in all but two genes. However, RSV has less than 50% of the same identity.

Table 1. A summary of significant Human Metapneumovirus (HMPV) outbreaks

Location	Population Affected	Description	Symptoms	Impact	Reference
United States	Pediatric population	The outbreak coincided with the seasonal peak of respiratory viruses.	Cold-like symptoms to severe respiratory discomfort	Renewed interest in vaccination and antiviral research	Mostafa et al., 2024
Canada	Indigenous communities	Large outbreak in remote areas.	Severe respiratory problems and hospitalisations	Highlighted challenges in remote healthcare response	Richardson et al., 2012
Australia	Elderly in care homes	Outbreak in long-term care facilities.	Respiratory distress, cough, and fever	High morbidity highlighted the susceptibility of the elderly to HMPV	Richardson et al., 2012
Japan	Children & immunocompromised	Notable rise in HMPV cases during winter.	Severe lower respiratory tract infections	Reinforced need for surveillance and potential vaccine development	Richardson et al., 2012
United States	Pediatric population	Outbreak in young children, including hospitalised patients.	Flu-like symptoms, pneumonia, bronchiolitis, wheezing	Increased understanding of respiratory diseases in children	Wisplinghoff et al., 2003
Global	General population	Lower HMPV prevalence during the COVID-19 pandemic due to health measures.	Similar to other respiratory illnesses	Demonstrated efficacy of masks and distancing in limiting HMPV spread	Tan et al., 2020
Netherlands	General population	Initially recognised, research conducted retrospectively.	Cough, nasal congestion, fever, breathing difficulties	Established HMPV as a significant global respiratory pathogen	van den Hoogen et al., 2001

Despite having the closest genetic kinship with APV subtype C, HMPV is commonly compared to RSV due to their shared biologic characteristics, such as their natural hosts. Features of the viruses RSV and HMPV share certain characteristics and belong to the Pneumoviridae subfamily. Both viruses are vulnerable to damage during handling, storage, and transportation. Additionally, both viruses cause cell cultures to produce syncytia, making them identical under an electron microscope and displaying similar cytopathic effects. In vitro, HMPV can only infect LLC-MK2 cells, Vero, and tertiary monkey kidney cells (tMK), but RSV can quickly multiply in a wide range of cell lines. Many HMPV isolates, unlike RSV, require trypsin in the culture media for efficient reproduction.

Virus Reproduction

HMPV replicates in the lung and the nasal tissues and mainly targets airway epithelial cells. Through G protein interactions, HMPV is thought to stick to the target cell by interacting with heparin sulfate and other glycosaminoglycans (Thammawat et al., 2008; El Najjar et al., 2016; Adamson et al., 2012). The HMPV F protein encodes the RGD (Arg-Gly-Asp) motif, which binds RGD-binding integrins as cellular receptors (Cseke et al., 2009; Cox et al., 2012). This promotes the fusion of the viral envelope and cell membrane in a pH-independent manner, most likely within endosomes (Cox et al., 2015; Yang et al., 2016; Schonalter et al., 2006). Only a few lineage F proteins show fusion that is dependent on low pH (Herfst et al., 2008). The M protein facilitates the budding of newly produced virions from the plasma membrane, enabling them to exit the host (Lamb et al., 2001).

Age-Related Burden

Children

In children under five, HMPV contributes to a number of lower respiratory tract infections (LRTIs), which include infections that result in bronchiolitis, pneumonia, and wheezing. It causes 5–10% of hospitalisations for pediatric acute respiratory infections (ARIs) and frequently manifests as symptoms like RSV, such as fever, cough, rhinorrhea, and respiratory distress. Particularly in infants under two years old, severe infections can cause hypoxia, necessitating hospitalisation and mechanical ventilation. Hospital admissions may be prolonged and disease severity increased by co-infections with bacterial pathogens, influenza, or RSV (Boivin et al., 2003).

Adults

These infections are typically mild in healthy adults, resembling the symptoms of the cold with a sore throat, cough, fever, and congestion of the nose. However, severe pneumonia, acute exacerbations of preexisting respiratory illnesses, and a higher rate of hospitalisations in the elderly and those with chronic disorders such as cardiovascular disease, asthma, and chronic obstructive pulmonary disease (COPD) are all possible outcomes of HMPV. HMPV outbreaks are a significant cause of morbidity and mortality in these populations (Aagaard et al., 2005).

Immuno-Compromised Patients

People with damaged immune systems, such as those receiving organ transplants, cancer patients receiving chemotherapy, hematopoietic stem cell transplants, and people with primary immune deficiencies, are very vulnerable to the risk of long-term, severe HMPV infections. When compared to immunocompetent people, these patients frequently have greater virus loads, greater fatality rates, and longer illness durations. In many cases, HMPV requires urgent care, mechanical ventilation, and antiviral treatments due to the increasing pneumonia, respiratory failure, and secondary bacterial infections it might cause. For this population, supportive care remains the primary therapeutic strategy, as no specific antiviral therapies are currently available (Shi et al., 2022).

Regional Trends and Global Distribution

Temperate Regions: Like RSV, seasonal outbreaks generally happen in late winter and early spring.

Tropical Regions: Peaks frequently coincide with the rainy season, and transmission patterns are less clear. Wealthy vs. Developing Countries: Although wealthy countries are better at diagnosing conditions, underreporting is still a problem in situations with limited resources (Shi et al., 2022).

Clinical Diagnosis and Presentation

From serious lower respiratory tract infections (LRTIs) like pneumonia, human metapneumovirus (HMPV) infections can cause a wide range of respiratory symptoms and bronchitis. Age, immunological status, and underlying medical conditions all affect the severity of symptoms (Aagaard et al., 2005).

Typical clinical signs and symptoms include:

- Mild Cases: Symptoms include low-grade fever, coughing, sneezing, sore throat, and nasal congestion, much like a regular cold.
- Moderate Cases: Especially in young children, symptoms may include dyspnea, wheezing, and a protracted cough.
- Severe Cases: These are frequent in immune-compromised people, the elderly, and babies. They can result in hypoxia, a high fever, respiratory distress, and abrupt respiratory failure that necessitates hospitalization.
- Complications: Immune-compromised people, severe HMPV infections can cause bacterial superinfections, worsening of asthma or COPD, and extended respiratory disease.

Difficulties in Diagnosis

Due to the limitations of conventional diagnostic testing and the clinical similarities with other respiratory viruses, diagnosing HMPV infections remains challenging. It is challenging to distinguish HMPV from other viruses based solely on clinical presentation due to the extensive overlap in symptoms between RSV, influenza, adenovirus, and rhinovirus. While pneumonia and exacerbations of chronic lung disease associated with HMPV can imitate influenza or bacterial infections in adults, bronchiolitis and pneumonia caused by HMPV in children can mimic RSV infections. The diagnosis and treatment plans are made more difficult by co-infections with other respiratory pathogens. The gold standard for HMPV identification is polymerase chain reaction (PCR) testing due to its high sensitivity and specificity. This is among the molecular methods that are employed in lab experiments (Shi et al., 2022). By detecting HMPV and other respiratory viruses simultaneously, multiplex RT-PCR panels increase the precision of diagnosis.

Laboratory Examination

It is less frequently employed due to its cross-reactivity with RSV and other paramyxoviruses, although it can detect antibodies specific to HMPV. Antibody formation happens later in the infection, making it unsuitable for acute diagnosis.

Detection Based on Antigens

Though their sensitivity is still lower than that of PCR-based techniques, emerging fast antigen tests hold promise for point-of-care diagnosis. Immune fluorescence studies and enzyme-linked immunosorbent assays (ELISAs) are being developed to enhance the speed of detection. Molecular testing remains the recommended approach, particularly for hospitalised patients and in outbreak situations, due to these diagnostic challenges. Improving quick point-of-care diagnostics for early detection and improved epidemic management is the goal of future research.

Monitoring and Surveillance

Integration with Respiratory Virus Surveillance: coordinating RSV and influenza programs with HMPV surveillance.

Global Health Policies: Developing nations must have easier access to diagnostic services (Huaman et al., 2025).

Campaigns for Public Awareness

Teaching the public and health care providers about HMPV Acute Respiratory Infections (ARIs), particularly in youngsters, the elderly with compromised immune systems, which are brought on by the human metapneumovirus (HMPV), continues to be a major worldwide health problem. The virus has a clear seasonal pattern and frequently co-occurs with influenza and RSV, which makes diagnosis more difficult and increases the cost of treatment. Rapid point-of-care tests are still necessary for efficient clinical management, even though improvements in diagnostic tools, particularly PCR-based molecular assays, have enhanced HMPV detection. Understanding the dynamics of viral development, transmission, and the influence of environmental variables on disease epidemics requires ongoing epidemiological surveillance. There is no particular antiviral treatment or approved vaccination for HMPV, despite its significant morbidity and economic burden. Nonetheless, medicinal research and vaccine development are advancing, with live attenuated vaccine candidates and monoclonal antibodies demonstrating promise in preclinical and early clinical trials. A multimodal strategy is needed to lessen the worldwide effect of HMPV, which includes:

- Ongoing research on viral pathogenesis and immune response.
- Better surveillance methods to monitor epidemics and guide public health regulation.
- The creation of potent vaccinations to shield high-risk groups from serious diseases.
- Public health efforts, including enhanced healthcare readiness during peak seasons, awareness campaigns, and infection control measures (Huaman et al., 2025).

Methods for Treatment and Prevention

Treatment for human metapneumovirus (HMPV) is currently supportive, as no specific antiviral medication is available. To prevent severe infections, research is focused on developing vaccines and customised antivirals for high-risk populations, including small children, adults, and those with weakened immune systems. Current Techniques for Management. Supportive Care:

- Oxygen therapy: For individuals experiencing severe respiratory distress or hypoxia. Although their effectiveness in treating HMPV is still under discussion, bronchodilators are occasionally administered to individuals experiencing bronchospasm or wheezing.
- Nutritional assistance and hydration: Crucial for avoiding dehydration, particularly in young infants.

Research Antivirals

- Ribavirin: A broad-spectrum antiviral used to treat RSV infections, it is being studied for HMPV; however, there is currently no clinical evidence to support its regular use. Preclinical research indicates that neutralising mAbs may aid in the management of severe HMPV infections. While several experimental mAbs have demonstrated in vitro activity, more clinical validation is necessary.
- Fusion inhibitors: Research is being done on medications that target the Protein, i.e., essential for the virus to enter host cells.
- Preventive Actions:
- Hand hygiene: Using soap and water to wash your hands properly helps prevent the spread of viruses. When seasonal epidemics occur, mask-wearing and social distancing are beneficial, particularly for healthcare professionals and individuals with compromised immune systems (Adivitiya et al., 2021).

Conclusion

Acute respiratory infections are a global health concern that are exacerbated by human metapneumovirus (HMPV), especially in children, adults, and older people with weakened immune systems. Frequently co-circulating with RSV and influenza, the virus exhibits a clear seasonal pattern, which makes diagnosis more challenging and increases the financial burden on healthcare. HMPV has a high rate of morbidity and a substantial financial impact, although there is no licensed vaccine or particular antiviral treatment. However, live attenuated vaccine candidates and monoclonal antibodies are demonstrating promise in preclinical and early clinical studies, suggesting that therapeutic research and vaccine development are moving forward. Increased research on viral pathogenesis and immune response, as well as improved surveillance methods to monitor outbreaks and inform public health policies, are all necessary to mitigate the worldwide impact of HMPV.

References

Aagaard, E., & Gonzales, R. (2005). Management of acute bronchitis in healthy adults. *Infectious disease clinics of North America*, *18*(4), 919.

Adamson, P., Thammawat, S., Muchondo, G., Sadlon, T., & Gordon, D. (2012). Diversity in glycosaminoglycan binding amongst hMPV G protein lineages. *Viruses*, *4*(12), 3785-3803.

Adivitiya, Kaushik, M. S., Chakraborty, S., Veleri, S., & Kateriya, S. (2021). Mucociliary respiratory epithelium integrity in molecular defense and susceptibility to pulmonary viral infections. *Biology*, *10*(2), 95.

Boivin, G., De Serres, G., Côté, S., Gilca, R., Abed, Y., Rochette, L., & Déry, P. (2003). Human metapneumovirus infections in hospitalized children. *Emerging infectious diseases*, *9*(6), 634.

Côté, S., Abed, Y., & Boivin, G. (2003). Comparative evaluation of real-time PCR assays for detection of the human metapneumovirus. *Journal of Clinical Microbiology*, *41*(8), 3631-3635.

Cox, R. G., Livesay, S. B., Johnson, M., Ohi, M. D., & Williams, J. V. (2012). The human metapneumovirus fusion protein mediates entry via an interaction with RGD-binding integrins. *Journal of Virology*, *86*(22), 12148–12160.

Cox, R. G., Mainou, B. A., Johnson, M., Hastings, A. K., Schuster, J. E., Dermody, T. S., & Williams, J. V. (2015). Human metapneumovirus is capable of entering cells by fusion with endosomal membranes. *PLoS pathogens*, *11*(12), e1005303.

Cseke, G., Maginnis, M. S., Cox, R. G., Tollefson, S. J., Podsiad, A. B., Wright, D. W., & Williams, J. V. (2009). Integrin αvβ1 promotes infection by human metapneumovirus. *Proceedings of the National Academy of Sciences*, *106*(5), 1566-1571.

Darniot, M., Pitoiset, C., Petrella, T., Aho, S., Pothier, P., & Manoha, C. (2009). Age-associated aggravation of clinical disease after primary metapneumovirus infection of BALB/c mice. *Journal of Virology*, *83*(7), 3323-3332.

Du, Y., Li, W., Guo, Y., Li, L., Chen, Q., He, L., & Shang, S. (2022). Epidemiology and genetic characterisation of human metapneumovirus in pediatric patients from Hangzhou, China. *Journal of Medical Virology*, *94*(11), 5401-5408.

Ebihara, T., Endo, R., Ma, X., Ishiguro, N., & Kikuta, H. (2005). Detection of human metapneumovirus antigens in nasopharyngeal secretions by an immunofluorescent-antibody test. *Journal of Clinical Microbiology*, *43*(3), 1138-1141.

El Najjar, F., Cifuentes-Muñoz, N., Chen, J., Zhu, H., Buchholz, U. J., Moncman, C. L., & Dutch, R. E. (2016). Human metapneumovirus induces reorganisation of the actin cytoskeleton for direct cell-to-cell spread. *PLoS pathogens*, *12*(9), e1005922.

Fouchier, R. A., Kuiken, T., Schutten, M., Van Amerongen, G., Van Doornum, G. J., Van Den Hoogen, B. G., & Osterhaus, A. D. (2003). Koch's postulates fulfilled for the SARS virus. *Nature*, *423*(6937), 240-240.

Freymuth, F., Vabret, A., Legrand, L., Lebon, P., Bach, N., Brouard, J., & Guillois, B. (2004). Le métapneumovirus humain. *Virologie*, *8*(6), 413-423.

Herfst, S., Mas, V., Ver, L. S., Wierda, R. J., Osterhaus, A. D., Fouchier, R. A., & Melero, J. A. (2008). Low-pH-induced membrane fusion mediated by human metapneumovirus F protein is a rare, strain-dependent phenomenon. *Journal of Virology*, *82*(17), 8891-8895.

Huaman Horna, D. E., & Sanchez Figueroa, C. A. (2025). Metapneumovirus humano: Un análisis bibliométrico de su detección, epidemiología y manifestaciones clínicas.

Kahn, J. S. (2006). Epidemiology of human metapneumovirus. *Clinical microbiology reviews*, *19*(3), 546-557.

Kuypers, J., Wright, N., Corey, L., & Morrow, R. (2005). Detection and quantification of human metapneumovirus in pediatric specimens by real-time RT-PCR. *Journal of Clinical Virology*, *33*(4), 299-305.

Lamb, R. A., & Kolakofsky, D. (2001). *Paramyxoviridae: the viruses and their replication* (No. Ed. 4, pp. 689-724).

Landry, M. L., Ferguson, D., Cohen, S., Peret, T. C., & Erdman, D. D. (2005). Detection of human metapneumovirus in clinical samples by immunofluorescence staining of shell vial centrifugation cultures prepared from three different cell lines. *Journal of Clinical Microbiology*, *43*(4), 1950-1952.

Lim, Y. K., Kweon, O. J., Kim, H. R., Kim, T. H., & Lee, M. K. (2020). Clinical features, epidemiology, and climatic impact of genotype-specific human metapneumovirus infections: long-term surveillance of hospitalized patients in South Korea. *Clinical Infectious Diseases*, *70*(12), 2683-2694.

Ling, R., Easton, A. J., & Pringle, C. R. (1992). Sequence analysis of the 22K, SH and G genes of turkey rhinotracheitis virus and their intergenic regions reveals a gene order different from that of other pneumoviruses. *Journal of General Virology*, *73*(7), 1709-1715.

Louie, J. K., Schnurr, D. P., Pan, C. Y., Kiang, D., Carter, C., Tougaw, S., & Trochet, G. (2007). A summer outbreak of human metapneumovirus infection in a long-term-care facility. *The Journal of infectious diseases*, *196*(5), 705-708.

Mackay, I. M., Bialasiewicz, S., Waliuzzaman, Z., Chidlow, G. R., Fegredo, D. C., Laingam, S., & Sloots, T. P. (2004). Use of the P gene to genotype human metapneumovirus identifies 4 viral subtypes. *The Journal of infectious diseases*, *190*(11), 1913-1918.

Maertzdorf, J., Wang, C. K., Brown, J. B., Quinto, J. D., Chu, M., de Graaf, M., & Fouchier, R. A. (2004). Real-time reverse transcriptase PCR assay for detection of human metapneumoviruses from all known genetic lineages. *Journal of clinical microbiology*, *42*(3), 981-986.

Mostafa, H. H., Fall, A., Norton, J. M., Sachithanandham, J., Yunker, M., Abdullah, O., & Klein, E. Y. (2024). Respiratory virus disease and outcomes at a large academic medical center in the United States: a retrospective observational study of the early 2023/2024 respiratory viral season. *Microbiology Spectrum*, *12*(10), e01116-24.

Palacios, G., Lowenstine, L. J., Cranfield, M. R., Gilardi, K. V., Spelman, L., Lukasik-Braum, M., & Lipkin, W. I. (2011). Human metapneumovirus infection in wild mountain gorillas, Rwanda. *Emerging infectious diseases*, *17*(4), 711.

Papenburg, J., & Boivin, G. (2010). The distinguishing features of human metapneumovirus and respiratory syncytial virus. *Reviews in medical virology*, *20*(4), 245-260.

Percivalle, E., Sarasini, A., Visai, L., Revello, M. G., & Gerna, G. (2005). Rapid detection of human metapneumovirus strains in nasopharyngeal aspirates and shell vial cultures by monoclonal antibodies. *Journal of Clinical Microbiology*, *43*(7), 3443-3446.

Richardson, K. L., Driedger, M. S., Pizzi, N. J., Wu, J., & Moghadas, S. M. (2012). Indigenous populations health protection: a Canadian perspective. *BMC Public Health*, *12*, 1-8.

Scheltinga, S. A., Templeton, K. E., Beersma, M. F. C., & Claas, E. C. J. (2005). Diagnosis of human metapneumovirus and rhinovirus in patients with respiratory tract infections by an internally controlled multiplex real-time RNA PCR. *Journal of clinical virology*, *33*(4), 306-311.

Schowalter, R. M., Smith, S. E., & Dutch, R. E. (2006). Characterization of human metapneumovirus F protein-promoted membrane fusion: critical roles for proteolytic processing and low pH. *Journal of virology*, *80*(22), 10931-10941.

Shi, H. J., Kim, N. Y., Eom, S. A., Kim-Jeon, M. D., Oh, S. S., Moon, B. S., & Eom, J. S. (2022). Effects of non-pharmacological interventions on respiratory viruses other than SARS-CoV-2: analysis of laboratory surveillance and literature review from 2018 to 2021. *Journal of Korean medical science*, *37*(21).

Skiadopoulos, M. H., Biacchesi, S., Buchholz, U. J., Riggs, J. M., Surman, S. R., Amaro-Carambot, E., & Murphy, B. R. (2004). The two major human metapneumovirus genetic lineages are highly related antigenically, and the fusion (F) protein is a major contributor to this antigenic relatedness. *Journal of virology*, *78*(13), 6927-6937.

Tan, J. Y., Conceicao, E. P., Sim, X. Y. J., Wee, L. E. I., Aung, M. K., & Venkatachalam, I. (2020). Public health measures during COVID-19 pandemic reduced hospital admissions for community respiratory viral infections. *The Journal of Hospital Infection*, *106*(2), 387.

Thammawat, S., Sadlon, T. A., Hallsworth, P. G., & Gordon, D. L. (2008). Role of cellular glycosaminoglycans and charged regions of viral G protein in human metapneumovirus infection. *Journal of virology*, *82*(23), 11767-11774.

Van den Hoogen, B. G., de Jong, J. C., Groen, J., Kuiken, T., de Groot, R., Fouchier, R. A., & Osterhaus, A. D. (2001). A newly discovered human pneumovirus isolated from young children with respiratory tract disease. *Nature medicine*, *7*(6), 719-724.

Wisplinghoff, H., Seifert, H., Tallent, S. M., Bischoff, T., Wenzel, R. P., & Edmond, M. B. (2003). Nosocomial bloodstream infections in pediatric patients in United States hospitals: epidemiology, clinical features and susceptibilities. *The Pediatric infectious disease journal*, *22*(8), 686-691.

Yang, H., He, H., Tan, B., Liu, E., Zhao, X., & Zhao, Y. (2016). Human metapneumovirus uses endocytosis pathway for host cell entry. *Molecular and Cellular Probes*, *30*(4), 231-237.

Yu, Q., Davis, P. J., Li, J., & Cavanagh, D. (1992). Cloning and sequencing of the matrix protein (M) gene of turkey rhinotracheitis virus reveal a gene order different from that of respiratory syncytial virus. *Virology*, *186*(2), 426-434.

Zhao, H., Feng, Q., Feng, Z., Zhu, Y., Ai, J., Xu, B., & Xie, Z. (2022). Clinical characteristics and molecular epidemiology of human metapneumovirus in children with acute lower respiratory tract infections in China, 2017 to 2019: A multicentre prospective observational study. *Virologica Sinica*, *37*(6), 874-882.

Chapter 3

Molecular Virology of Human Métapneumovirus (HMPV)

Nidhi Rani[1,*]
Rita Saini[2]
Shivanand Patil[2]
Abhishek Kumar Mishra[3]
and Thakur Gurjeet Singh[1]
[1]Chitkara College of Pharmacy, Chitkara University, Punjab, India
[2]Department of Pharmacy, Shree Dev Bhoomi Institute of Education, Science and Technology, Pondha, Dehradun, Uttarakhand, India
[3]Medpharm, Place - Durham, NC, USA

Abstract

The Human Metapneumovirus (HMPV) is a single-stranded RNA virus that primarily causes respiratory tract infections in adolescents, the elderly, and immunocompromised people. It is generally responsible for bronchitis, pneumonia, asthma, and chronic obstructive pulmonary disease (COPD) in some severe cases. The virus was first isolated in 2001, with further study on molecular virology. According to the virology investigations, the virus has a negative-sense RNA genome that codes for nine proteins. Further, the virus enters the host by interacting with heparan sulphate peptidoglycans present on the cell surface, where it replicates its RNA genome, generates new viral proteins, is released via budding, and infects other cells. The study also depicted that HMPV interacts with host immune cells and interferes with interferon

* Corresponding Author's Email: nidhiprajapati8@gmail.com

In: Human Metapneumovirus
Editors: Anjali Sharma, Vishnu Mittal, Devkant Sharma et al.
ISBN: 979-8-90134-063-9

production. The virology studies are helpful in the development of new treatments and vaccines for HMPV.

Keywords: human metapneumovirus, immunocompromised, bronchitis, pneumonia, asthma, chronic obstructive pulmonary disease, virology

List of Abbreviations

HMPV	Human Metapneumovirus
COPD	Chronic Obstructive Pulmonary Disease
RTI	Respiratory Tract Infection
LRTI	Lower Respiratory Tract Infection
URTI	Upper Respiratory Tract Infection
HRSV	Human Respiratory Syncytial Virus
RT-PCR	Reverse Transcription Polymerase Chain Reaction
RNA	Ribonucleic Acid
RdRP	RNA-dependent RNA Polymerase
NGS	Next Generation Sequencing
GAGs	Glycosaminoglycans
HS	Heparin Sulfate
mAbs	Monoclonal Antibodies
ARI	Acute Respiratory Infection
IFN	Interferon
F	Fusion protein
G	Glycoprotein
SH	Small Hydrophobic protein
M	Matrix protein
M2	Matrix 2 protein (includes M2-1 and M2-2)
N	Nucleoprotein
P	Phosphoprotein
L	RNA-dependent RNA Polymerase (Large protein)
DNA	Deoxyribonucleic Acid
TC-PCR	Transcriptase-PCR
PERCH	Pneumonia Aetiology Research for Child Health
KFSH	King Faisal Specialist Hospital
HGH	Hamad General Hospital.

Introduction

According to the World Health Organization (WHO), respiratory tract infections (RTIs) are the leading cause of death in low-income countries and rank second globally among children under five. Viruses cause the majority of upper and lower RTIs (LRTI and URTI), although the culprit is sometimes never found (Hermos et al., 2010). Paramyxovirus, also known as HMPV, is a newly discovered respiratory virus that has drawn considerable interest because of its effects on the health of patients and therapeutic developments. A significant global respiratory infection, HMPV can cause symptoms or none at all in an infected person (Gaunt et al., 2011). HMPV infection is widespread because by the age of five, almost all children are seropositive. Preceding estimations of the proportion of severe pediatric infections in the lower respiratory tract linked to HMPV fluctuate between 5% to 25%; these variations are probably due to different age groups assessed, different geographic regions under study, seasonal variations in HMPV circulation, and methodological variations (Williams et al., 2010).

The first discovery of HMPV was made in the Netherlands in 2001 by van Den Hoogen et al., who isolated the virus from a young child who was displaying symptoms similar to an HRSV infection (Panda et al., 2014). Pune reported the country's first HMPV case in 2004. Other studies with children as the study population have been carried out in India in the cities of Lucknow, New Delhi, and Vellore (Hindupur et al., 2022). Vanden Hoogen *et al.,* initially described HMPV after isolating the virus from 28 clinically unrelated children (27 of whom were ≥5 years old) with a variety of respiratory tract illnesses. Serological studies revealed that by the time they were five years old, every Dutch child had contracted the infection. According to serological research, all Dutch children were infected by the time they were five years old. Although no comprehensive clinical data were included, the clinical symptoms of these infected infants included illnesses extending from inconsequential respiratory matters to bronchiolitis and pneumonia (Boivin et al., 2002). Despite its recent discovery, the virus has most likely been spreading throughout human groups for a long time. It mainly affects older adults, people with underlying medical issues, and children under five. HMPV typically strikes before the age of five. Although HMPV can recur, symptoms are often modest following an initial infection. In 2010, Williams et al., carried out a second survey comparing reported and population-based HMPV infection cases in children admitted to hospitals.

In two US states, the researchers performed two years of population-wide prospective surveillance for HMPV infection in children under five years of age who had an acute respiratory disease or fever and were brought to the hospital. Swab-obtained nasal and throat tissues were genotyped and put through real-time testing using the reverse transcription (RT) polymerase chain reaction. The overall yearly prevalence of hospitalisations related to HMPV per 1000 children aged ≥5 years was 1.2 (95% CI: 0.9–1.6), with 42 (3.8%) out of 1104 children testing positive for the virus. Children aged 6–11 months had the second-highest rate (2.9 / 1000 [95% CI, 1.4–4.7]), behind infants aged 0–5 months (4.9 / 1000 [95% CI, 2.9–7.2]). HMPV infection was associated with a lower annual hospitalisation incidence than respiratory virus infection. However, it was similar to that of influenza and parainfluenza virus infection across all age groups. The average age of hospitalised HMPV-infected children was 6 months. Most often, children infected with HMPV were diagnosed with asthma, pneumonia, and bronchiolitis. It is concluded that HMPV had a population prevalence comparable to that of influenza and parainfluenza viruses, and it was found in 3.8% of kids admitted with ARI or delirium (Williams et al., 2010).

Devanthan and his colleagues have confirmed the above survey through a follow-up investigation based on the community of HMPV-infected patients. The incidence, genetic variety, systemic lineages, and clinical manifestations of hMPV infections in South Indian children under five are all clarified by the current study. A 2.5% incidence rate was found in 4519 samples that were analysed for hMPV, which was similar to research conducted in Spain between 2014 and 2021 (Anand et al., 2020). The positive rate for various viral respiratory infections was 21.75% (129 of 583), which was low (50.7%) in comparison to studies conducted in eastern India and high (7.1–13.0%) in comparison to comparable studies conducted in southern India. In children with ARI, viral infection rates range from 21.9% to 44.7%, according to research from China and Nepal (Pinana et al., 2023). In Puducherry, India, the hMPV genotypes A (A2.1, A2.2.1, A2.2.2) and B (B1, B2) co-circulate, according to phylogenetic analysis, which is consistent with results from other nations.

A2.2.1 and A2.2.2, in particular, demonstrated slow development over time in the A2.2 lineages, which was detected for the first time in India in the present investigation. Similarities were found between these strains and isolates from Japan in 2018 and the USA in 2010 (Hindupur et al., 2022). The link between hMPV and bronchiolitis and pneumonia—the latter of which is more severe in children younger than one year old who have previously experienced coughing episodes—is highlighted. Numerous hMPV progenitors are shown to co-circulate in Puducherry, and continuous changes in local strains are noted. To our knowledge, our results are the first to identify two separate hMPV sub-clusters (A2.2.1 and A2.2.2) under the A genotype in India.

Spread of HMPV

Touching infected objects or coming into close contact with an infected individual can spread HMPV. Examples include inhaling and exhaling, kissing, embracing, shaking hands, and putting your hand on things like toys, doorknobs, phones, or keyboards. The incubation period for HMPV can range from one to five days, depending on the individual. The virus can quickly spread across the respiratory tract after infecting the nasopharyngeal mucosa. The inflammatory process also causes monocytes and lymphocytes to pierce the airway endothelium. Pulmonary inflammation, which presents as fever, coughing, dyspnoea, and mucus production, is the outcome of these reactions together (Jain, 2025). Even though hMPV infections have become more common recently and have impacted healthcare facilities all over the world, there are currently no effective medications or commercially available vaccines for managing or preventing hMPV infections (Soto et al., 2018).

Molecular Virology: The Structure and Genes of a Virus

HMPV relates to the Pneumoviridae group and the genus Metapneumovirus. Approximately 13,280–13,378 nucleotides make up the encapsulated virus's one-stranded, non-segmented, negative-sense RNA pattern. The genes are further wrapped by a leader sequence at the 30' end and an auxiliary sequence at the 50' end, confirming Kumar *et al.,* (2018). The various methods by which these proteins impact the immunity of the host are unknown (Soto et al., 2018). According to Kumar *et al.,* (2018), the virus's genetic profile consists of 13,350 nucleotides and comprises RNA-dependent RNA polymerase (L), tiny hydrophobic molecule (SH), glycoprotein (G), fused protein (F), matrix proteins; (M2-1 and M2-2), phosphoprotein (P), the nucleoprotein (N), and a matrix protein (M).

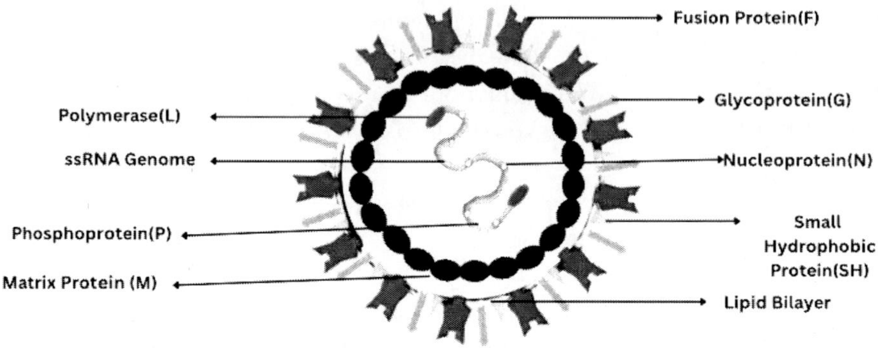

Figure 1. A block diagram of the human metapneumovirus (HMPV). The attachment glycoprotein (G), fusion protein (F), and small hydrophobic protein (SH) of the virus protrude on the virion surface. In contrast, the matrix protein (M) covers the inside of the lipid bilayer envelope. The negative sense of the viral single-stranded RNA genome is surrounded by the phosphoprotein (P), RNA-dependent RNA polymerase (L), and nucleoprotein (N).

The outer layer of the virion exposes three glycoproteins: the fusion (F) amino acids, the extensively glycosylated G protein content, and the small hydrophobic (SH) protein. To help the virus evade the host's antiretroviral defences, the SH protein may regulate recipient membrane permeability and suppress type I IFN signalling. However, its precise function is unresolved (Gaunt et al., 2011). The G and F protein molecules, which are vital to the virus's integration and passage into the host cell with the heparin sulfate proteoglycan receptors, are also evident on the virion covering. For propagating nucleic acids, the F gene promises to be a great choice because of its significant fraction maintenance (Mohamed et al., 2014). As the F and G components have implications for HMPV multiplication and host immunological action, they may be exploited by immunisations, monoclonal antibody therapies, and antiviral medications (Papenburg et al., 2013). Figure 1 demonstrates the complete HMPV virus structure. According to Ganguly et al., (2025), this matrix protein (M) creates a layer underneath the virus envelope in addition to aiding in its development and assembly. There are two proteins, M2-1 and M2-2, which are encoded by the second M (M2) gene. Whilst the M2-2 protein regulates a balance among transcriptional stages in the host cytosol and viral genome repetition, the M2-1 protein is required for the extended generation of viral mRNA and the efficacy of RNA-dependent RNA polymerase (RdRP). HMPV has been divided into two types, A and B, both of which are further split into A1 and A2 and B1 and B2. A2a,

A2b, and A2c are extra subsets of A2 (Parida et al., 2024). In an outbreak, one genotype typically becomes prevailing; however, both potentially co-circulate at the same time. The membrane glycoproteins of the virus have been categorised based on their degree of diversity. The G protein is highly varied, with only 30–35% of the subtypes sharing the same sequence, while the F protein is generally conserved across HMPV types, with a sequence identity of 94–98% (Hermos et al., 2010).

Role of HMPV Fusion Protein and Heparan Sulfate Interactions in Adherence and Infection of HMPV

The majority of paramyxoviruses express two main glycoproteins on their surface: fusion (F) and accessory proteins. The paramyxovirus attachment protein is type II integral cell membrane protein HN, H, or G. Although the attachment protein is required for virus attachment and subsequent membrane fusion in the Paramyxoviridae subfamily, it is interesting to note that studies have shown that some members of the Pneumoviridae subfamily can still spread infection even in the absence of the attachment protein (Chang et al., 2012). Moreover, African green monkeys may be effectively infected by a mutant virus lacking the G protein, indicating that the HMPV F protein can carry out both the attachment and fusion processes *in vivo* (Biacchesi et al., 2005). The HMPV F protein is a reliable predictor of human infection. Many different types of surface carbohydrates are expressed by most cells and mediate adhesion, proliferation, and signalling, among other functions. Based on their composition, glycosaminoglycans (GAGs) are often divided into six groups: heparin, chondroitin sulfate, dermatan sulfate, keratan sulfate, hyaluronic acid, and heparan sulfate (HS) (Prydz et al., 2000). The GAG that is most commonly involved in virus-cell communications is HS. It has been demonstrated that several herpesviruses attach to HS, which is also essential for the primary attachment of additional viruses, HIV and influenza. Almost all kinds of cells express integrins, which are cellular matrix proteins that bind with a variety of functions, such as controlling motility, tissue growth, and cell adhesion (Barczyk et al., 2010). Additionally, it was recently discovered that the $\alpha v\beta 1$ integrin is vital for the transmission of HMPV infection.

The study investigates the role of GAGs and the integrin $\alpha v\beta 1$ in HMPV infection using the wild-type strain of HMPV, a modified virus without the G protein, with a mutant virus without G and SH (Cseke et al., 2009).

Additionally, it was demonstrated that the G and SH proteins are not crucial for viral interaction and that F is the key viral cause for HMPV interaction. Lastly, it is shown that HMPV F exclusively relates to heparan sulphate and that HS is a crucial component of the HMPV binding receptor complex. It has been established that the main entrance factor of HMPV is its fusion protein, which facilitates membrane fusion and virus-cell interaction. Notably, the data show that the dependence on HS for infection is caused by HS connections with the F protein rather than the G protein as previously suggested (Wyde et al., 2004). Since other human diseases in the same family employ the binding protein for this function, HMPV differs from other paramyxoviruses. It utilises the F protein as its prime viral protein in cellular addition.

Diagnosis of HMPV

The four main techniques for diagnosing respiratory viral infections are serological analysis, RNA or DNA detection, antigen detection, and virus isolation by culture. Prior research has employed reverse transcription-PCR (RT-PCR), serological analysis, and virus isolation by culture to diagnose hMPV infections. effective practical method for detecting hMPV in respiratory samples is a real-time PCR test, which also determines the seasonal distribution and percentage of hMPV outbreaks (Pabbaraju et al., 2007 & Ebihara et al., 2005).

Home Care and Prevention of HMPV

It is essential to take preventive action against HMPV, especially in high-risk groups. Infections can be controlled by maintaining hand hygiene, the use of masks and the isolation of infected persons (Iragamreddy et al., 2025). There has been a recent surge in interest in medicinal plants used to treat respiratory viruses, particularly human metapneumovirus, because of the numerous adverse effects of synthetic medications. Many plants' bioactive chemicals like kaempferol, flavonoids, alkaloids, rotenone, terpenoids, vanillic acid, and phenolic compounds are utilised in the treatment of HMPV infections by blocking RNA polymerase and replication. They also strengthen the human immune system and help prevent HMPV viral infections (Ganguly et al., 2025). Anti-HMPV plant extract medicine is also becoming more and more well-liked as a safe and reasonably priced substitute for conventional antiviral drugs. Nutritional supplements with anti-oxidant and anti-inflammatory qualities, such as quercetin and resveratrol, have been helpful in reducing inflammation and oxidative stress in the fight against a number of illnesses (Komaravelli et al., 2015).

Treatment

HMPV does not currently have an approved antiviral treatment. Supportive measures are the treatment's mainstay. For patients who have a fever, antipyretic drugs such as ibuprofen and acetaminophen (paracetamol) are used (Iragamreddy et al., 2025). If the patient seems desiccated and not able to stand oral hydration, intravenous hydration is advised. Furthermore, patients may require further oxygen support and hospitalisation if HMPV results in acute respiratory failure (Jain, 2025). The most effective method of treating any viral infection is vaccination. Numerous attempts have already been made to create vaccines specific to HMPV, and the majority of these aim to target the virus's most immunogenic protein, the fusion protein.

Morbidity and Epidemiology

HMPV has been found on every continent and is distributed throughout the world. In temperate regions, the closing weeks of winter and spring are when HMPV is most prevalent, and the peak of prevalence at any given location usually happens at the same period as or after the crowning of RSV activity. HMPV has been found all year long in many places; however, at lower concentrations in the final days of spring (Kahn, 2006). Other factors, for instance, the child's age and the frequency of further chronic infections, finally decide the severity of the illness, which varies from a modest cough to unadorned pneumonia. HMPV was found to be more common among children born preterm or with any other chronic airway disease, including asthma, than other comparable respiratory viruses like RSV (Chang et al., 2012).

Even while re-infection can occur during maturity, a noteworthy share of progenies (90–100%) had been contaminated by the age of 5–10 years, according to several seroprevalence studies. Although it occurs at a younger rate—roughly 3.5% of adults with LRTI test diagnostic for HMPV infection—

HMPV infection is found in people of all ages except toddlers (Wilkhoo et al., 2025). In North America, the prevalence of severe hospitalised illness associated with HMPV is similar to that of influenza and the combined effects of parainfluenzas 1, 2, and 3. According to estimates, HMPV caused acute lower respiratory illnesses in 14.2 million kids below the age of five worldwide in 2018, leading to 643000 hospital admissions and 7700 in-hospital deaths. Similarly, another study with people from both hemispheres indicated that the burden of HMPV was significantly higher in the northern hemisphere than in the southern hemisphere. It is unclear, though, how strain variation affects illness severity, and it varies widely (Kumar et al., 2018).

Immunosuppression and HMPV

Immunocompromised individuals are susceptible to respiratory diseases caused by the human metapneumovirus, although HMPV infection in immunocompromised animals has not been previously modelled. One popular illustration of respiratory viral infections is the cotton-tufted rat, Sigmoidin hispidus. To figure out if impairment influences HMPV adverseaetiology and perhaps an anti-HMPV antiviral immunoglobulin would mitigate any negative adverse effects, the researchers created an immunodeficient cotton rat model to study HMPV infection. In addition to suppressing HMPV copying, immunised cotton rats fed anti-HMPV antibody MPV467 observed diminished chemokine production and lung disease. On the fifth day after infection, sick animals had higher pulmonary and nasal HMPV titers than healthy animals. On days 7 and 9 after infection, HMPV was still found in the debilitated animals' respiratory tracts, implying that the virus had grown for a long time. MPV467 doses safeguarded the top and bottom bronchial tracts from HMPV illness. According to Yim et al., (2023), these findings imply that immune-suppressed cotton rats are a valuable tool for researching the pathogenesis of HMPV and assessing treatments.

Features of HMPV That Are Clinical and Epidemiological

Badawy et al., carried out a clinical study in 2012. This study was conducted on male and female candidates. The elderly critical care facilities of KFSH and HGH, as well as internal male and female medical wards, were used to select 189 patients in total. Periodic workups were carried out on patients who came with suspected viral infections throughout February 2011 and January 2012. A Seeplex aerial virus testing kit was used to examine the respiratory swabs. The detection methods used were shell vial amplification, a quick culture method that uses monoclonal antibodies (mAbs) of aspirate fluid or nasal wash, direct fluorescent antibody labelling, and transcriptase-PCR (TC-PCR) for virus identification. The investigation found that 61 (32.3%) out of the 189 respiratory samples had respiratory viruses, and eight (13.1%) out of the sixty-one samples had HMPV. Seasonal variation was seen in HMPV. Six patients (75%) who tested positive for HMPV had significant medical conditions beforehand. When we employed the shell vial cells with mAbs, the authors found that non-Hodgkin lymphoma patients with the related isolated virus had a plaque of infected cells employing tiny syncytial forms. The remaining seven cases, however, showed isolated contaminated cells. The findings of shell vial cultures using mAbs or direct fluorescent antibody labelling were compared to all RT-PCR data from HMPV-positive individuals. According to the study's findings, HMPV is a dangerous illness that puts immunocompromised individuals at a significant risk of morbidity and death. A number of diagnostic tests could be required to confirm the identification of HMPV.

Future Directions for HMPV Research

By recognising the warning signs for serious illness, knowing the genetic and immunological traits of HMPV-infected persons may enable tailored treatment approaches. Each patient's peculiar DNA makeup or prone response profile can be used to design antiviral medication (Shanil et al., 2025).

The swift detection and therapy of HMPV infections rely on the development of fast, reliable, and reasonably priced diagnostic instruments. Technology known as next-generation sequencing (NGS) offers promise for boosting surveillance and revealing new vistas on the evolution of viruses.

Sturdy Vaccination Strategies are imperative that a global vaccination be devised that offers persistent protection against every type of HMPV. Because mRNA vaccines have previously been beneficial in other domains, these technologies are anticipated to be essential to the construction of the HMPV vaccine (Ren et al., 2015).

Impact of HMPV Over Time

Additionally, there is a pressing need for research on the ongoing effects of HMPV infections, namely their connection to the onset of pneumonia and chronic obstructive pulmonary disease (COPD).

Conclusion

In conclusion, the human metapneumovirus (HMPV), which has developed into a deadly respiratory disease, primarily affects young kids and individuals with deteriorated immune systems. Given its high frequency and ability to cause severe lower respiratory tract infections, as demonstrated by its almost universal early childhood seropositivity, it is imperative to comprehend its epidemiology, molecular virology, and pathogenesis. Despite its current findings, the infection has most likely been in human populations for a very long time. It has greatly increased the burden of respiratory infections and hospitalisations worldwide. Our ability to prevent and control HMPV infections is seriously compromised by the absence of licensed vaccines and targeted antiviral treatments. With further investigation into the assembly of the virus, host interactions (particularly the role of the fusion protein and heparan sulphate), and the development of diagnostic tools and treatment strategies, including plant-based remedies and vaccination programs, the impact of this important respiratory virus may be mitigated. Future research initiatives are crucial to fighting the sickness and death linked with this frequent respiratory virus, reducing the sickness and death linked with this frequent respiratory virus, and improving public health outcomes. These include research on the longstanding significances of HMPV infection, the creation of a universal vaccine, tailored medical strategies, and sophisticated diagnostic tools.

References

Anand, M., & Nimmala, P. (2020). Seasonal incidence of respiratory viral infections in Telangana, India: utility of a multiplex PCR assay to bridge the knowledge gap. *Tropical medicine & international health : TM & IH*, *25*(12), 1503–1509.

Badawy, E. S., Rahman, S. M. A., Yousef, M. S., Bukhary, S. Z. (2012). Molecular diagnosis of human metapneumovirus. *Egypt J Intern Med,* 24, 47–50.

Barczyk, M., Carracedo, S., & Gullberg, D. (2010). Integrins. *Cell and tissue research*, *339*(1), 269–280.

Biacchesi, S., Pham, Q. N., Skiadopoulos, M. H., Murphy, B. R., Collins, P. L., & Buchholz, U. J. (2005). Infection of nonhuman primates with recombinant human metapneumovirus lacking the SH, G, or M2-2 protein categorises each as a nonessential accessory protein and identifies vaccine candidates. *Journal of virology*, 79(19), 12608–12613.

Boivin, G., Abed, Y., Pelletier, G., Ruel, L., & Moisan, D., et al., (2002). Virological Features and Clinical Manifestations Associated with Human Metapneumovirus: A New Paramyxovirus Responsible for Acute Respiratory-Tract Infections in All Age Groups. *The Journal of Infectious Diseases*, 186, 13304.

Chang, A., Masante, C., Buchholz, U. J., & Dutch, R. E. (2012). Human Metapneumovirus (HMPV) Binding and Infection Are Mediated by Interactions between the HMPV Fusion Protein and Heparan Sulfate. *Journal of Virology*, 86(6), 3230-3243.

Cseke, G., Maginnis, M. S., Cox, R. G., Tollefson, S. J., Podsiad, A. B., Wright, D. W., Dermody, T. S., & Williams, J. V. (2009). Integrin alphavbeta1 promotes infection by human metapneumovirus. *Proceedings of the National Academy of Sciences of the United States of America*, 106(5), 1566–1571.

Ebihara, T., Endo, R., Ma, X., Ishiguro, N., & Kikuta, H. (2005). Detection of human metapneumovirus antigens in nasopharyngeal secretions by an immunofluorescent-antibody test. *Journal of clinical microbiology*, *43*(3), 1138–1141.

Ganguly, P., Konar, A., DS, S., Ghosh, P., Chakraborty, A., Garai, P., & Mukherjee, R. (2025). Plant-based approach in the treatment of HMPV virus. *YMER*, 24(3), 545556.

Gaunt, E. R., Jansen, R. R., Poovorawan, Y., Templeton, K. E., Toms, G. L., & Simmonds, P. (2011). Molecular epidemiology and evolution of human respiratory syncytial virus and human metapneumovirus. *PloS one*, *6*(3), e17427.

Hermos, C. R., Vargas, S. O., & McAdam, A. J. (2010). Human metapneumovirus. *Clinics in laboratory medicine*, *30*(1), 131–148.

Hindupur, A., Menon, T. & Dhandapani, P. (2022). Molecular investigation of human metapneumovirus in children with acute respiratory infections in Chennai, South India, from 2016–2018. *Braz J Microbiol,* 53, 655661. .

Hindupur, A., Menon, T., & Dhandapani, P. (2022). Molecular investigation of human metapneumovirus in children with acute respiratory infections in Chennai, South India, from 2016-2018. *Brazilian journal of microbiology : [publication of the Brazilian Society for Microbiology]*, *53*(2), 655–661.

Iragamreddy, V. R. (2025). Human Metapneumovirus (HMPV): A Comprehensive Review of its Impact on Pediatric and General Populations. *International journal for multidisciplinary research,* 7(4), 250134972.

Jain, S. (2025). Human Metapneumovirus: An Overview of Its Impact on Human Health. *International journal of pharmaceutical sciences,* 3(1), 16701673.

Kahn J. S. (2006). Epidemiology of human metapneumovirus. *Clinical microbiology reviews*, *19*(3), 546–557.

Komaravelli, N., Kelley, J. P., Garofalo, M. P., Wu, H., Casola, A., & Kolli, D. (2015). Role of dietary antioxidants in human metapneumovirus infection. *Virus research*, *200*, 19–23.

Kumar, P., & Srivastava, M. (2018). Prophylactic and therapeutic approaches for human metapneumovirus. *VirusDis.* 29, 434–444.

Miyakawa, R., Zhang, H., Brooks, W. A., Prosperi, C., Baggett, H. C., et al., (2025). Epidemiology of human metapneumovirus among children with severe or very severe pneumonia in high pneumonia burden settings: the Pneumonia Etiology Research for Child Health (PERCH) study experience. *Clinical microbiology and Infection,* 31, 441-450.

Mohamed, M. S. E., Reiche, S., Jacobsen, S., Thabit A. G., Badary, M. S., Brune, W., Schweiger, B., & Osman, A. H. (2014). Molecular Analysis of Human Metapneumovirus Detected in Patients with Lower Respiratory Tract Infection in Upper Egypt. *International Journal of Microbiology*. 11, 290793.

Pabbaraju, K., Wong, S., McMillan, T., E. Lee, B., & Fox, J. D. (2007). Diagnosis and epidemiological studies of human metapneumovirus using real-time PCR. *Journal of clinical virology*, 40(3), 186192.

Panda, S., Mohakud, N. K., Pena, L., & Kumar, S. (2014). Human metapneumovirus: review of an important respiratory pathogen. *International journal of infectious diseases*, 25, 4552.

Papenburg, J., Carbonneau, J., Isabel, S., Bergeron, M. G., Williams, J. V., Serres, G. D., Hamelin, M. E., & Boivin, G. (2013). Genetic diversity and molecular evolution of the major human metapneumovirus surface glycoproteins over a decade. *Journal of Clinical Virology,* 58(3), 541547.

Parida, P., Shetty, U., Parida, P., Varamballi, P., Mukhopadhyay, C., & N, S. (2024). Molecular detection and genotyping of HMPV in patients with severe acute respiratory infection in India. *Annals of medicine*, *56*(1), 2398719.

Piñana, M., González-Sánchez, A., Andrés, C., Abanto, M., Vila, J., Esperalba, J., Moral, N., Espartosa, E., Saubi, N., Creus, A., Codina, M. G., Folgueira, D., Martinez-Urtaza, J., Pumarola, T., & Antón, A. (2023). The emergence, impact, and evolution of human metapneumovirus variants from 2014 to 2021 in Spain. *The Journal of infection*, 87(2), 103–110.

Prydz, K., & Dalen, K. T. (2000). Synthesis and sorting of proteoglycans. *Journal of cell science*, *113 Pt 2*, 193–205.

Ren, J., Phan, T., & Bao, X. (2015). Recent vaccine development for human metapneumovirus. *The Journal of general virology*, *96*(Pt 7), 1515–1520.

Shanil, P. M., & Jasmin, K. F. (2025). Human metapneumovirus: Unraveling the innovations and horizons. *World journal of pharmaceutical and medical research*, 11(2), 116-123.

Soto, J. A., Gálvez, N. M. S., Benavente, F. M., Pizarro-Ortega, M. S., Lay, M. K., Riedel, C., Bueno, S. M., Gonzalez, P. A., & Kalergis, A. M. (2018). Human Metapneumovirus: Mechanisms and Molecular Targets Used by the Virus to Avoid the Immune System. *Frontiers in immunology*, *9*, 2466.

Wilkhoo, H. S., Islam, A. W., Wilkhoo, H. S., Hussain, S., Singh, B., & Kadam, S. R. (2025). Clinical Insights and Advancements in Human Metapneumovirus management and Prognosi. *Discoveries*, 13(1), e204.

Williams, J. V., Edwards, K. M., Weinberg, G. A., Griffin, M. R., Hall, C. B., Zhu, Y., Szilagyi, P. G., Wang, C. K., Yang, C. F., Silva, D., Ye, D., Spaete, R. R., & Crowe,

J. E., Jr (2010). Population-based incidence of human metapneumovirus infection among hospitalized children. *The Journal of infectious diseases*, *201*(12), 1890–1898.

Wyde, P. R., Moylett, E. H., Chetty, S. N., Jewell, A., Bowlin, T. L., & Piedra, P. A. (2004). Comparison of the inhibition of human metapneumovirus and respiratory syncytial virus by $NMSO_3$ in tissue culture assays. *Antiviral research*, 63(1), 51–59.

Yim, K. C., Mousa, J. J., Blanco, J. C. G., Kim, S., & Boukhvalova, M. S. (2023). Human Metapneumovirus (hMPV) Infection and MPV467 Treatment in Immunocompromised Cotton Rats *Sigmodon hispidus*. *Viruses*, *15*(2), 476.

Chapter 4

Pathogenesis and Clinical Manifestations of Human Metapneumovirus Infections (HMPV)

Sandeep Singh[1]
Gaurav Gupta[2,3,*]
and Pallavi[4]
[1]Adesh Institute of Pharmacy and Biomedical Sciences, Adesh University, Bathinda, Punjab, India
[2]Centre for Medical and Bioallied Health Sciences Research, Ajman University, Ajman, UAE
[3]Centre for Research Impact and Outcome, Chitkara College of Pharmacy, Chitkara University, Punjab, India
[4]Amity Institute of Pharmacy, Amity University, Rajasthan, Jaipur, India

Abstract

Human metapneumovirus is a prime cause of respiratory tract infections. Compared to other infections, the intensity and clinical manifestations of pneumonia related to HMPV have not been well investigated. The human metapneumovirus, or hMPV, has been discovered worldwide since 2001. HMPV is a prevalent pulmonary ailment, particularly in newborns and babies. The virus may cause asthma with infections of the lower and upper respiratory tract. Additionally, there are at least two primary hMPV genotypes in circulation throughout the epidemics. It is debatable if these genotypes correlate with different serotypes. When children have acute respiratory tract infections, HMPV is the primary cause of hospitalisation, accounting for five to ten per cent of all admissions. Children infected with HMPV might develop severe asthma and

---

* Corresponding Author's Email: gauravpharma25@gmail.com

In: Human Metapneumovirus
Editors: Anjali Sharma, Vishnu Mittal, Devkant Sharma et al.
ISBN: 979-8-90134-063-9

bronchiolitis. The symptoms resemble those brought on by the respiratory syncytial virus in humans. Initial hMPV infection often occurs in early infancy, despite frequent reinfections throughout life. You may be more susceptible to a dangerous hMPV infection if you were born prematurely, are young, have had a nosocomial infection in the past, or have long-term lung, heart, or brain issues. In terms of mortality and fatality, the latest discovered HMPV seems just as dangerous as HRSV. Because hMPV is a severe respiratory infection, it is crucial to understand its pathophysiology and molecular mechanisms that lead to severe illness to develop an effective hMPV vaccine. Clinical characteristics were unable to differentiate HMPV-associated pneumonia from other infections consistently. HMPV-related pneumonia was less critical than bacterial and mature RSV pneumonia, although it was comparable to or worse than other prevalent illnesses.

Keywords: respiratory tract infections, pneumonia, pathogenesis, severe, human metapneumovirus

Abbreviations

HMPV	Human Metapneumovirus
HRSV	Human respiratory syncytial virus
ARTIs	Acute respiratory tract infections
AMPVs	Avian Metapneumovirus
PCR	Polymerase chain reaction
RT-PCR	Reverse transcriptase polymerase chain reaction
LRTI	Lower respiratory tract infection
URI	Upper respiratory tract infection
COPD	Chronic obstructive pulmonary disease
ILI	Influenza-like illness
HIV	Human immunodeficiency virus
CPEs	Cytopathic effects
VLPs	Virus-like particles
LLC-MK2	Rhesus monkey kidney epithelial cells
Th	Helper T cell.

Introduction

The most significant risks to public health globally are that ARTIs produce a high risk of human morbidity and death (Feng et al., 2024). Several developing or novel respiratory infections causing human illness were discovered at the start of the twenty-first century, including coronavirus, critical acute respiratory syndrome, and HMPV. Single-stranded, encapsulated, RNA-negative-sense viruses are known as metapneumoviruses (Hamelin et al., 2004; Shafagati & Williams, 2018). Metapneumoviruses, which belong to the Pneumoviridae family, are found in both humans (AMPVs or avian metapneumoviruses) and birds. AMPV and human metapneumovirus are Bird and human respiratory tract infections caused by closely related viruses that have a similar genetic structure (Jesse et al., 2022).

Genotyping investigations have revealed that human metapneumovirus strains are separated into four sub-lineages, with two major lineages, A1 and A2, and B1 and B2 (Mackay et al., 2004, Principi et al., 2006). In 2001, Van den Hoogen et al., reported that a new agent in the Netherlands, found in nasopharyngeal aspirates from toddlers and babies who were hospitalised for respiratory conditions, included human metapneumovirus (HMPV). That virus was distinct from other regular respiratory viruses since it was not detectable by PCR-dependent methods using viral primers specific to the genome or immunological testing using virus-specific antibodies. Prior to the identification of genomic sequence segments using molecular biology technology, the genetic characterisation of this agent was unclear. Dutch researchers used a method called randomly primed PCR to extract the genetic sequence of this unidentified disease. This virus was termed human metapneumovirus because, according to limited sequencing data, it appears to be closely associated with avian pneumovirus, a member of the Metapneumovirus genus (hMPV) (Kahn, 2006; Van den Hoogen et al., 2001; Pata & Kristeva, 2025).

Structure and Genetic Variability of HMPV

Genus Metapneumovirus, subfamily Pneumoviridae, and family Paramyxoviridae, is the sole human virus (Amer., 2016). The single-stranded RNA virus known as HMPV has a genomic size of about 13 kilobases. Nine encoded proteins by eight genes in the genome: M2-1/M2-2 (two proteins are encoded by same gene), matrix protein (M), fusion protein (F), nucleoprotein (N), phosphoprotein (P), small water insoluble protein (SH), glycoprotein (G), and large protein (L) (Yang et al., 2024). Like all other members of its family, HMPV is an enveloped virus with a negative single-stranded, non-segmented RNA genome and a helical capsid (Principi & Esposito, 2014). Two distinct hMPV groups and subgroups have been identified by genetic studies on the virus; more recently, evidence has indicated that there are several lineages. (Mackay et al., 2004, Bastien et al., 2004). Amino acid changes are caused by the highest degree of nucleotide polymorphism in the human metapneumovirus attachment glycoprotein. The sequence alteration of the hMPV G gene has been linked to immunological pressure. (Ludewick et al., 2005). Upon genetic evaluation of both G and F proteins, human metapneumovirus strains were divided into two subgroups (A and B) and four genotypes (A1, A2, B1, and B2) (Principi & Esposito, 2014).

Epidemiology

HMPV infections affect a diverse variety of individuals worldwide, with children under five, immunocompromised adults, and the elderly being most susceptible (Amrutkar et al., 2025). Children in their initial few months of life had the incidence rates of HMPV, which was found in six per cent of hospitalised children, seven per cent of children detected in external patient clinics, with 7% of children seen in the emergency unit. Overall, there was a 1 in 1,000 chance of hospitalisation for hMPV infection in children under five years old, a 3 in 1,000 risk for babies younger than six months, and a 2 in 1,000 chance for children between six and eleven months old (Principi & Esposito., 2014).

Seroprevalence studies have shown that, although reinfection can occur throughout adulthood, a significant portion (90-100%) of children are infected by the time they are five to ten years old (Van den Hoogen et al., 2001; Panda et al., 2014). Among the respiratory diseases that hMPV can co-infect include influenza A, influenza B, bocavirus, enterovirus, rhinovirus, parainfluenza virus, coronavirus, and RSV (Panda et al, 2014; Pilger et al., 2011; Fathima et al., 2012). According to certain studies, seasonal division of HMPV prevalence may be influenced by meteorological conditions, such as air speed, relative humidity, temperature, and the duration of sunshine (Ye et al., 2023). The winter-spring season was when most viral activity was seen in temperate regions, whereas the spring-summer season was when it was documented in subtropical regions (Hamelin et al., 2004).

Pathogenesis of HMPV

Droplet precautions, such as maintaining a physical separation of at least 6 feet, are advised since transmission occurs through direct contact with secretions and fomites. Incubation typically lasts four to nine days, followed by a surge in viral shedding that lasts for nearly one to two weeks. A person remains infected from day two to fourteen; however, the virus may persist in the lungs for weeks (Pata & Kristeva, 2025). After being injected into the nasopharyngeal mucosa, the virus can swiftly disseminate throughout the respiratory system (Porwal et al., 2025). Cynomolgus macaques, cotton rats, and BALB/c mice are among the animal models used to study the immunogenicity and pathophysiology of hMPV infection. After intranasal hMPV exposure in cotton rats and BALB/c mice, the virus titer in the nasal turbinate peaks on the second day, while in lung homogenates, it peaks from day 4 to day 5 (Darniot et al., 2005). In contrast to BALB/c mice, which exhibit a more prolonged sickness with biphasic hMPV serotype B viral replication, the majority of small animal screening methods show respiratory system viral clearance by day 21. Rats seem to be asymptomatic; however, mice show respiratory problems and weight loss on days 5–7 following infection (Alvarez & Tripp, 2005; Hermos et al., 2010). Furthermore, hMPV infection increases myofibroblast thickness near the epithelium of the airways, as well as cellular debris staining (Principi et al., 2006).

HMPV significantly harms the airway epithelium, according to samples obtained by bronchoalveolar lavage in four days of virus being discovered in nasal secretions of children suffering from acute respiratory disease (Vargas et al., 2004). In the presence of hemosiderin-loaded macrophages, a large number of neutrophils, and noticeable mucus, infection of airway epithelial cells results in necrosis, ciliacytophthoria, cell deterioration, and red cytoplasmic inclusions (Principi et al., 2006). In fact, there have been several focal lesions where inflammation of the lung parenchyma has been linked to the presence of HMPV proteins. This suggests that (i) host immunity activation is restricted to areas where the virus replicates, and (ii) the Extent of respiratory participation is closely linked to viral spread in the respiratory tract (Kuiken et al., 2004) as with other respiratory viral diseases. The contaminated cells cause respiratory symptoms such as mucus hyperproduction and bronchial hyper-responsivity, which are caused by an inflammatory response shown by cellular infiltration of perivascular and parabrachial. Additional pathological findings involve the presence of foamy macrophages and degraded epithelial cells, detached ciliary tufts, intra-alveolar hemosiderin and rounded red cytoplasmic inclusions (Vargas et al., 2004).

Clinical Manifestations of Human Metapneumovirus Infections

Patients of various ages have been documented to exhibit several clinical signs and symptoms related to minor upper respiratory tract infections to severe illnesses requiring hospitalisation, including human metapneumovirus infections. Adults infected with hMPV typically experience minor respiratory symptoms similar to a typical cold, including coughing, hoarseness, sore throat, rhinorrhea, and occasionally fever); Hospitalised juvenile patients with medical disorders, immunocompromised, and elderly individuals who are at risk are more likely to get hMPV disease (Falsey et al., 2003; Stockton et al., 2002; Wilbrink et al., 2002). A group of these patients has been observed to demonstrate a range of symptoms affecting the uppermost with lower respiratory region, such as rhinorrhea, coughing, wheezing, and dyspnea. The diagnosis may result in some individuals being admitted to critical care units, which might include everything from pneumonia to bronchitis and rhinosinusitis. Furthermore, there have been cases of otitis media, conjunctivitis, diarrhoea, vomiting, rash, febrile seizures, and feeding issues (Boivin et al., 2002, Peiris et al., 2003, van den Hoogen et al., 2003, Boivin et al.,2003, Esper et al., 2003).

Lower Respiratory Tract Disease

According to several studies, hMPV causes a sizable portion of lower respiratory tract infection in newborns and young children and is another one of the most prevalent sources of bronchiolitis in childhood, behind RSV (Chano et al., 2005, Freymouth et al., 2003; Laham et al., 2004, Mullins et al., 2004, Sasaki et al., 2005, Viazov et al., 2003). Geographical location and season affect the prevalence of human metapneumovirus-associated LRTI in youngsters. Most research (Bastien et al., 2003, Esper et al., 2004, McAdam et al., 2004, Williams et al., 2004) estimate incidences between 5 and 15%; nevertheless, other investigations have observed higher rates (Maggi et al., 2003; Dollner et al., 2004). There is no discernible difference between clinical signs of infection of RSV and hMPV in young children. A hMPV infection manifested as fever, tachypnea, coughing, hypoxia, and abnormalities of chest radiographs, including hyperinflation, infiltrates and peribronchial cuffing. Young children seldom appear to have an asymptomatic hMPV infection.

Only one out of 86 asymptomatic children (1.2%) in the Williams et al., trial tested positive for hMPV, suggesting that LRT is caused in part by hMPV (Bastien et al., 2003; Esper et al., 2004; McAdam et al., 2004; Williams et al., 2004) Hospitalisation for LRTI linked to hMPV in newborns and young children is common. Ten per cent of LRTI hospitalisations are probably caused by hMPV, which, after RSV, is the second most frequent cause of LRTI that requires hospitalisation (Bastien et al., 2003; Esper et al., 2004; McAdam et al., 2004; Williams et al., 2004). Common diagnoses for hospitalised children who test positive for human metapneumovirus are bronchiolitis, bronchitis and pneumonia. The sickness linked to hMPV does not have any symptoms that are distinct to any one infection. This is clear now, newborns & young children are the paediatric population's most vulnerable groups to serious illness caused by either hMPV or RSV, even though some studies indicate that the mean age for hMPV-linked LRTI is slightly higher than for respiratory syncytial virus-linked LRTI. Effective medicines and immunisation initiatives must target this patient population (Esper et al., 2004; Pelletier et al., 2002).

Infection of the Upper Respiratory Tract

Like more human respiratory viruses, hMPV is linked to the Upper respiratory tract. Although different studies have different definitions of URI, hMPV may be to blame for 5–15% of cases of pediatric URI. In a recent study, Williams et al., looked at respiratory samples from children with URI who were 5 years old and had stomatitis, otitis media (OM), coryza, conjunctivitis, or pharyngitis during a 20-year period. These children had no prior virological diagnosis. URIs associated with hMPV were found in 1–5% of 2,000 samples analysed through real-time Reverse transcriptase-PCR. From year to year, this was different. Overall, hMPV was linked with a lower percentage of URIs than RSV, adenovirus, influenza virus, & parainfluenza viruses. In a study,

50% of children with URI connected to hMPV had otitis media (Williams et al., 2006).

hMPV in the Population of Adults

In adults, asthma and COPD are connected with ILI, bronchitis, and pneumonia (Falsey et al., 2006). Compared to children, adults probably have lower overall rates of hMPV illness. Adults of all ages can develop an illness linked to hMPV (Falsey et al., 2003). 3.4% of people suffering from respiratory tract illnesses had hMPV, according to Falsey et al., 158 controls with no respiratory issues did not test positive for hMPV (Falsey et al., 2006). hMPV was uncommon in people with acute respiratory infections who were previously healthy and who were examined throughout the course of three months in San Francisco, California; however, this could be because of the study's short duration.(Louie et al., 2005) Elderly persons with hMPV were more likely to have dyspnea than young adults. It's unclear how hMPV contributes to COPD flare-ups. People with acute exacerbations of COPD have been found to have hMPV (Hamelin et al., 2005; Rohde et al., 2005). However, a causal involvement may be challenging to define because the length of it is uncertain. It is uncertain if patients with COPD shed viruses. Further study is needed to definethe involvement of hMPV in COPD (Louie et al., 2005).

Infection in the Immunocompromised Person

Serious and protracted infections in the immunocompromised host can result from hMPV. The identification of hMPV in immunocompromised individuals. Numerous case reports & short case sequences have reported persons with severe pulmonary disease (Cane et al., 2003, Esper et al., 2004, Larcher et al., 2005, Martino et al.,). Numerous case reports & short case sequences have reported persons with severe pulmonary disease (Cane et al., 2003, Esper et al., 2004, Larcher et al., 2005, Martino et al., 2005, Pelletier et al., 2002). In a research of lung transplant patients, nine out of twenty-five individuals who were examined over the course of a year tested positive for hMPV at least once. Numerous deaths were reported. Since many of these people had concurrent bacterial or fungal illnesses, it is challenging to identify the symptoms of hMPV illness that they exhibit. In a prospective 4-year analysis of individuals with haematological malignancy infections, a positive hMPV test result was found in 9% of respiratory tract infection episodes of 22 people who were diagnosed positive for hMPV, 16 (73%) had received a hematopoietic stem cell transplant. Eight of the twenty hMPV-individuals who first experienced URI symptoms went on to develop LRTI. Two of the three patients who passed away from hMPV-associated LRTI also had concurrent bacterial infections. One patient died within a month of the onset of LRTI, and the sole pathogen found in that patient was hMPV. Two different virus strains were revealed to have infected an immunocompromised child with hMPV twice over a 10-month period. It is challenging to detect whether the hMPV-linked illness was more or less critical in children with HIV than in children in the absence of HIV, since there were so few children in the research. However, children infected with HIV have been confirmed to have HMPV (Williams et al., 2005; Madhi et al., 2003).

Diagnosis of HMPV Infections

Several methods are now available for detecting hMPV in clinical samples. RT-PCR, often referred to as real-time PCR or conventional PCR, appears to be the most crucial method, as it is faster and more sensitive than other methods. The remarkable nucleotide similarity across the four subgroups and ability to determine genotype causing infection after amplicon sequence have made N, P, F, or L genes the focus of PCR techniques often (Mackay et al., 2004; Maertzdorf et al., 2004, Cote S et al., 2003, Mackay et al., 2003) Although cell culture is another option for diagnosis, hMPV growth is meticulous. It often takes over 14 days for cytopathic effects (CPEs) to manifest. The late discovery of hMPV in 2001 may be partially attributed to this slow increase. Vero (green African monkey) cells and tertiary LLC-MK2 (monkey kidney cells) are primary cell lines utilised for viral growth.

The various CPEs seen after inoculation include focal rounding, cell death, and syncytial forms resembling hRSV (Boivin et al., 2002; Deffrasnes et al., 2005; Hamelin et al., 2004). Unlike the other cell lines, human bronchial cells (16HBE140) do not require exogenous trypsin and have also been successfully employed for hMPV identification (Ingram RE et al., 2006). Lastly, serological testing can only make a diagnosis after the fact. Because paediatric infections are so common, it is necessary to collect early and convalescent serum samples. A seroconversion that results in a quadruple enhancement in antibody titers is required to determine the latest infection.

Currently available serologic diagnostics include ELISA and immunofluorescence tests that use either viral recombinant proteins or hMPV-contaminated cells (Ebihara et al., 2003; Wolf et al., 2003; Ebihara et al., 2004).

Management and Treatment Strategies

The majority of hMPV infection therapies now on the market are supportive. Nonetheless, several studies have proposed the use of fusion inhibitors, immunoglobulin, ribavirin, and short-interfering RNA in the treatment and management of hMPV contamination. Rodent and non-human primate models have been used to evaluate a number of hMPV vaccine candidates. None has been tested on human volunteers yet, despite their encouraging results. When tested in mice, a heat-inactivated viral vaccine against hMPV increased the incidence of pulmonary illness, suggesting potential issues (Wyde et al., 2003, Kitanovski et al., 2013, Hamelin et., al., 2010, Ulbrandt et al., 2006, Corti et al., 2013, Deffrasness et al., 2008, Deffrasnes et al., 2008, Darniot et al., 2012). It has been demonstrated that T cell epitope vaccines lessen immunomodulation caused by hMPV challenge. Mice given a human metapneumovirus cytotoxic T cell determinant vaccination generate less Th1 & Th2 type cytokines after an hMPV challenge than mice not given the vaccine (Herd et al., 2006).

By mimicking features of the viral surface of both subgroups A and B, a recent study investigated hMPV VLPs as a possible vaccine candidate. Mice exposed to both homologous and heterologous strains showed a strong humoral immune response to these VLPs. Even though an hMPV-VLP vaccine seems like a good plan, A vaccination that is effective against every hMPV subgroup will require more investigation. The introduction of plasmid-dependent reverse genetics technology significantly facilitated the development of a live vaccine to prevent hMPV infection (Smith, 2007). In a recent study, a living attenuated vaccine lineage of hMPV was developed through modifying the glycosylation site in protein F. Even when tested 56 days after inoculation, the vaccine was shown to provide full protection against a homologous virus challenge and moderate protection from a heterologous viral infection. All of these results suggest that a deeper understanding of the molecular pathophysiology of hMPV is necessary before developing an effective vaccine to prevent it (Liu et al., 2013).

Future Perspectives

The prevention of hMPV transmission still depends on infection control measures, including wearing masks, maintaining hand hygiene, and separating individuals with the infection from others. Education campaigns can increase knowledge and reduce the stigma associated with respiratory illnesses. Effective vaccines, such as live-attenuated, inactivated, & subunit-based formulations, must be developed immediately to lessen the worldwide impact of HMPV. Pan-pneumovirus vaccines offer cross-protective immunity against both HMPV and RSV and have been the subject of recent research, which might transform preventative methods. Researchers are investigating substances that could efficiently inhibit viral replication while minimising host cell toxicity as part of their ongoing search for novel antiviral drugs and identifying reliable biomarkers correlated with the severity and progression of disease. Cost-effective preventive and treatment strategies remain crucial, especially in environments with limited resources.

Conclusion

Human metapneumovirus is a common but poorly understood respiratory infection that can seriously impair the health of immunocompromised, elderly, and pediatric patients. Even with their improvements, current diagnostic techniques still have drawbacks in terms of cost-effectiveness, speed, and accessibility, particularly in resource-constrained environments. Our ability to quickly detect and treat hMPV infections could be significantly enhanced by the development of rapid, point-of-care diagnostic methods. Looking ahead, there are encouraging opportunities for better treatment of hMPV infections through the combination of cutting-edge molecular tools, enhanced surveillance systems, and creative therapeutic approaches. Reducing the impacts of sickness will require increasing public health awareness and implementing early diagnosis procedures. Although experimental antiviral therapies, such as ribavirin and monoclonal antibodies, show promise, the majority of current therapy options are supportive and centre on oxygen therapy and hydration.

References

Alvarez, R., & Tripp, R. A. (2005). The immune response to human metapneumovirus is associated with aberrant immunity and impaired virus clearance in BALB/c mice. *Journal of Virology*, 79(10), 5971–5978.

Amer, H. M. (2016). Molecular epidemiology of human metapneumovirus in Riyadh Province, Saudi Arabia. *Journal of Molecular Microbiology and Biotechnology*, 26(6), 414–421.

Amrutkar, M. S. S., Marwah, M. N., Kedari, M. C. C., Sati, M. T. S., Kumar, M. V., & Dilip, M. B. S. (2025). *Seasonal trends and global impact of human metapneumovirus: a review of current research*, 5(2), 152–157.

Bastien, N., Ward, D., Van Caeseele, P., Brandt, K., Lee, S. H., McNabb, G., Klisko, B., Chan, E., & Li, Y. (2003). Human metapneumovirus infection in the Canadian population. *Journal of Clinical Microbiology*, 41, 4642–4646.

Bastien, N., Liu, L., Ward, D., Taylor, T., & Li, Y. (2004). Genetic variability of the G glycoprotein gene of human metapneumovirus. *Journal of Clinical Microbiology*, 42(8), 3532–3537.

Boivin, G., De Serres, G., Cote, S., et al., (2003). Human metapneumovirus infections in hospitalized children. *Emerging Infectious Diseases*, 9, 634–640.

Cane, P. A., van den Hoogen, B. G., Chakrabarti, S., Fegan, C. D., & Osterhaus, A. D. (2003). Human metapneumovirus in a haematopoietic stem cell transplant recipient with fatal lower respiratory tract disease. *Bone Marrow Transplantation*, 31, 309–310.

Chano, F., Rousseau, C., Laferriere, C., Couillard, M., & Charest, H. (2005). Epidemiological survey of human metapneumovirus infection in a large pediatric tertiary care center. *Journal of Clinical Microbiology*, 43, 5520–5525.

Cote, S., Abed, Y., & Boivin, G. (2003). Comparative evaluation of real-time PCR assays for detection of the human metapneumovirus. *Journal of Clinical Microbiology*, 41, 3631–3635.

Darniot, M., Petrella, T., Aho, S., Pothier, P., & Manoha, C. (2005). Immune response and alteration of pulmonary function after primary human metapneumovirus (hMPV) infection of BALB/c mice. *Vaccine*, 23(36), 4473–4480.

Darniot, M., Schildgen, V., Schildgen, O., Sproat, B., Kleines, M., Ditt, V., et al., (2012). RNA interference in vitro and in vivo using Dsi RNA targeting the nucleocapsid N mRNA of human metapneumovirus. *Antiviral Research*, 93, 364–373.

Deffrasnes, C., Cote, S., & Boivin, G. (2005). Analysis of replication kinetics of the human metapneumovirus in different cell lines by real-time PCR. *Journal of Clinical Microbiology*, 43, 488–490.

Deffrasnes, C., Hamelin, M. È., & Boivin, G. (2007). Human metapneumovirus. *Seminars in Respiratory and Critical Care Medicine*, 28(2), 213–221.

Deffrasness, C., Hamelin, M. E., Prince, G. A., & Boivin, G. (2008). Identification and evaluation of a highly effective fusion inhibitor for human metapneumovirus. *Antimicrobial Agents and Chemotherapy*, 52, 279–287.

Dollner, H., Risnes, K., Radtke, A., & Nordbo, S. A. (2004). Outbreak of human metapneumovirus infection in Norwegian children. *Pediatric Infectious Disease Journal*, 23, 436–440.

Ebihara, T., Endo, R., Kikuta, H., et al., (2003). Seroprevalence of human metapneumovirus in Japan. *Journal of Medical Virology*, 70, 281–283.

Ebihara, T., Endo, R., Kikuta, H., et al., (2004). Human metapneumovirus infection in Japanese children. *Journal of Clinical Microbiology*, 42, 126–132.

Esper, F., Boucher, D., Weibel, C., Martinello, R. A., & Kahn, J. S. (2003). Human metapneumovirus infection in the United States: clinical manifestations associated with a newly emerging respiratory infection in children. *Pediatrics*, 111, 1407–1410.

Esper, F., Martinello, R. A., Boucher, D., Weibel, C., Ferguson, D., Landry, M. L., & Kahn, J. S. (2004). A 1-year experience with human metapneumovirus in children aged 5 years. *Journal of Infectious Diseases*, 189, 1388–1396.

Falsey, A. R., Erdman, D., Anderson, L. J., & Walsh, E. E. (2003). Human metapneumovirus infections in young and elderly adults. *Journal of Infectious Diseases*, 187, 785–790.

Falsey, A. R., Criddle, M. C., & Walsh, E. E. (2006). Detection of respiratory syncytial virus and human metapneumovirus by reverse transcription polymerase chain reaction in adults with and without respiratory illness. *Journal of Clinical Virology*, 35, 46–50.

Fathima, S., Lee, B. E., May-Hadford, J., Mukhi, S., & Drews, S. J. (2012). Use of an innovative web-based laboratory surveillance platform to analyze mixed infections between human metapneumovirus (hMPV) and other respiratory viruses circulating in Alberta (AB), Canada (2009–2012). *Viruses*, 4(11), 2754–2765.

Feng, Y., He, T., Zhang, B., Yuan, H., & Zhou, Y. (2024). Epidemiology and diagnosis technologies of human metapneumovirus in China: a mini review. *Virology Journal,* 21(1), 59.

Freymouth, F., Vabret, A., Legrand, L., Eterradossi, N., Lafay-Delaire, F., Brouard, J., & Guillois, B. (2003). Presence of the new human metapneumovirus in French children with bronchiolitis. *Pediatric Infectious Disease Journal*, 22, 92–94.

Hamelin, M. È., Abed, Y., & Boivin, G. (2004). Human metapneumovirus: a new player among respiratory viruses. *Clinical Infectious Diseases*, 38(7), 983–990.

Hamelin, M. E., Cote, S., Laforge, J., Lampron, N., Bourbeau, J., Weiss, K., Gilca, R., DeSerres, G., & Boivin, G. (2005). Human metapneumovirus infection in adults with community-acquired pneumonia and exacerbation of chronic obstructive pulmonary disease. *Clinical Infectious Diseases*, 41, 498–502.

Hermos, C. R., Vargas, S. O., & McAdam, A. J. (2010). Human metapneumovirus. *Clinics in Laboratory Medicine*, 30(1), 131–148.

Ingram, R. E., Fenwick, F., McGuckin, R., Tefari, A., Taylor, C., & Toms, G. L. (2006). Detection of human metapneumovirus in respiratory secretions by reverse-transcriptase polymerase chain reaction, indirect immunofluorescence, and virus isolation in human bronchial epithelial cells. *Journal of Medical Virology*, 78, 1223–1231.

Jesse, S. T., Ludlow, M., & Osterhaus, A. D. (2022). Zoonotic origins of human metapneumovirus: A journey from birds to humans. *Viruses*, 14(4), 677.

Kahn, J. S. (2006). Epidemiology of human metapneumovirus. *Clinical Microbiology Reviews*, 19, 546–557.

Kuiken, T., van den Hoogen, B. G., van Riel, D. A., Laman, J. D., van Amerongen, G., Sprong, L., Fouchier, R. A., & Osterhaus, A. D. (2004). Experimental human metapneumovirus infection of cynomolgus macaques results in virus replication in ciliated epithelial cells and pneumocytes with associated lesions. *American Journal of Pathology*, 164, 1893–1900.

Mackay, I. M., Bialasiewicz, S., Waliuzzaman, Z., Chidlow, G. R., Fegredo, D. C., Laingam, S., et al., (2004). Use of the P gene to genotype human metapneumovirus identifies 4 viral subtypes. *The Journal of Infectious Diseases*, 190(11), 1913–1918.

Maertzdorf, J., Wang, C. K., Brown, J. B., et al., (2004). Real-time reverse transcriptase PCR assay for detection of human metapneumoviruses from all known genetic lineages. *Journal of Clinical Microbiology*, 42, 981–986.

Panda, S., Mohakud, N. K., Pena, L., & Kumar, S. (2014). Human metapneumovirus: review of an important respiratory pathogen. *International Journal of Infectious Diseases*, 25, 45–52.

Pata, R., & Kristeva, J. (2025). Human Metapneumovirus Infections: A Comprehensive Review of Diagnosis and Management. *Current Trends in Internal Medicine*, 8, 238.

Pilger, D. A., Cantarelli, V. V., Amantea, S. L., & Leistner-Segal, S. (2011). Detection of human bocavirus and human metapneumovirus by real-time PCR from patients with respiratory symptoms in Southern Brazil. *Memórias do Instituto Oswaldo Cruz*, 106, 56–60.

Porwal, S., Malviya, R., Sridhar, S. B., Shareef, J., & Wadhwa, T. (2025). Global Impact of hMPV Virus: Transmission, Pathogenesis, Diagnostic and Treatment. *Diagnostic Microbiology and Infectious Disease*, 116809.

Principi, N., & Esposito, S. (2014). Paediatric human metapneumovirus infection: epidemiology, prevention and therapy. *Journal of Clinical Virology*, 59(3), 141–147.

Principi, N., Bosis, S., & Esposito, S. (2006). Human metapneumovirus in paediatric patients. *Clinical Microbiology and Infection*, 12(4), 301–308.

Van den Hoogen, B. G., de Jong, J. C., Groen, J., Kuiken, T., de Groot, R., Fouchier, R. A., & Osterhaus, A. D. (2001). A newly discovered human pneumovirus isolated from young children with respiratory tract disease. *Nature Medicine*, 7(6), 719–724.

Chapter 5

Human Metapneumovirus (HMPV) in the Pediatric Population

Anand Singh Chouhan[1]
Vinay Jain[1,*]
Ankita Verma[1]
and Garima Maurya[2]

[1]ShriRam College of Pharmacy, Banmore, MP, India
[2]Maharana Pratap College of Pharmaceutical Sciences, Kanpur, UP, India

Abstract

One important respiratory pathogen influencing the paediatric population worldwide is human metapneumovirus (HMPV). Originally discovered in 2001, HMPV is connected to bronchiolitis, pneumonia, and aggravation of children's asthma in acute respiratory tract infections (ARTIs). It is a major cause of hospitalisation in young children and newborns and has clinical parallels with respiratory syncytial virus (RSV). By the time they are five, almost all children have HMPV; severe cases arise in individuals with underlying medical problems or compromised immune systems. With a seasonal rhythm, HMPV mostly circulates in late winter and early spring. With occasional death in high-risk categories, it greatly adds to paediatric morbidity. Given the restrictions of conventional viral culture techniques, diagnosis mostly depends on molecular techniques such as RT-PCR. There isn't any particular antiviral treatment or vaccination available right now; management is still supportive. The epidemiology, clinical presentation, and diagnostic difficulties of HMPV in children are covered in this

[*] Corresponding Author's Email: vinni77@gmail.com

In: Human Metapneumovirus
Editors: Anjali Sharma, Vishnu Mittal, Devkant Sharma et al.
ISBN: 979-8-90134-063-9

chapter. It draws attention to the socioeconomic load and the necessity of better preventive actions, including the creation of vaccines. Furthermore, the value of surveillance initiatives and possible therapeutic developments are discussed in order to lessen the effect of HMPV on young healthcare systems.

Keywords: Human Metapneumovirus (HMPV), pediatric respiratory infections, bronchiolitis, pneumonia, epidemiology, viral burden, RT-PCR diagnosis, seasonal variation, immunocompromised children

List of Abbreviations

HMPV	Human Metapneumovirus
RTI	Respiratory Tract Infection
LRTI	Lower Respiratory Tract Infection
URTI	Upper Respiratory Tract Infection
RSV	Respiratory Syncytial Virus
PCR	Polymerase Chain Reaction
RT-PCR	Reverse Transcription Polymerase Chain Reaction
ICU	Intensive Care Unit
WHO	World Health Organization
CDC	Centres for Disease Control and Prevention
mAbs	Monoclonal Antibody
ELISA	Enzyme-Linked Immunosorbent Assay
IgG	Immunoglobulin G
IgM	Immunoglobulin M
RNA	Ribonucleic Acid
DNA	Deoxyribonucleic Acid
CDC	Centres for Disease Control and Prevention
NIH	National Institutes of Health
FDA	Food and Drug Administration
CI	Confidence Interval
OR	Odds Ratio
NP	Nasopharyngeal
ICU	Intensive Care Unit
Ag	Antigen
Ab	Antibody
WHO	World Health Organisation

AI Artificial Intelligence (if discussed in surveillance or prediction contexts)
SARS- CoV-2 Severe Acute Respiratory Syndrome Coronavirus 2 (if used for comparison)
EUA Emergency Use Authorisation (for future vaccines/ antivirals)
R&D Research and Development.

Introduction

First found in the Netherlands in 2001, the non-segmented, negative-stranded RNA virus Human Metapneumovirus (HMPV) belongs to the Pneumoviridae family (Sharma et al., 2025). Especially in newborns, young children, immunocompromised people, and the elderly, it is acknowledged as a major etiological agent of acute respiratory tract infections (ARTIs). Another main cause of paediatric respiratory infections, respiratory syncytial virus (RSV), has clinical and epidemiological characteristics similar to those of HMPV. But unlike RSV, HMPV stays underdiagnosed because of low clinical awareness and the need for molecular diagnostics tools for validation (Cox et al., 2012; Hamelin et al., 2006). Mostly occurring in the winter and early spring (Kahn et al., 2011), HMPV infections show a biennial epidemic trend (Jain et al., 2023).

Lower respiratory tract infections (LRTIs) in children under five years of age account for a significant fraction of hospital visits (Schmidt and Varga, 2018). By the age of five, almost all children show serological evidence of past HMPV exposure; reinfections are somewhat prevalent throughout life (Karron et al., 2013). Beyond hospital stays, HMPV causes outpatient visits, emergency department visits, and antibiotic usage because of its clinical similarity to bacterial pneumonia (Biacchesi et al., 2004). Although the disease load is high, there are no approved vaccinations or particular antiviral treatments for HMPV. Mostly supportive, current treatment consists of hydration, oxygen therapy, and symptomatic relief (Herd et al., 2006). Targeting medicines and vaccines is still a major focus of research since it emphasises the need for improved surveillance and preventive plans (Hamelin et al., 2004). Emphasising the need for future research and intervention techniques, this chapter investigates the epidemiology, clinical symptoms, and difficulties related to HMPV diagnosis and management (Skiadopoulos et al., 2006).

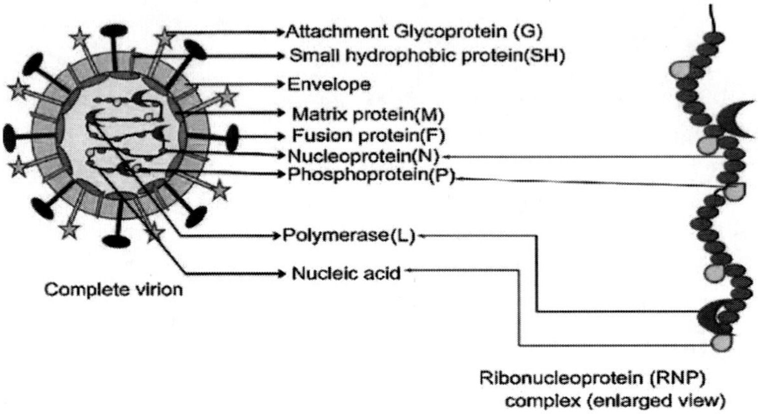

Figure 1. Structure of Human Metapneumovirus (HMPV).

Human Metapneumovirus (HMPV), an enveloped, negative-sense single-stranded RNA virus of the Pneumoviridae family, with structural composition shown in Figure 1. Particularly in infants, elderly people, and immunocompromised patients, the virus is a major cause of respiratory infections (Yi et al., 2005). Figure 1 The picture shows the whole structure of a paramyxovirus, with its most important parts highlighted. The envelope has attachment glycoprotein (G) and tiny hydrophobic protein (SH) on its outer surface. The matrix protein (M) and the fusion protein (F) make up the inner layer. The ribonucleoprotein (RNP) complex inside the virus has nucleoprotein (N), phosphoprotein (P), polymerase (L), and nucleic acid (RNA). The larger image of the RNP complex shows exactly how these intracellular proteins are arranged around the genetic material. This is important for viral replication and transcription (Skiadopoulos et al., 2006).

Structural Components

- Fusion Protein (F): Essential for viral entry into host cells by mediating membrane fusion. Plays a role in syncytium formation and virus infectivity.
- Glycoprotein (G): Facilitates viral attachment to host cell receptors. A major determinant of viral tropism.
- Short Hydrophobic (SH) Protein: Its function is not fully understood, but it is thought to be involved in immune evasion.

- Matrix Protein (M): Provides structural integrity and helps in virus assembly and budding.
- RNA Polymerase (RNAP) Complex: Comprises essential proteins responsible for viral RNA replication and transcription.

Significance of HMPV Structure

Development of focused antiviral treatments and vaccines depends on an awareness of the framework of HMPV. While the RNAP complex is being investigated for antiviral medicine design, the F and G proteins are the main targets for vaccination development. Globally common respiratory pathogen affecting children, especially young children under five years of age, Human Metapneumovirus (HMPV). First discovered in 2001, it belongs to the Pneumoviridae family and is somewhat similar to the respiratory syncytial virus (RSV). In pediatric patients, HMPV is a main cause of acute respiratory tract infections (ARTIs), bronchiolitis, and pneumonia, causing a great morbidity and healthcare load (Banerjee and Barik, 2012). Seasonal fluctuations in HMPV infections mostly affect temperate areas and circulate late winter and early spring. Studies show that almost all children have HMPV by the age of five; Seroprevalence rates approach 100%. Often found in association with RSV, influenza, and adenoviruses (Agapov & Holtzman, 2009; Skiadopoulos et al., 2006), the virus causes 5–15% of ARTIs in hospitalised pediatric patients (Jain et al., 2023). Mostly through respiratory droplets and direct touch with contaminated surfaces, HMPV is transmitted.

Severe disease is more likely to strike premature infants, immunocompromised children, and those with chronic lung or cardiac disease (Van Den Hoogen et al., 2004). Increased transmission rates are caused in part by socioeconomic variables, including overcrowding and poor healthcare access (Wyde et al., 2005). Studies find that for lower respiratory tract infections (LRTIs), HMPV accounts for around 10–20% of pediatric hospitalisations. With co-infections aggravating disease severity, severe cases sometimes call for oxygen support and critical care (Williams et al., 2004; Panda et al., 2014). Although mortality is still low, among high-risk populations, including children with immunodeficiency diseases or congenital cardiac disease, it is somewhat noteworthy (Schildgen et al., 2008). Mostly by means of RT-PCR tests, routine molecular surveillance has enhanced HMPV identification. Multiple HMPV genotypes (A1, A2, B1, B2) have been found by surveillance studies; these co-circulate and develop over time (Schmidt and Varga, 2018). Preventive policies serve to lower transmission by means of hand cleanliness and infection control practices (Biacchesi et al., 2004). Still, the lack of an approved vaccination or antiviral treatment emphasizes the importance of ongoing research and development (Mackey et al., 2006).

Clinical Manifestations and Disease Spectrum of Human Metapneumovirus (HMPV)

In paediatric populations all over, human metapneumovirus (HMPV) is a major contributor to acute respiratory tract infections (ARTIs). Affecting the lower and upper respiratory systems, the virus mostly causes moderate cold-like symptoms to severe pneumonia. Factors include the child's age, immunological function, and the existence of underlying medical disorders, which define the degree of the illness (Xepapadaki et al., 2004).

Mild to Moderate Respiratory Symptoms: Like the common cold, most HMPV infections in young children show mild to moderate symptoms. Among these are: Fever, Cough and Nasal Congestion, Sore Throat and Hoarseness, Fatigue and Malaise (Zhang et al., 2016).

Lower Respiratory Tract Infections (LRTIs): More severe forms of HMPV might cause major lower respiratory problems that call for hospitalisation. These consist of: Bronchiolitis, Pneumonia, and Asthma Exacerbation (Falsely et al., 2003).

Severe Cases in High-Risk Populations: Children with compromised immune systems, early birth, and chronic illnesses are more likely to have severe disease progression. Severe cases could include: Respiratory Failure, Secondary Bacterial Infections, and Intensive Care Admission (Watanabe et al., 2005).

Diagnosis and Detection Techniques of HMPV

Differentiating Human Metapneumovirus (HMPV) from other respiratory diseases and guaranteeing appropriate patient management depends on the diagnosis used. From genetic tests to serological and culture-based approaches (Schickli et al., 2005), several laboratory techniques are at hand for identifying

HMPV. Effective treatment and virus epidemiological tracking depend on early, precise detection.

Reverse Transcription Polymerase Chain Reaction (RT-PCR): Given its great sensitivity (95–99%) and specificity (98–100%) (24), RT-PCR is regarded as the gold standard for HMPV detection. It acts by magnifying viral RNA taken from nasopharyngeal swabs or aspirates. The most dependable test for both clinical and scientific uses, since this method lets one identify the virus even in low viral load patients (Bastien et al., 2003). RT-PCR's availability in low-resource environments is limited, nevertheless, since it calls for specific laboratory equipment and qualified staff (McAdam et al., 2004).

Real-Time Quantitative PCR (qPCR): An improved variation of RT-PCR called qPCR lets doctors evaluate the degree of infection by allowing the quantification of viral load. With a sensitivity of roughly 92–98% and a specificity above 97% (Agapov et al., 2009), the method provides its quick processing time and capacity to identify several viruses in one test make it extensively employed in research institutes and hospitals. Still, it calls for costly chemicals and qualified experts, much like RT-PCR.

Immunofluorescence Assay (IFA): Using fluorescently labelled antibodies, IFA—an antigen-based technique—detects HMPV proteins in respiratory secretions. Results of this fast diagnostic instrument come within a few hours. Its sensitivity is much less than RT-PCR, though, ranging between 60 and 80%, which increases the false negative rate (Schildgen et al., 2011). The test also calls for well-preserved materials and qualified staff members to view the findings under a fluorescence microscope.

Enzyme-Linked Immunosorbent Assay (ELISA): ELISA is a serological technique for identifying antibodies particular to HMPV in blood samples. Particularly helpful for epidemiological studies, this approach clarifies HMPV frequency across various groups. ELISA is not useful for early-stage diagnosis, though, since antibodies build slowly following an infection. ELISA's sensitivity falls between 70 to 85%, hence it is more of a complement than a main diagnostic tool (Sharma et al., 2025).

Viral Culture Method: Cell culture methods allow HMPV to be separated, especially in LLC-MK2 cells, where the virus generates a distinct cytopathic effect. Viral culture is slow, though, and requires five to ten days for results; it is therefore not suitable for regular clinical use. The detection rate for viral culture is relatively low, ranging from 50-70%, and it requires specialised biosafety conditions. These restrictions mean that it is mostly employed in research rather than in regular diagnosis.

Loop-Mediated Isothermal Amplification (LAMP): One new method for quick and reasonably priced HMPV detection is LAMP. Under isothermal circumstances, it increases viral RNA; results are seen 30 to 60 minutes. LAMP has a sensitivity of 85–95%, which makes it more appropriate for resource-limited environments than RT-PCR, while comparable. Given its simplicity and cost, this approach has significant promise for the next HMPV diagnosis.

Disease Burden and Hospitalisation Trends

Often necessitating hospitalisation, especially in newborns, young children, and immunocompromised patients, Human Metapneumovirus (HMPV) is a main cause of acute respiratory tract infections (ARTIs) in paediatric patients. Comparable to Respiratory Syncytial Virus (RSV) and Influenza, the illness burden of HMPV adds greatly to paediatric morbidity globally. Healthcare planning and resource allocation depend on an awareness of the trends in hospitalisation and degree of HMPV infection (Agapov and Holtzman, 2009). With annual outbreaks mostly occurring during late winter and early spring, HMPV accounts for 5–25% of paediatric ARTIs.

Nearly all children are exposed to HMPV by the age of five, according to a comprehensive study; serious infections arise in 10–15% of cases, mostly in those with underlying medical disorders such as congenital heart disease, asthma, or prematurity (Huck et al., 2006). Studies estimate that viral respiratory infections account for 10–20% of paediatric hospital admissions, including HMPV. According to a sizable cohort research, HMPV-related problems cause roughly 6–7 per 1,000 children under five years to need hospitalisation yearly. Among high-risk populations, ICU admission rates for severe HMPV cases vary from 5-12%; the overall mortality rate is 1-3% (Pena et al., 2011). Children with HMPV often spend 4–6 days in a hospital; severe cases span more than 10 days. Estimates of the financial cost of HMPV-related hospitalisations range from $3,000 to $20,000 per patient, depending on the degree of severity and ICU need (Semple et al., 2005).

Preventive Strategies and Management of HMPV in Paediatric Patients

Human Metapneumovirus (HMPV) is a leading cause of respiratory infections in children. Effective prevention and management strategies can reduce disease severity and complications (Williams et al., 2004). Infection control measures play a critical role in preventing the spread of Human Metapneumovirus (HMPV). Frequent handwashing with soap and water significantly reduces virus transmission, while proper respiratory hygiene—such as covering the mouth while coughing or sneezing—minimises the risk of spreading the virus. Additionally, regular disinfection of surfaces and toys, particularly in day-care centres and hospitals, helps prevent outbreaks. Avoiding exposure to risk factors is also essential; for instance, reducing contact with second-hand smoke decreases respiratory complications, and avoiding crowded places during peak viral seasons lowers the risk of infection. Exclusive breastfeeding for the first six months has been shown to strengthen an infant's immunity against respiratory infections (Watanabe et al., 2005). Although there is currently no licensed vaccine available for HMPV, research efforts continue toward vaccine development. Monoclonal antibodies targeting HMPV are under investigation for use in high-risk groups, offering a potential avenue for future protection.

Management strategies for HMPV infection are primarily supportive. Symptomatic treatment includes adequate hydration, the use of antipyretics to manage fever, and oxygen therapy in severe cases. In patients experiencing wheezing, nebulised bronchodilators may be considered, although their effectiveness remains uncertain. Hospitalisationis required for children presenting with severe respiratory distress, hypoxia, or dehydration (Xepapadaki et al., 2004), and close monitoring is essential for high-risk populations such as premature infants and immunocompromised children (Bastien et al., 2003). Experimental and adjunctive therapies, including antiviral treatments, are currently undergoing clinical trials, but they are not yet a part of standard care (Mackay et al., 2006). Corticosteroids are generally not recommended unless the patient has underlying conditions such as asthma.

Future Perspectives: Vaccine Development and Therapeutics for HMPV

Human Metapneumovirus (HMPV) remains a significant cause of pediatric respiratory infections. Advancements in vaccine development and therapeutic strategies offer hope for future prevention and treatment (Boivin et al., 2007). Research is focused on live-attenuated vaccines that mimic natural infection to induce immunity. Inactivated vaccines are being explored for safer immunisation, especially in high-risk children. Recombinant vaccines using viral proteins to stimulate an immune response are in preclinical trials. Fusion (F) protein-based vaccines are a major target due to their role in viral entry (Martinello et al., 2002). mRNA vaccine platforms, similar to those used for COVID-19, are under investigation for HMPV. Viral vector vaccines aim to provide long-lasting immunity by delivering HMPV antigens (Almajhdi and Farrag, 2013).

Neutralising monoclonal antibodies targeting the HMPV F protein are in clinical trials. These mAbs could be used for prophylaxis in high-risk infants and immunocompromised patients. Small-molecule inhibitors targeting viral replication are being studied. RNA interference (RNAi) therapies offer a novel approach to suppress HMPV infection. Cytokine-based treatments aim to regulate immune responses and prevent severe inflammation. Combination therapies with antivirals and immune modulators are being explored for severe cases. Human metapneumovirus (HMPV) is a significant pathogen causing acute respiratory tract infections in children, leading to notable socioeconomic impacts (Garcia-Garcia et al., 2006).

Case Study of HMPV Infection in Pediatric Patients (2005-2025)

Cases from 2005-2010 – Early Identifications and Limited Diagnosis

During this period, HMPV infections in children were primarily diagnosed through clinical symptoms and early molecular techniques like RT-PCR and serological tests. There were only a few antiviral choices; thus, treatments were essentially supportive. Few cases needed hospitalisation; most had mild to moderate severity. Table 1 shows clinical case data from 2005 to 2010, concentrating on how early diagnoses were made and how few diagnostic methods were used in paediatric patients. There are three cases in the table that involve kids between the ages of 1.5 and 3. Fever, cough, stuffy nose, sore throat, and minor breathing problems were some of the most common symptoms. There were other ways to diagnose the virus, including RT-PCR, chest X-ray, nasopharyngeal swab, viral culture, and serological assays. Most of the treatments were supportive, such as giving fluids, oxygen therapy, and fever reducers. All of the patients got better; however, it took them between 4 and 7 days. Table 1 shows that there were just a few diagnostic and therapeutic procedures recognizing clinical cases, but they were effective (2Schildgen et al., 2011).

Table 1. Cases from 2005-2010 –
Early identifications and limited diagnosis

Case No.	Year	Age/Gender	Symptoms	Diagnosis Method	Treatment Given	Outcome
1	2005	2 years Male	Fever, cough, nasal congestion	RT-PCR, chest X-ray	Supportive care, hydration	Recovered in 7 days
2	2007	3 years Female	Sore throat, hoarseness, fatigue	Nasopharyngeal swab, viral culture	Symptomatic treatment	Symptoms resolved in 5 days
3	2010	1.5 years Male	Persistent cough, mild breathing difficulty	Serological test	Oxygen therapy, antipyretics	Hospitalised for 4 days, recovered

Cases from 2011-2015 – Advancements in Diagnosis and Management

Improved molecular testing (RT-PCR and viral antigen identification) between 2011 and 2015 produced earlier and more reliable diagnosis of HMPV in children. Oxygen therapy for moderate cases and bronchodilator use also rose during this time. Still, serious infections in newborns needed ICU hospitalisations. Table 2 shows paediatric cases from 2011 to 2015, which shows how both diagnostic methods and clinical care have improved. Patients were between 6 months and 5 years old and had symptoms such as lethargy, wheezing, high fever, trouble breathing, and a stuffy nose, as seen in Table 2. More advanced diagnostic technologies were used, such as RT-PCR, auscultation, chest X-rays, viral antigen assays, and nasal swab tests. Depending on how bad the case was, treatments included hydration, bronchodilators, ICU care, oxygen support, and therapy for symptoms. In all cases, the outcomes were good, and the recovery times were between 5 and 8 days. Table 2 shows that diagnosis and focused management have improved since previous years (Debiaggi et al., 2006).

Table 2. Cases from 2011-2015 – Advancements in diagnosis and management

Case No.	Year	Age/Gender	Symptoms	Diagnosis Method	Treatment Given	Outcome
1	2011	4 years, Female	Fatigue, nasal congestion, mild wheezing	RT-PCR, auscultation	Hydration, bronchodilators	Symptoms improved in 6 days
2	2013	6 months, Male	High fever, respiratory distress	Chest X-ray, viral antigen test	ICU care, oxygen support	Required hospitalisation for 8 days
3	2015	5 years, Female	Runny nose, cough, fever	Nasal swab test	Antipyretics, rest	Recovery in 5 days

Cases from 2016-2020 – Increase in Severe Cases and ICU Admissions

Increasingly severe HMPV cases in young children in 2016–2020 resulted in higher ICU admissions. Introduced were advanced diagnostic instruments, including CT scans and nasopharyngeal PCR. Though no particular antiviral therapy was readily available, treatment plans included oxygen therapy, bronchodilators, and antiviral studies (Deffrasnese et al., 2008). Table 3 shows clinical cases from 2016 to 2020. It shows that the symptoms got worse and the number of ICU admissions went up. Table 3 shows that kids between the ages of 2.5 and 4 had symptoms that ranged from mild fever and sore throat to more serious problems such as wheezing, tiredness, and trouble breathing. Nasopharyngeal PCR, viral antigen tests, and full clinical exams were some of the ways that doctors figured out what was wrong. Some instances were treated with supportive care, while others needed to go to the ICU and have oxygen assistance. In the worst circumstances, recovery durations could last up to 10 days. Table 3 shows that there was an increase in acute respiratory presentations and the requirement for more advanced medical care during this time (Debiaggi et al., 2006).

Table 3. Cases from 2016-2020 –
Increase in severe cases and ICU admissions

Case No.	Year	Age/Gender	Symptoms	Diagnosis Method	Treatment Given	Outcome
1	2016	3 years, Male	Wheezing, fever, cough	Nasopharyngeal PCR	Oxygen therapy, bronchodilators	Symptoms subsided in 7 days
2	2018	2.5 years, Female	Cough, mild fever, sore throat	Viral antigen test	Supportive care	Recovery in 6 days
3	2020	4 years, Male	Difficulty breathing, fever, fatigue	RT-PCR, clinical examination	ICU admission, oxygen support	Hospitalised for 10 days, recovered

Cases from 2021-2025 (January) – Advancements in Treatment and Vaccine Trials

Table 4. Cases from 2021-2025 (January) –
Advancements in treatment and vaccine trials

Case No.	Year	Age/ Gender	Symptoms	Diagnosis Method	Treatment Given	Outcome
1	2021	3 years, Female	Fever, cough, nasal congestion	RT-PCR, lung imaging	Antiviral therapy, nebulization	Full recovery in 7 days
2	2023	6 months, Male	Severe breathing distress, high fever	Viral culture, CT scan	ICU support, oxygen therapy	Hospitalised for 12 days, survived
3	2025 (Jan)	2 years, Female	Runny nose, sore throat, cough	PCR testing	Symptomatic care, hydration	Recovery in 5 days

Vaccine trials and antiviral medication have started in the most recent time (2021–2025), which will help to control severe HMPV infections. Although supportive care is still vital, the use of nebulization and focused antiviral medications has shown improved rates of recovery and shortened ICU stays (Biere et al., 2010). Table 4 shows the number of paediatric respiratory cases reported from 2021 to January 2025. It shows how treatment methods have improved and how vaccine trial assistance has been added. Table 4 shows that individuals between the ages of 6 months and 3 years had symptoms like fever, stuffy nose, trouble breathing, and sore throat. RT-PCR, PCR testing, lung imaging, viral culture, and CT scans were some of the diagnostic methods used, which shows that case identification has gotten better. Compared to past years, treatments were better. They included antiviral therapy, nebulization, and ICU-level assistance when needed. All of the patients got better, but some had to stay in the hospital for up to 12 days. Table 4 shows how therapy techniques and early diagnosis have continued to improve during the vaccine trial period (Boivin et al., 2011).

Conclusion

Human Metapneumovirus (HMPV) is still a major and widespread cause of acute respiratory tract infections in children all over the world. HMPV has been known about for decades, but it still causes a lot of problems for people, especially babies, young children, and people with weak immune systems. The virus can cause a wide range of ailments, from minor upper respiratory infections to serious lower respiratory tract diseases like pneumonia and bronchiolitis. The high number of hospitalisations owing to HMPV-related problems, especially during seasonal outbreaks, shows how important it is to have good diagnostic, therapeutic, and preventive strategies. There are no licensed vaccinations or particular antiviral treatments for HMPV right now, which makes it harder to manage. Supportive care is the major treatment. Without focused interventions, prevention mostly depends on conventional public health policies like keeping respiratory hygiene, encouraging handwashing, lowering exposure to established risk factors like tobacco smoke, and isolating affected people when possible. These methods are helpful, but they don’t totally stop the spread, especially in places where the danger is high, such as childcare centres and paediatric hospital wards. The HMPV genome, how it causes disease, and how it avoids the immune system are becoming better understood. This is opening up new possibilities for both vaccine and treatment development. Recent progress in making monoclonal antibodies that target HMPV surface glycoproteins has shown promise in preclinical testing, which means they could be used in the future to protect high-risk groups. Also, recent research into small-molecule antivirals that stop HMPV from replicating gives us hope that specific therapeutic options will be available in the future. Along with these efforts, various vaccine candidates are being studied, including live-attenuated, subunit, and vector-based vaccines. Some of these candidates are even moving on to early-phase clinical trials. To effectively prevent and treat HMPV infections, we need to take a variety of approaches. Continued epidemiological surveillance, global cooperation, and funding for research on paediatric viruses are all necessary to keep an eye on new strains and learn more about how diseases spread in different parts of the world. Also, adding HMPV to normal diagnostic panels in healthcare settings could help doctors find and treat it more quickly, which could make the disease less severe and shorten hospital stays. In conclusion, HMPV is still a dangerous respiratory virus for kids, but more and more research is being done that makes us hopeful for the future. If we keep doing research, put money into making vaccines and antivirals, and stick to public health measures, it is possible that the burden of HMPV in kids will be much less in the years to come.

References

Agapov, E. and Holtzman, M. J. (2009). Human metapneumovirus: a newly emerging paramyxovirus infection in children. *Current Opinion in Pediatrics*, 21(1): 85–90.

Almajhdi, F. N. and Farrag, M. A. (2013). Human metapneumovirus: current knowledge and future directions. *Acta Virologica*, 57(3): 213–222.

Banerjee, S. and Barik, S. (2012). Respiratory syncytial virus and human metapneumovirus: similarities and differences. *Clinical and Vaccine Immunology*, 19(4): 428–435.

Bastien, N., Ward, D., Van Caeseele, P., Brandt, K., Lee, S. H. S., McNabb, G. and Li, Y. (2003). Human metapneumovirus infection in the Canadian population. *Journal of Clinical Microbiology*, 41(10): 4642–4646Biacchesi, S., Skiadopoulos, M. H., Yang, L., Lamirande, E. W., Tran, K. C., Murphy, B. R., Collins, P. L. and Buchholz, U. J. (2004). Recombinant human metapneumovirus lacking the small hydrophobic SH and/or attachment G glycoprotein: Deletion of G yields a promising vaccine candidate. *Journal of Virology*, 78(23): 12877–12887.

Biere, B., Bauer, B. and Schweiger, B. (2010). Differentiation of influenza B virus lineages Yamagata and Victoria by real-time PCR. *Journal of Clinical Microbiology*, 48(4): 1425–1427.

Boivin, G., De Serres, G., Hamelin, M. E., Côté, S., Argouin, M., Tremblay, G. and Déry, P. (2007). An outbreak of severe respiratory tract infection due to human metapneumovirus in a long-term care facility. *Clinical Infectious Diseases*, 44(9): 1152–1158.

Boivin, G., Mackay, I. and Sloots, T. P. (2011). Human metapneumovirus infections. In: Richman, D. D., Whitley, R. J. and Hayden, F. G. (Eds.), *Clinical Virology* (3rd ed., pp. 933–949). Washington, DC: ASM Press.

Cox, R. G., Levendosky, K. F., Johnson, M., Evers, T. J., Lazarus, M. A., Johnson, T. R. and Williams, J. V. (2012). Respiratory syncytial virus and human metapneumovirus fusion proteins induce similar neutralizing antibody responses but strikingly different protection in aged mice. *Journal of Virology*, 86(11): 6378–6387.

Debiaggi, M., Canducci, F., Sampaolo, M., Marinozzi, M. C. and Principi, N. (2006). Persistent respiratory infections by human metapneumovirus in children with underlying diseases: report of three cases. *Journal of Clinical Virology*, 35(2): 202–204.

Deffrasnes, C., Hamelin, M. E. and Boivin, G. (2008). Presence of human metapneumovirus RNA in the brain of an immunocompromised child with fatal encephalitis. *Journal of Clinical Microbiology*, 46(1): 331–333.

Esper, F., Boucher, D., Weibel, C., Martinello, R. A. and Kahn, J. S. (2005). Human metapneumovirus infection in young children in the United States: results of a 2-year prospective study. *Journal of Infectious Diseases*, 191(4): 503–506.

Falsey, A. R., Erdman, D., Anderson, L. J. and Walsh, E. E. (2003). Human metapneumovirus infections in young and elderly adults. *New England Journal of Medicine*, 349(1): 5–14.

García-García, M. L., Calvo, C., Rey, C., Díaz, M., Molinero, M., Pozo, F. and Casas, I. (2006). Human metapneumovirus infections in hospitalized children and adults: comparison with other respiratory viruses. *Journal of Clinical Virology*, 35(1): 93–99.

Hamelin, M. E., Abed, Y. and Boivin, G. (2004). Human metapneumovirus: A new player among respiratory viruses. *Clinical Infectious Diseases*, 38(7): 983–990.

Hamelin, M. E., Prince, G. A., Gomez, A. M., Kinkead, R. and Boivin, G. (2006). Human metapneumovirus infection induces long-term pulmonary inflammation associated with airway obstruction in mice. *Journal of Infectious Diseases*, 193(12): 1634–1642.

Herd, K. A., Mahalingam, S., Mackay, I. M., Nissen, M. D., Sloots, T. P. and Tindle, R. W. (2006). Vaccination with virus-like particles composed of the human metapneumovirus matrix and fusion proteins induces humoral and cellular immunity in mice. *Virology*, 347(1): 127–139.

Huck, B., Scharf, G., Neumann-Haefelin, D., Puppe, W., Weigl, J. and Falcone, V. (2006). Novel human metapneumovirus sublineage. *Emerging Infectious Diseases*, 12(1): 147–150.

Jain, S., Sharma, P., Dhakad, K. and Jain, V. (2023). Design, optimization, and characterization of herbal gel for facial application. *Asian Journal of Pharmaceutics*, 17(3): 486.

Kahn, J. S., Schnell, M. J., Buonocore, L. and Rose, J. K. (2001). Recombinant vesicular stomatitis virus expressing an influenza virus hemagglutinin provides protective immunity against influenza virus infection. *Journal of Virology*, 75(15): 6775–6779.

Karron, R. A., Buchholz, U. J. and Collins, P. L. (2013). Live-attenuated respiratory syncytial virus vaccines. *Current Topics in Microbiology and Immunology*, 372: 259–284.

Mackay, I. M., Bialasiewicz, S., Jacob, K. C., McQueen, E., Arden, K. E., Nissen, M. D. and Sloots, T. P. (2006). Genetic diversity of human metapneumovirus over 4 consecutive years in Australia. *Journal of Infectious Diseases*, 193(12): 1630–1633.

Martinello, R. A., Esper, F., Weibel, C., Ferguson, D. and Kahn, J. S. (2002). Human metapneumovirus and exacerbations of chronic obstructive pulmonary disease. *Journal of Infectious Diseases*, 186(3): 385–388.

McAdam, A. J., Hasenbein, M. E., Feldman, H. A., Cole, S. E., Offermann, M. K., Riley, A. M. and Sandora, T. J. (2004). Human metapneumovirus in children tested at a tertiary-care hospital. *Emerging Infectious Diseases*, 10(4): 700–705.

Osterhaus, A. D., Fouchier, R. A. and Kuiken, T. (2004). The aetiology of SARS: Koch's postulates fulfilled. *Nature*, 423(6937): 240–240.

Panda, S., Mohakud, N. K., Pena, L. and Kumar, S. (2014). Human metapneumovirus: review of an important respiratory pathogen. *International Journal of Infectious Diseases*, 25: 45–52. Papenburg, J., Hamelin, M. E. and Boivin, G. (2012). Human metapneumovirus: Review of clinical relevance and host immune response. *Journal of Infection*, 64(2): 111–118.

Peña, R. C., Wong, D. T. and Kim, J. Y. (2011). Human metapneumovirus infection: mechanisms and clinical implications. *Current Opinion in Pulmonary Medicine*, 17(3): 244–250.

Schickli, J. H., Kaur, J., Ulbrandt, N., Spaete, R. R. and Tang, R. S. (2005). An S101P substitution in the human metapneumovirus L protein increases fidelity of the polymerase activity and attenuates virus replication in hamsters. *Journal of Virology*, 79(12): 7764–7772.

Schildgen, O., Müller, A., Allander, T., Mackay, I. M., Völz, S., Kupfer, B. and Simon, A. (2008). Human metapneumovirus: lessons learned over the first decade. *Clinical Microbiology Reviews*, 21(2): 275–289.

Schildgen, O., Simon, A. and Williams, J. V. (2007). Animal models for human metapneumovirus (HMPV) infections. *Veterinary Research*, 38(1): 117–126.

Schildgen, V., Pieper, M., Khalfaoui, S. and Schildgen, O. (2011). Human metapneumovirus replicates in the lower respiratory tract of immunocompetent mice and induces pneumonia. *Journal of Virology*, 85(8): 4039–4049. Schmidt, M. E. and Varga, S. M. (2018). Immunological responses to respiratory syncytial virus infection and the development of vaccines. *Microbiology and Molecular Biology Reviews*, 82(3): e00068-17.

Semple, M. G., Cowell, A., Dove, W., Greensill, J., McNamara, P. S., Halfhide, C. and Smyth, R. L. (2005). Dual infection of infants by human metapneumovirus and human respiratory syncytial virus is strongly associated with severe bronchiolitis. *Journal of Infectious Diseases*, 191(3): 382–386.

Sharma, P., Shivhare, P. and Jain, V. (2025). Hydrotropy as a tool for enhancing mefenamic acid solubility: A comprehensive study. *Indian Journal of Pharmaceutical Education and Research*, 59(1 Suppl): Article 92.

Skiadopoulos, M. H., Biacchesi, S., Buchholz, U. J., Amaro-Carambot, E., Surman, S. R., Collins, P. L. and Murphy, B. R. (2006). Individual contributions of the human metapneumovirus F, G, M2-1, and M2-2 proteins to virus replication and pathogenesis. *Journal of Virology*, 80(4): 1167–1174.

Skiadopoulos, M. H., Biacchesi, S., Buchholz, U. J., Amaro-Carambot, E., Surman, S. R., Collins, P. L. and Murphy, B. R. (2006). The two major human metapneumovirus genetic lineages are highly related antigenically and the fusion (F) protein is a major contributor to this antigenic relatedness. *Journal of Virology*, 80(1): 120–128.

van den Hoogen, B. G., Herfst, S., Sprong, L., Cane, P. A., Forleo-Neto, E., de Swart, R. L., Osterhaus, A. D. and Fouchier, R. A. (2004). Antigenic and genetic variability of human metapneumoviruses. *Emerging Infectious Diseases*, 10(4): 658–666.

von Linstow, M. L., Høgh, M. and Høgh, B. (2008). Clinical and epidemiologic characteristics of human metapneumovirus and respiratory syncytial virus infections in children. *European Journal of Pediatrics*, 167(9): 1125–1130.

Watanabe, M., Ito, H. and Okuno, Y. (2005). Human metapneumovirus in young children with respiratory tract infection in Japan. *Pediatrics International*, 47(4): 416–419.

Williams, J. V. (2010). The clinical presentation and outcomes of human metapneumovirus infection. *Clinical Infectious Diseases*, 50(8): 1223–1230.

Williams, J. V., Harris, P. A., Tollefson, S. J., Halburnt-Rush, L. L., Pingsterhaus, J. M., Edwards, K. M. and Wright, P. F. (2004). Human metapneumovirus and lower respiratory tract disease in otherwise healthy infants and children. *New England Journal of Medicine*, 350(5): 443–450.

Wyde, P. R., Chetty, S. N., Jewell, A. M., Schoonover, S. L. and Piedra, P. A. (2005). Comparison of the inhibition of human metapneumovirus and respiratory syncytial virus by ribavirin and immune serum globulin in vitro. *Antiviral Research*, 65(1): 51–58.

Xepapadaki, P., Psarras, S., Bossios, A., Tsolia, M., Gourgiotis, D., Liapi-Adamidou, G. and Papadopoulos, N. G. (2004). Human metapneumovirus as a causative agent of acute bronchiolitis in infants. *Journal of Clinical Virology*, 30(3): 267–270.

Yi, J., Cheon, D. S., Kang, J. H., Kim, J. M., Chung, Y. S. and Lee, J. S. (2005). Detection and molecular characterization of human metapneumovirus in children with acute respiratory illness. *Archives of Virology*, 150(3): 521–531.

Zhang, Y., Zhu, Y., Zhu, H., Zhang, X., Wang, D. and Lu, H. (2016). Clinical and epidemiological characteristics of human metapneumovirus infection in children hospitalized for acute respiratory infection. *Journal of Clinical Virology*, 76: 14–19.

Chapter 6

Advances in Diagnostic Approaches for Human Metapneumovirus (HMPV)

Mirunalini Gobinath[1]
R. Soundarya[2]
Tejaswini Reddy Jeeru[3]
Naina Mohamed Pakkir Maideen[4,5,*]
and Mohd Aftab Siddiqui[6,†]
[1]Department of Pharmacognosy and Phytopharmacy, JSS College of Pharmacy, JSS Academy of Higher Education and Research, Ooty, Tamil Nadu, India
[2]Department of Pharmaceutics, JSS College of Pharmacy, JSS Academy of Higher Education and Research, Mysuru, Karnataka, India
[3]Department of Pharmaceutical Chemistry, JSS College of Pharmacy, JSS Academy of Higher Education & Research, Ooty, Tamil Nadu, India
[4]Clinical Associate Professor of Pharmacology, College of Medicine, Mohammed Bin Rashid, University of Medicine and Health Sciences, Dubai. UAE
[5]Dubai Health, Dubai, UAE
[6]Faculty of Pharmacy, Integral University, Lucknow, U. P., India

Abstract

Human metapneumovirus (HMPV) is a significant respiratory pathogen associated with upper and lower respiratory tract infections, particularly in young children, immunocompromised patients, and the elderly. Due to the nonspecific clinical presentation of HMPV infections, accurate and timely diagnosis is crucial for effective disease management and

---

* Corresponding Author's Email: nmmaideen@dubaihealth.ae
† Corresponding Author's Email: aftab.uzaiz@gmail.com

In: Human Metapneumovirus
Editors: Anjali Sharma, Vishnu Mittal, Devkant Sharma et al.
ISBN: 979-8-90134-063-9

epidemiological surveillance. Traditional diagnostic methods, including viral culture and serology, have limited sensitivity and are time-consuming. Recent advancements in molecular diagnostics have revolutionised the detection of HMPV. Real-time polymerase chain reaction (RT-PCR) has emerged as the gold standard due to its high sensitivity and specificity. Multiplex PCR panels enable the simultaneous detection of multiple respiratory pathogens, improving diagnostic efficiency. Additionally, loop-mediated isothermal amplification (LAMP) offers a rapid and cost-effective alternative, particularly in resource-limited settings. Emerging technologies, such as next-generation sequencing (NGS) and CRISPR-based diagnostics, are further enhancing detection capabilities and enabling strain differentiation. Point-of-care testing (POCT) also gains prominence, allowing for rapid bedside diagnosis and timely clinical decision-making. Immunochromatographic assays, while less sensitive, provide immediate results, which are critical in outbreak settings. The integration of artificial intelligence (AI) in diagnostic interpretation is an emerging frontier, promising increased accuracy and efficiency. This chapter explores the evolution of HMPV diagnostic methodologies, highlighting the strengths and limitations of each approach. It also discusses future perspectives in diagnostic innovations, including biosensor-based detection and machine learning applications.

Keywords: human metapneumovirus (HMPV), molecular diagnostics, RT-PCR & LAMP, next-generation sequencing, point-of-care testing, artificial intelligence in virology

List of Abbreviations

AI	artificial intelligence
HMPV	human metapneumovirus
NGS	next-generation sequencing
mNGS	metagenomics NGS
PCR	polymerase chain reaction
RT-PCR	reverse transcriptase polymerase chain reaction
RT-qPCR	real-time quantitative RT-PCR
LAMP	loop-mediated isothermal amplification
RT-LAMP	reverse transcriptase LAMP
POCT	point of care testing
ORF	open reading frames

CRISPR	Clustered Regularly Interspaced Short Palindromic Repeats
ICTV	International Committee on Taxonomy of Viruses
NAAT	nucleic acid amplification test
LOD	limit of detection
ML	machine learning
SVM	support vector machines
DL	deep learning
ANN	artificial neural networks
CNN	convolutional neural networks
SAS	specificity of the antigen system
ICA	immunochromatographic tests
LF	lateral flow
RT-RPA	reverse transcriptase recombinase polymerase amplification
WGS	whole genome sequencing
cDNA	complementary DNA
CRG	Centre for Genomic Regulation
AINU	AI of the nucleus
SMOTE	synthetic minority oversampling technique
STORM imaging	Stochastic Optical Reconstruction Microscopy Imaging.

Introduction

Human metapneumovirus (HMPV) is an RNA virus that belongs to the subfamily *Pneumoviridae* and family *Paramyxovirus,* which are closely linked to respiratory syncytial virus, parainfluenza virus, and other respiratory viruses. In recent years, it has created an impact by re-emerging and causing outbreaks in certain parts of the world. It is a common respiratory virus that was known before in the year 2001, which infects individuals in a seasonal pattern, mostly in the winter. But recently, it has gained concern because it affects vulnerable groups such as young children, immunocompromised patients, and the elderly. Clinical manifestations caused by HMPV are likely flu or flu-like symptoms with wheezing or bronchiolitis that could range from mild to moderate and severe respiratory illness (Porwal et al., 2025). So far, there is no antiviral medication or vaccine licensed for the treatment and cure of HMPV infection. In addition, with the incubation period of 3-5 days, they could rapidly spread through respiratory droplets of infected people, airborne, and through close contact with contaminated areas. It is also observed that the pediatric population who are infected by HMPV have incomplete recovery due to weaker immunity and have a chance for relapses of the disease at later ages. Thus, accurate and timely diagnosis is required for early and quick detection of infection and epidemiological surveillance in order to prevent disease severity, transmission, and outbreaks (Gálvez et al., 2021).

Current diagnostic methods that are used have poor results due to lower specificity, sensitivity, and being time-consuming. Early diagnosis of the infection would minimise the outbreak and assist in effective, timely treatment and preventative strategies. Therefore, to overcome this problem, novel diagnostic approaches that are advanced should be developed for accuracy, precision, and rapid monitoring of the disease. Some instances of breakthroughs in novel diagnostic approaches that have ameliorated detection sensitivity are RT-PCR (reverse transcriptase polymerase chain reaction), RT-qPCR (real-time quantitative RT-PCR), mNGS (metagenomics next generation sequencing), loop-mediated isothermal amplification (LAMP), reverse transcription loop-mediated isothermal amplification (RT-LAMP), CRISPR-Cas technologies, etc. (Akingbola et al., 2025). The HMPV genome contains eight gene nucleotides that encode nine open reading frames (ORF) and three surface glycoproteins, such as the fusion (F) protein, which is the main target of antibodies, the attachment (G) protein, and the small hydrophobic (SH) protein. The strains of HMPV belong to two important lineages, i.e., A and B, which are further sub-categorised into A1, A2, B1, and B2. In phylogenetic analysis, subgroup A2 is further classified as A2a and A2b; these clades are used in influenza viruses and the ICTV (International Committee on Taxonomy of Viruses) (Kulkarni et al., 2025). Thus, a thorough understanding of pathophysiology is essential for the diagnosis of the disease. This chapter deals with advances in current diagnostic approaches to metapneumovirus in humans.

Traditional Diagnostic Methods

Traditional techniques are used to diagnose HMPV or any other viral infection at the early stage. This assists in the development of infection control strategies and prevents epidemic breakouts. Some instances of conventional diagnostic techniques include viral cultures, RT-PCR, RT-qPCR, multiplex PCR, serological tests, immunofluorescence assays, enzyme assays, etc. Even in modern days, RT-PCR is a gold standard diagnostic tool to detect HMPV and other specific viral infections. PCR tests provide improved specificity and sensitivity, but the critical problem that has been faced is carry-over or amplicon contamination, even in experienced laboratories. In some cases, serological tests are difficult due to the highly conserved amino acid sequences of the protein F in HMPV as well as RSV, which makes it challenging to identify HMPV-specific antibodies. Thus, various novel molecular methods, such as probing the nucleic acid of the virus, could detect HMPV (Feng et al., 2024). In comparison with other traditional methods like viral cultures or the use of direct fluorescent-labelled antibodies, multiplex RT-PCR detects respiratory viruses more accurately. But in order to decrease amplification efficiency, primers and probes are used in detection. In other words, traditional techniques such as viral cultures or immunological assays have more specificity and are hence used as reference standards. On the other hand, PCR-based methods are used due to their speed, versatility, sensitivity, safety, and cost-effective approach (Costa-Filho et al., 2025).

Molecular Diagnostics

RT-PCR

It is a kind of NAAT (Nucleic Acid Amplification Test). In case of any viral diagnosis in the current days, including the SARS-CoV, the reverse transcriptase polymerase chain reaction has been the standard procedure for identification and diagnosis; HMPV is not an exception to that as well. Employing the identification of the target genes of HMPV P, N, F, and M via amplification of the corresponding DNA following the conversion of RNA to complementary DNA or cDNA, via reverse transcription, diagnosis is carried out in this process (J. S. Lee et al., 2021).

Multiplex PCR

Also called mRT-PCR, it works by producing unique amplicons for different target sequences. These amplicons are made by conjugating several primers into one PCR tube. Optimum designing is ensured to achieve a uniform working annealing temperature for primer pairs. Various amplicons are identified by using different types of fluorescent dyes. It is more advantageous than common RT-PCR, as it can detect an array of respiratory viruses in one single sample run. Compared to a 54.6% sensitivity of the rRT-PCR technique, this technique has a sensitivity of almost 100% with an impressive 96% selective specificity of the different viruses (Tai et al., 2021).

Nucleic Acid Isothermal Amplification Methods

LAMP

LAMP, or loop-mediated isothermal amplification, is the most used variant of nucleic acid isothermal amplification techniques, which was discovered in the year 2000 by a Japanese team. LAMP uses online primer design employing the software Primer-Explorer v4. The processes include designing 4 targeting pairs specifically for M genes, then 2 different RT-LAMP reactions are designed to specifically detect and isolate between the A and B subspecies of the virus (Zhang et al., 2024). LAMP has shown a significant level of sensitivity towards the detection of the virus compared to RT-PCR methods, being almost 10-fold more sensitive, as the LOD (limit of detection) of LAMP is around 4.33 copies and 3.53 copies of A and B types of HMPV per microliter of sample. LAMP is simpler than RT-PCR methods due to its usage of 65 degrees Celsius throughout the process. Omitting the need for complex thermal management, amplifications can even be seen with the naked eye, further making the process simpler. Despite all these advantages, LAMP is still a very expensive procedure and has a higher probability of getting false positive results (Li et al., 2023).

Virus Isolation

Viral culture and isolation have always been the backbone of traditional diagnostic techniques of all kinds of viral infections and are used as the gold standard for all viral identifications. In this, usually LLC-MK2, human Chang conjunctiva cell lines, and feline kidney cells are used for culturing of viruses. In HMPV, particularly, LLC-MK2 cells are used abundantly (Yao et al., 2025). The isolation is done in 2 steps: incubation of the positive HMPV samples with the cell monolayer for 2-3 days, followed by serological evaluation or molecular detection for the antigens or viral nucleic acid. Although it is regarded as the ‘gold standard,’ it does have disadvantages like the requirement of trained personnel, time constraints, high cost, instrumental burden, and low rate of isolation of HMPV (Jeong et al., 2020).

Recombinase-Aided Amplification (RAA)

It is an easily operable thermostatic amplification method that is newly added to the list; it boosts simplicity, ease of operation, low-maintenance equipment, and high amplification output. It is highly employed in the cases of infection and newly identified pathogens' field diagnosis, where complicated equipment and time are major constraints. It requires only 15 minutes of runtime at 39 degrees Celsius, even though it is highly useful in rapid and emergency detection of HMPV in the fields, but it does have a low sensitivity, making it unreliable in a hospital setting (He et al., 2021).

Metagenomics Next-Generation Sequencing (mNGS)

It is a new, high-throughput technique for diagnosing, identifying and gene sequencing new and emerging pathogens. As new viruses emerge, it is difficult to identify them, but mNGS can be employed to do that as well as to amplify the viral genome accurately, and Sanger sequencing of Illumina tools is used for the reverse transcription of RNA to cDNA. From earlier data it is seen that this technique is useful for detecting the full genome sequence of HMPV from 15 out of 25 samples and can successfully detect HMPV in 20 among those 25 patients, so with a sensitivity of 80%, it is safe to say that even though it is a specific and promising technique, the sensitivity is yet to be fully unlocked (Gao et al., 2024).

Emerging Diagnostic Technologies

Emerging technology for Human Metapneumovirus (HMPV) is an important aspect in gaining the knowledge and management of HMPV-induced respiratory infections. As HMPV has been established as an important pathogen among children and the immunocompromised population, advances in the development of innovative diagnostic methods for timely identification and treatment are urgently needed (Costa-Filho et al., 2025). New developments, such as molecular methods like polymerase chain reaction (PCR), next-generation sequencing, and quick antigen tests, have enhanced sensitivity and specificity to allow healthcare providers to detect HMPV infections more precisely and effectively (Krüger et al., 2025). Such technologies not only contribute to the rapid detection of active infections but also help with epidemiological studies by monitoring virus strains and determining transmission patterns. In addition, incorporation of these diagnostic techniques into practice can greatly contribute to improved patient outcomes through early intervention and customised therapeutic approaches, ultimately decreasing the impact of respiratory diseases linked with HMPV (Nema et al., 2024). Novel treatments, like opting for natural products that prevent viral infections, were trending. For instance, in studies related to COVID-19 and dengue viral infection, *Nigella sativa* and *Carica papaya* extracts have potential antiviral and immunomodulatory components to halt the disease (Maideen et al., 2023, 2025).

Next-Generation Sequencing (NGS) for Comprehensive HMPV Genome Analysis

HMPV, a member of the Pneumoviridae, is an important cause of respiratory disease in susceptible individuals. Classical genotyping of HMPV has centred mostly on the sequencing of the fusion (F) and attachment (G) glycoprotein genes. The G gene, however, specifically bears high immune pressure and has high genetic heterogeneity. Although this diversity is useful in grouping the strains into two major genetic lineages (A and B) and four sublineages (A1, A2, B1, and B2), it does not necessarily capture the virus's evolutionary epidemiological patterns. On the other hand, whole genome sequencing (WGS) through the next-generation sequencing NGS is a more detailed technique that considers complete genomic data and thus offers insight into HMPV evolution, transmission dynamics, and outbreak patterns. WGS can also assist in the creation of better diagnostic tools and guide future therapeutic approaches (Houldcroft et al., 2017).

Whole Genome Sequencing of HMPV Using MinION Nanopore Technology

To overcome the shortfalls of conventional HMPV genotyping, which frequently does not reflect complete viral diversity because of intense variability in genes such as the G gene, a new whole-genome sequencing technique based on MinION Nanopore technology was devised and validated. This focused method uses thoughtfully designed degenerate primers to amplify the complete HMPV genome from clinical specimens from all sublineages with extensive coverage, including the highly variable G gene (Groen et al., 2022). The approach applies multiplex PCR with overlapping amplicons and takes advantage of the affordable, portable MinION platform for sequencing. Validation proved consistent genome recovery even from low RNA levels (Ct values up to 25), with robust performance in both reference strains and clinical specimens. In contrast to conventional NGS platforms and untargeted metagenomics, this MinION-based assay provides improved sensitivity, specificity, and even genome coverage. Overall, the strategy is a potent advance for HMPV molecular epidemiology, with broader implications for respiratory virus surveillance, outbreak investigation, and diagnostic development (Kaminski et al., 2021).

Role of Artificial Intelligence in Diagnostics

Machine learning (ML) and deep learning (DL) are powerful tools to analyse complex and massive biological datasets that are struggling to be handled by traditional statistical methods. Technologies like next-generation sequencing (NGS) led to data explosions in genomic data sets, but these are challenging due to their high dimensionality, noise heterogeneity, and small sample sizes. These issues can be overcome with the help of ML, which performs with labelled data, i.e., supervised learning used for classification and regression (e.g., mapping gene expressions to diseases), and with unlabeled data, i.e., Unsupervised learning used to find natural groupings or patterns (e.g., clustering gene sequences) (Filippis & Foysal, 2025). Semi-supervised learning is the combination of both supervised and unsupervised learning. It uses a small amount of labelled data and a large amount of unlabeled data. Hence, useful when there is a scarcity of labelled data but abundant unlabeled data. It has been successfully applied in image recognition, natural language processing, medical prognosis, speech recognition, and fraud detection.

A standard ML pipeline flow diagram in biology: data collection → preprocessing → model training → model testing → application to new data (Tang et al., 2019). Neural networks, Support Vector Machines (SVMs), Gaussian processes, and principal component analysis are some of the common ML techniques. Deep learning, a subset of machine learning powered by artificial neural networks (ANNs), excels in handling complex datasets. Applying supervised, unsupervised, or semi-supervised approaches. Convolutional neural networks (CNNs), a specific type of deep learning model, analyse histopathological images to assess viral loads within tissues. By mimicking the structure of the human brain, these techniques enhance diagnostic accuracy while accelerating the process, thereby reducing the likelihood of false negatives and positives (Shi et al., 2025).

AI-Driven Approaches for HMPV Detection

JIVI.AI: (https://www.jivi.ai/), which is an AI-enabled risk assessment tool that evaluates HMPV risk levels using smartphones. The system identifies cellular heterogeneity with nanoscale images (Carnevali et al., 2024). The functionality of AINU involves advanced microscopic integration along with STORM imaging, which is employed to produce ultra-high-resolution views of cells. Detection of microscale patterns could recognise subtle changes in structural biology that are as small as 20 μm. It employs detecting infections before any emergence of pre-clinical symptoms and assists in effective differentiation of healthy and diseased cells in either cancer or infection-related cells with high-precision technology. AINU could be a game changer in virology diagnostics and precision medicine applications (Edgar et al., 2022).

Genomic Analysis Using AI

Viruses have the tendency to mutate and evolve in a short span, which makes it difficult to analyse their genomes for vaccine development and even diagnosis. In this case, incorporating AI algorithms would aid in outbreak tracking, analysing viral genomes to identify mutated patterns and predict new variants and strains. These technologies would also help in phylogenetic analysis and create viral lineage trees for better tracking, development, and dispersal of strains among various populations. Machine learning models analyse global sequencing data to detect any presence of infection or an outbreak in a certain population or region. Furthermore, incorporating AI in viral diagnostics would speed up the process of detecting infected individuals, creating personalised treatment strategies, and rapidly developing next-generation vaccines (Shriwas et al., 2024).

Conclusion

Though there is a surge of HMPV detection tools, the need for accessible, scalable, cost-effective, and resource-limited diagnostic tools, which include portable devices, is crucial to offer convenience and high sensitivity for quick and early diagnosis to prevent the outbreak. Rapid diagnosis could offer a path to discover vaccines for viral strains or mutations. Integration of AI, DL, and ML in clinical diagnostics of viral disease could help address current challenges faced in viral diagnosis by enabling timely decisions and treatment options during the outbreak. Therefore, it is important for all healthcare practitioners to stay updated with the latest diagnostic tools and AI-enabled functions for accurate and precise diagnostic interpretations.

References

Akingbola, A., Adegbesan, Abiodun, TundeAlao, Samuel, Adewole, Olajumoke, Ayikoru, Comfort, Benson, Akpevwe Emmanuella, Shekoni, Mayowa, & and Chuku, J. (2025). Human Metapneumovirus: An emerging respiratory pathogen and the urgent need for improved Diagnostics, surveillance, and vaccine development. *Infectious Diseases*, 57(3), 304–310.

Carnevali, D., Zhong, L., González-Almela, E., Viana, C., Rotkevich, M., Wang, A., Franco-Barranco, D., Gonzalez-Marfil, A., Neguembor, M. V., Castells-Garcia, A., Arganda-Carreras, I., & Cosma, M. P. (2024). A deep learning method that identifies cellular heterogeneity using nanoscale nuclear features. *Nature Machine Intelligence*, 6(9), 1021–1033.

Costa-Filho, R. C., Saddy, F., Costa, J. L. F., Tavares, L. R., & Castro Faria Neto, H. C. (2025). The Silent Threat of Human Metapneumovirus: Clinical Challenges and Diagnostic Insights from a Severe Pneumonia Case. *Microorganisms*, 13(1).

Edgar, R. C., Taylor, B., Lin, V., Altman, T., Barbera, P., Meleshko, D., Lohr, D., Novakovsky, G., Buchfink, B., Al-Shayeb, B., Banfield, J. F., de la Peña, M., Korobeynikov, A., Chikhi, R., & Babaian, A. (2022). Petabase-scale sequence alignment catalyses viral discovery. *Nature*, 602(7895), 142–147.

Fellmann, C., Gowen, B. G., Lin, P.-C., Doudna, J. A., & Corn, J. E. (2017). Cornerstones of CRISPR–Cas in drug discovery and therapy. *Nature Reviews Drug Discovery*, 16(2), 89–100.

Feng, Y., He, T., Zhang, B., Yuan, H., & Zhou, Y. (2024). Epidemiology and diagnosis technologies of human metapneumovirus in China: A mini review. *Virology Journal*, 21(1), 59.

Filippis, R. de, & Foysal, A. A. (2025). Machine Learning-Based Detection of Human Metapneumovirus (HMPV) Using Clinical Data. *Open Access Library Journal*, 12(4).

Gálvez, N. M. S., Andrade, C. A., Pacheco, G. A., Soto, J. A., Stranger, V., Rivera, T., Vásquez, A. E., & Kalergis, A. M. (2021). Host Components That Modulate the Disease Caused by hMPV. *Viruses*, 13(3).

Gao, Q., Li, L., Su, T., Liu, J., Chen, L., Yi, Y., Huan, Y., He, J., & Song, C. (2024). A single-center, retrospective study of hospitalized patients with lower respiratory tract infections: Clinical assessment of metagenomic next-generation sequencing and identification of risk factors in patients. *Respiratory Research*, 25(1), 250.

Groen, K., van Nieuwkoop, S., Meijer, A., van der Veer, B., van Kampen, J. J. A., Fraaij, P. L., Fouchier, R. A. M., & van den Hoogen, B. G. (2022). Emergence and Potential Extinction of Genetic Lineages of Human Metapneumovirus between 2005 and 2021. *mBio*, 14(1), e02280-22.

He, Y., Chen, W., Fan, J., Fan, S., Ding, H., Chen, J., & Yi, L. (2021). Recombinase-Aided Amplification Coupled with Lateral Flow Dipstick for Efficient and Accurate Detection of Porcine Parvovirus. *Life*, 11(8).

Houldcroft, C. J., Beale, M. A., & Breuer, J. (2017). Clinical and biological insights from viral genome sequencing. *Nature Reviews Microbiology*, 15(3), 183–192.

Irfan, M., Iftikhar, M. A., Yasin, S., Draz, U., Ali, T., Hussain, S., Bukhari, S., Alwadie, A. S., Rahman, S., Glowacz, A., & Althobiani, F. (2021). Role of Hybrid Deep Neural Networks (HDNNs), Computed Tomography, and Chest X-rays for the Detection of COVID-19. *International Journal of Environmental Research and Public Health*, 18(6).

Jeong, S., Park, M.-J., Song, W., & Kim, H.-S. (2020). Advances in laboratory assays for detecting human metapneumovirus. *Annals of Translational Medicine*, 8(9), 608.

Kaminski, M. M., Abudayyeh, O. O., Gootenberg, J. S., Zhang, F., & Collins, J. J. (2021). CRISPR-based diagnostics. *Nature Biomedical Engineering*, 5(7), 643–656.

Kodani, M., Martin, A., Mixson-Hayden, T., Drobeniuc, J., Gish, R. R., & Kamili, S. (2013). One-step real-time PCR assay for detection and quantitation of hepatitis D virus RNA. *Journal of Virological Methods*, 193(2), 531–535.

Krüger, N., Laufer, S. A., & Pillaiyar, T. (2025). An overview of progress in human metapneumovirus (hMPV) research: Structure, function, and therapeutic opportunities. *Drug Discovery Today*, 104364.

Kulkarni, D., Cong, B., Ranjini, M. J. K., Balchandani, G., Chen, S., Liang, J., Gordon, L. G., Meulen, A. S., Wang, X., Li, Y., Osei-Yeboah, R., Templeton, K., & Nair, H.

(2025). The global burden of human metapneumovirus-associated acute respiratory infections in older adults: A systematic review and meta-analysis. *The Lancet Healthy Longevity*, 6(2).

Lee, J. S., Ahn, J. J., Kim, S. J., Yu, S. Y., Koh, E. J., Kim, S. H., Sung, H. S., Huh, J. W., & Hwang, S. Y. (2021). POCT Detection of 14 Respiratory Viruses Using Multiplex RT-PCR. *BioChip Journal*, 15(4), 371–380.

Lee, S., Park, J. S., Woo, H., Yoo, Y. K., Lee, D., Chung, S., Yoon, D. S., Lee, K.-B., & Lee, J. H. (2024). Rapid deep learning-assisted predictive diagnostics for point-of-care testing. *Nature Communications*, 15(1), 1695.

Li, Z., Sinha, A., Zhang, Y., Tanner, N., Cheng, H.-T., Premsrirut, P., & Carlow, C. K. S. (2023). Extraction-free LAMP assays for generic detection of Old World Orthopoxviruses and specific detection of Mpox virus. *Scientific Reports*, 13(1), 21093.

Maideen, N. M. P., Balasubramanian, R., Gobinath, M., Rafiullah, M., & Muthusamy, S. (2023). Therapeutic Potentials of Black Seeds (Nigella sativa) in the Management of COVID-19 -A Review of Clinical and In-silico Studies. *Anti-Infective Agents*, 21(1), 14–23.

Maideen, N. M. P., Balasubramanian, R., Shanmugam, A., Gobinath, M., & Hussain, M. H. J. (2025). A Review of Potentials of Carica Papaya Leaves in Dengue Viral Infection – Insights of Clinical and Preclinical Studies. *Drug Research*, 75, 49–59.

Matsuzaki, Y., Takashita, E., Okamoto, M., Mizuta, K., Itagaki, T., Katsushima, F., Katsushima, Y., Nagai, Y., & Nishimura, H. (2009). Evaluation of a New Rapid Antigen Test Using Immunochromatography for Detection of Human Metapneumovirus in Comparison with Real-Time PCR Assay. *Journal of Clinical Microbiology*, 47(9), 2981–2984.

Nema, R. K., Singh, S., Singh, A. K., Sarma, D. K., Diwan, V., Tiwari, R. R., Mondal, R. K., & Mishra, P. K. (2024). Protocol for detection of pathogenic enteric RNA viruses by regular monitoring of environmental samples from wastewater treatment plants using droplet digital PCR. *Science in One Health*, 3, 100080.

Porwal, S., Malviya, R., Sridhar, S. B., Shareef, J., & Wadhwa, T. (2025). Global impact of hMPV virus: Transmission, pathogenesis, diagnostic and treatment. *Diagnostic Microbiology and Infectious Disease*, 112(3), 116809.

Qian, W., Huang, J., Wang, T., He, X., Xu, G., & Li, Y. (2021). Visual detection of human metapneumovirus using CRISPR-Cas12a diagnostics. *Virus Research*, 305, 198568.

Ribeiro, B. V., Cordeiro, T. A. R., Oliveira e Freitas, G. R., Ferreira, L. F., & Franco, D. L. (2020). Biosensors for the detection of respiratory viruses: A review. *Talanta Open*, 2, 100007.

Satapathy, T., Satapathy, A., Satapathy, A., Yadav, N., Chandrakar, M. C. M., & Chandrakar, K. (2025). Recent outbreaks of Human Metapneumovirus (HMPV): Prevention, Diagnosis and Therapeutic insights. *Journal of Drug Delivery and Therapeutics*, 15(2), Article 2.

Sharafeldin, M., & Davis, J. J. (2021). Point of Care Sensors for Infectious Pathogens. *Analytical Chemistry*, 93(1), 184–197.

Shi, S., Lin, H., Jiang, L., Zeng, Z., Lin, C., Li, P., Li, Y., & Yang, Z. (2025). Development of a respiratory virus risk model with environmental data based on interpretable machine learning methods. *Npj Climate and Atmospheric Science*, 8(1), 1–11.

Shriwas, P. K., Sundaravadivazhagan, B., & Patil, Y. M. (2024). Role of AI in Diagnosis of Viral Infection. In J. M. Chatterjee, R. Sujatha, & S. K. Saxena (Eds.), *Role of Artificial Intelligence, Telehealth, and Telemedicine in Medical Virology* (pp. 31–51). Springer Nature.

Tai, C. C., Tsai, C. H., Huang, Y. H., Lee, C. L., Chen, H. P., & Chan, Y. J. (2021). Detection of respiratory viruses in adults with respiratory tract infection using a multiplex PCR assay at a tertiary center. *Journal of Microbiology, Immunology and Infection*, 54(5), 858–864.

Tang, B., Pan, Z., Yin, K., & Khateeb, A. (2019). Recent Advances of Deep Learning in Bioinformatics and Computational Biology. *Frontiers in Genetics*, 10.

Xu, Y., & Li, Z. (2020). CRISPR-Cas systems: Overview, innovations and applications in human disease research and gene therapy. *Computational and Structural Biotechnology Journal*, 18, 2401–2415.

Yao, Z., Li, J., Shi, Y., Sun, T., Yang, X., Mao, J., Quan, R., Wang, D., Wang, D., Zhou, J., Liu, J., Chu, J., & Hou, L. (2025). Isolation and identification of a subtype C avian metapneumovirus in chickens in Jiangsu, China. *Microbial Pathogenesis*, 202, 107394.

Zhang, X., Zhao, Y., Zhu, X., Tian, W., & Zhang, C. (2024). Rapid detection of four major HFMD-associated enteroviruses by multiplex HiFi-LAMP assays. *Analytical and Bioanalytical Chemistry*, 416(8), 1971–1982.

Chapter 7

Therapeutic Strategies for Human Metapneumovirus (HMPV)

Vaishali Kamboj
Nikhil
Akash Jain
and Jasmine Chaudhary*
M. M. College of Pharmacy, M. M. (Deemed to be University), Mullana, Ambala, Haryana, India

Abstract

Human Metapneumovirus (HMPV) is a significant viral pathogen that causes acute respiratory infections (ARIs), particularly affecting small children, the elderly, and immunocompromised individuals. Infections caused by HMPV exhibit a spectrum of severity, ranging from minor upper respiratory tract symptoms to more serious conditions, including bronchiolitis and pneumonia. Human Metapneumovirus (HMPV) exhibits seasonal peaks in late winter and spring, with two primary genotypes (A and B) that vary in geographical distribution. No vaccine or antiviral treatment has been approved, and the health impact continues to be substantial. The present treatment exclusively comprises supportive interventions, including oxygen therapy and hydration. Monoclonal antibodies targeting the fusion protein, together with certain experimental antivirals, represent promising yet developmental techniques. Epidemiological studies indicate that HMPV accounts for around 5-10% of acute respiratory infection hospitalisations in children and presents significant hazards to older persons with chronic respiratory

* Corresponding Author's Email: jasdream17@gmail.com

In: Human Metapneumovirus
Editors: Anjali Sharma, Vishnu Mittal, Devkant Sharma et al.
ISBN: 979-8-90134-063-9

conditions. Advancements in the ability of HMPV detection have been achieved by the recent development of RT-PCR; currently, diagnostic methods encounter accessibility constraints in resource-limited environments. Live attenuated strains, subunit vaccines derived from prefusion F proteins, and mRNA-based vaccination platforms are now in the preclinical phase. Addressing genetic heterogeneity and the virus's adaptive abilities helps them escape immune detection, which will cause a significant hurdle. Fundamental to these initiatives, non-pharmaceutical interventions such as proper personal hygiene and seclusion continue to be the most effective strategies for controlling transmission. The proposed methodologies emphasise the development of remedies for this global health concern through a multidisciplinary strategy that integrates virology, immunology, public health policy, and precision medicine.

Keywords: HMPV, therapies, strategies, transcription, monoclonal antibodies

List of Abbreviations

HMPV	Human Metapneumovirus
RSV	Respiratory Syncytial Virus
ARIs	Acute Respiratory Infections
COPD	Chronic Obstructive Pulmonary Disease
ARDS	Acute Respiratory Distress Syndrome
RTI	Respiratory Tract Infection
LRTI	Lower Respiratory Tract Infection
RT-PCR	Reverse Transcriptase/Transcription Polymerase Chain Reaction
NAAT	Nucleic Acid Amplification Test
ELISA	Enzyme-Linked Immunosorbent Assay
IVIG	Intravenous Immunoglobulin
mAb(s)	Monoclonal Antibody(ies)
RNA	Ribonucleic Acid
F protein	Fusion Protein
N protein	Nucleoprotein
P protein	Phosphoprotein
M protein	Matrix Protein
L protein	Large protein (RNA-dependent RNA polymerase)
ECMO	Extracorporeal Membrane Oxygenation
HFNC	High Flow Nasal Cannula

CPAP	Continuous Positive Airway Pressure
BiPAP	Bilevel Positive Airway Pressure
ICU	Intensive Care Unit
RNP	Ribonucleoprotein
NK cells	Natural Killer cells
Th1/Th2	T-helper cell type 1/type 2
TNF	Tumour Necrosis Factor
mRNA	Messenger Ribonucleic Acid
HRSV	Human Respiratory Syncytial Virus
DFA	Direct Fluorescent Antibody
OTC	Over-the-Counter
PCR	Polymerase Chain Reaction
SARS-CoV-2	Severe Acute Respiratory Syndrome Coronavirus 2
WHO	World Health Organisation
CDC	Centres for Disease Control
PPE	Personal Protective Equipment
NCBI	National Centre for Biotechnology Information
NREVSS	National Respiratory and Enteric Virus Surveillance System

Introduction

Human Metapneumovirus (HMPV), which covers a wide range of respiratory illnesses, ranging from mild upper respiratory tract infections to bronchiolitis and pneumonia, captured global attention. HMPV was identified in 2001 as a significant contributor to Acute Respiratory Infections (ARIs). Chronic respiratory problems notably affect vulnerable groups, including small children, the elderly (Carter et al., 2006), and immunocompromised individuals (Thompson et al., 2023), resulting in heightened morbidity and mortality rates worldwide.

Similar to HMPV, RSV is another significant pathogen in respiratory infections, exhibiting both genetic and clinical similarities (Kozopas, 2024). The infection pathway is via the respiratory system, resulting in inflammation and destruction to the respiratory epithelium, potentially causing severe respiratory distress in the human population. Virus transmission may occur by direct contact with bodily fluids, contaminated surfaces, or infectious droplets during human interaction. HMPV exhibits a characteristic seasonality, with maxima occurring in late winter and spring in temperate regions (Sousa

Paulino et al., 2023). The two principal genotypes (A and B), along with their corresponding sublineages, exhibit regionally distinct virulence and prevalence. Lifelong inadequate immunity resulting from natural infection leads to recurrent infections throughout life. Researchers state that nearly every individual encounters HMPV by the age of five, marking a significant advancement in the understanding of respiratory diseases beyond influenza and RSV (Yan-a, 2009).

Epidemiological studies reveal an agreement that HMPV is responsible for 5-10% of hospital admissions for acute respiratory infections in children aged 5 years. The senior population, especially those aged 65 and above, faces a substantial risk of pneumonia and exacerbated chronic obstructive pulmonary disease (COPD) requiring hospitalisation. Human Metapneumovirus (HMPV) was detected in 8% of paediatric patients in Egypt with acute respiratory infections, with a greater incidence in children aged 2 to 24 months. Similar reporting has been noted in India during community-oriented surveillance at seasonal peaks. Besides direct healthcare costs associated with HMPV, considerable resources are devoted to inpatient care, outpatient consultations, and productivity losses stemming from the condition (Chatterjee et al., 2021). This chapter outlines HMPV and its historical epidemiology, while clarifying the clinically susceptible patient categories and the therapeutic challenges associated with the disease (Vinci et al., 2018).

Clinical Manifestations and Complications

The manifestations of HMPV infections significantly differ based on a patient's age, immune system robustness, and overall health condition. Symptoms include cough, rhinorrhoea, sore throat, fever, and weariness (Parameshwari et al., 2024). Progression to the lower respiratory tract may result in bronchiolitis or pneumonia, potentially leading to wheezing and acute respiratory distress syndrome (ARDS) (Krishnan et al., 2019). Aggravated newborns may have hypoxia, cyanosis and retractions of the chest wall. Infants may experience dehydration and bacterial infections. Geriatric patients experience prolonged hospitalisations or necessitate intensive care. The clinical diagnostic distinction of HMPV is complicated by the presence of other respiratory infections, including RSV. Advanced diagnostic techniques such as RT-PCR are essential for accurate detection (Khan et al., 2024).

Current Gaps in Treatment and Prevention

Despite the clinical significance of HMPV, there are currently no authorised vaccines or targeted antiviral therapies available. Currently, only supportive management is utilised, which includes oxygen therapy for hypoxic patients, antipyretic agents for patients with fever and wheezing is managed by nebulisers or inhalers (Satapathy et al., 2025). Small molecule inhibitors and monoclonal antibodies targeting the fusion protein remain in the developing phase but exhibit promise as experimental therapies. The absence of effective antiviral drugs highlights critical deficiencies in therapeutic alternatives. Preventative strategies are largely non-specific and consist of hand hygiene, utilisation of masks during current epidemics, environmental cleaning and disinfection and patient isolation within healthcare settings (Ahmed, 2025). Efforts are underway to develop vaccines employing live attenuated or recombinant viral proteins; however, these approaches remain in the experimental phase. Epidemiological studies require more advanced monitoring systems to guide public health interventions (Elemuwa et al., 2025).

Pathophysiology and Immunology

Infection with HMPV results in severe disease impacting the respiratory system due to the evasion of host immune systems and the exploitation of host cellular machinery. The virus's structural characteristics, coupled with replication dynamics and the host's immunological response, determined its pathogenesis (Geiser et al., 2021). Infection with HMPV results in severe disease impacting the respiratory system by circumventing host immune responses and exploiting host cellular mechanisms. The virus's structural characteristics, replication dynamics, and the host's immunological response determined its pathogenicity.

Viral Structure and Genome

Human Metapneumovirus (HMPV) is classified under the Pneumoviridae family as an enveloped, single-stranded, negative-sense RNA virus. HMPV contains a genome of 13.3 kb in length, comprising nine primary genes: nucleoprotein (N), phosphoprotein (P), matrix protein (M), fusion protein (F), and RNA-dependent RNA polymerase (L) (Pan et al., 2019). The N protein envelopes viral RNA, creating a ribonucleoprotein (RNP) complex that functions as a template for replication and transcription. Cryo-EM has demonstrated that the C-terminal domain of P can dynamically interact with RNA encapsidated by N. This engages the silencing L/P polymerase complex for genomic silencing, which is crucial for the formation of cytoplasmic inclusion bodies that serve as loci for viral replication (Mäkinen & Hafrén, 2014, Wei et al., 2023).

Mechanism of Infection and Replication Cycle

Glycosaminoglycans or integrins facilitate the attachment of HMPV to the host cell. Subsequently, the viral envelope merges with the host membrane. The subsequent stages in the replication of HMPV are as follows:

1. The F protein facilitates membrane fusion for HMPV entry.
2. The L/P complex facilitates the production of viral RNA and conducts genome replication. The disruption of actin microfilaments in the early phases of infection increases the synthesis of viral proteins and the secretion of virions.
3. During the assembly and release phases, newly produced virion particles are expelled from the apical surface of infected cells. In comparison to RSV, HMPV exhibits a diminished capacity to release virions at the apical surface (Soto et al., 2018).

Replication attains its zenith between 48 and 72 hours post-infection. During this period, inclusion bodies facilitate the synchronised synthesis of viral components.

Host Immune Response to HMPV

Human metapneumovirus (HMPV) affects both innate and adaptive immunity by infecting the host, resulting in dysfunctional alveolar macrophages that hinder bacterial clearance and promote inflammation through the release of neutrophilic enzymatic molecules and oxidative byproducts (Kinder et al., 2020, Malaer & Mathew, 2020). Severe infections impede NK cell cytotoxicity through receptor interference. In adaptive immunity, CD8+ T cells facilitate viral elimination but may induce immunopathology if they remain, whereas an imbalance between Th1 and Th2 responses is associated with the severity of bronchiolitis (Kolli et al., 2012). Neutralising antibodies, particularly those targeting the pre-fusion F protein, inhibit viral entry; nonetheless, reinfection remains feasible due to inadequate protection (Gálvez et al., 2021). Human Metapneumovirus (HMPV) circumvents host defences by inhibiting interferon signalling via TBK1 suppression and microRNA, inducing epigenetic silencing (H3K27me3) to diminish IL-1β production, commandeering the cytoskeleton to facilitate dissemination and inhibit phagocytosis, and employing antigenic variation in surface proteins such as the F protein to evade antibody detection (Ou et al., 2023).

Supportive Care and Symptomatic Management

Human Metapneumovirus (HMPV) infections are associated with less severe symptoms in the upper respiratory tract and more severe consequences in the lower respiratory tract, potentially leading to pneumonia and acute respiratory distress syndrome (ARDS) (Mishra et al., 2025). Currently, there are no antiviral medications or vaccines available for HMPV. Nonetheless, a degree of supportive care is essential. This section examines the role of supportive care in conjunction with self-medication, including antipyretics such as acetaminophen and ibuprofen, which are effective in alleviating fever and its associated symptoms. Additionally, it covers decongestants, cough suppressants, and honey for children over 12 months, as well as the importance of rest and hydration. It also addresses more advanced interventions, such as oxygen delivery via nasal cannula or face mask for patients experiencing mild hypoxemia who necessitate low to moderate oxygen therapy. The High Flow Nasal Cannula (HFNC) has been shown to improve cognitive function and reduce inflammation, oxidative stress, and other pulmonary issues in severely infected patients undergoing respiratory failure, and mechanical breathing includes Non-Invasive Ventilation, which allows for respiration without intubation, using CPAP or BiPAP in more severe cases of the illness. Supportive treatment for HMPV infection is critical for symptom management, preventing complications, and boosting the immune response. For patients, the primary focus is symptomatic care, as the illness typically resolves spontaneously. As a last resort, venovenous ECMO may be used in cases of refractory hypoxemia that do not respond to traditional ventilation. This approach provides external oxygenation to the body while allowing the lungs to rest and repair. A case study demonstrated the successful use of this approach in treating severe ARDS caused by HMPV infection (Hengst et al., 2008). In severe cases, particularly among high-risk populations such as young children, the elderly, and individuals with weakened immune systems, prompt and effective supportive measures are crucial.

The fluid intake must be adequate to prevent dehydration induced by fever, tachycardia, or poor oral intake. In young newborns with severe infections, oral rehydration salts may be required to rectify electrolyte imbalances. Hospitalised individuals who are severely dehydrated or have difficulty drinking fluids may need intravenous fluids. Rest is crucial for the proper functioning of the immune system and the efficient battle against the infection (Pipitò et al., 2025). Avoid all forms of exertion during the recovery phase to avoid exacerbating symptoms and prolonging the healing process. These modest regimens can significantly aid persons with mild to moderate disease (Mattoli & Schmidt, 2023). Supportive therapy in HMPV patients primarily focuses on preventing secondary bacterial infections, which can exacerbate the clinical course of the condition. Immediate action requires carefully monitoring for symptoms of dehydration, increasing distress, and low oxygen saturation, all of which necessitate further intervention. Today's medicine allows pneumonia to be caused by either a viral or bacterial infection, and excessive non-antineoplastic medications require specific intervention to control their use (Lin et al., 2023).

Antiviral Therapies for hMPV

Because there are no proven antiviral therapies or vaccines for human metapneumovirus (HMPV), supportive care is the primary mode of treatment. Ribavirin, a guanosine analogue, suppresses viral RNA synthesis by depleting GTP through the inhibition of IMPDH, generating mutagenesis, and interrupting replication (He et al., 2023). Laboratory tests verify its efficacy both in vitro and in animal models, indicating increased survival and lower inflammation. In practice, the combination of ribavirin with intravenous immunoglobulin (IVIG) has been shown to be beneficial in the treatment of individuals with weakened immunity (Raza et al., 2007). Nonetheless, these are not large-scale trials, which leaves some limitations on their use due to side effects such as anaemia, teratogenic effects, and the emergence of resistant strains.

Further Investigational Antiviral Research

Investigations aimed at discovering novel antivirals for HMPV have revealed some potential candidates:

- Inhibitors: Pharmaceuticals targeting the HMPV Fusion Protein (F) inhibitors aim to block viral entry, while small molecules identified via computational methods disrupt RNA polymerase activity (Tacke et al., 2017).
- Natural resources: Researchers have examined natural compounds, including resveratrol analogues, for their potential as antivirals due to their ability to modify the host's immune response and impede virus reproduction (Dubey et al., 2025; Zhang et al., 2025). The utilisation of these chemicals may facilitate the advancement of novel therapies; nonetheless, further data from clinical studies is required.

Combination Treatments Using Immunomodulators

Combination therapies incorporating immunomodulators offer potential benefits in managing HMPV-induced immunopathology.

- Ribavirin + IVIG: Ribavirin in conjunction with IVIG may equilibrate viral suppression and immunological modulation (Wyles et al., 2015)
- Anti-inflammatory agents: Corticosteroids and anti-TNF biologics may mitigate inflammation, although their application necessitates careful management to prevent immunosuppression (Snape et al., 2023)
- Experimental combinations: Innovative treatments, such as triacetylresveratrol combined with checkpoint inhibitors, are under investigation for their dual antiviral and immunoregulatory properties (Pol et al., 2016)

Monoclonal Antibodies and Immunotherapy

The use of monoclonal antibodies (mAbs) and passive immunotherapy highlights gaps in the available advanced treatment options. This section discusses the development of HMPV-specific monoclonal antibodies (mAbs), including the cross-reactivity of RSV antibodies, as well as all preclinical and clinical studies, and prospects for passive immunotherapy.

Advances in the Development of HMPV-Specific Monoclonal Antibodies

Because of its importance in viral entry, the HMPV fusion (F) protein is a popular target for neutralising monoclonal antibodies. Notable mAbs such as MPV364 target site III on the prefusion F protein, providing effective neutralisation across HMPV genotypes without RSV cross-reactivity (Mousa et al., 2018). Other antibodies targeting sites IV and V demonstrate improved neutralising ability (Xiao et al., 2019).

Cross-Reactivity with Respiratory Syncytial Virus (RSV) Antibodies

The F proteins of HMPV and RSV exhibit structural similarities that facilitate cross-reactive antibody responses. Specific cross-reactive antibodies, such as 17E10 and MPE8, identify conserved epitopes of HMPV and RSV. Conversely, RSV-specific monoclonal antibodies like palivizumab are ineffective against HMPV. These findings underscore the need for more targeted strategies.

Preclinical and Clinical Evaluations of Monoclonal Antibodies

Preclinical studies have demonstrated the robust in vitro and in vivo efficacy of monoclonal antibodies, such as MPV364 and 17E10, which markedly decrease viral loads and pathogenesis in animal models (Chu et al., 2020).

Although HMPV-related antibodies have not yet progressed to late-stage clinical trials, safety and dosing considerations are informed by parallels with therapeutics for RSV, such as nirsevimab. Evaluation of wide-reaching cross-reactivity vascular binding site pharmacokinetics for dual-target candidates is currently underway. For patients who are immunocompromised, passive immunotherapy provides rapid protective effects. Enhanced activity of immune clearance while moderating inflammation due to the use of Fc-engineered antibodies may result from modifying the Fc region. However, the expense and risks associated with Fcγ receptors pose difficulties (West et al., 2023). Innovative delivery utilising mRNA-encoded antibodies within lipid nanoparticles demonstrates potential for prolonged efficacy and economical manufacture, possibly maintaining antibody levels for weeks following treatment (Koizumi et al., 2023).

Drug Repositioning for HMPV Treatment

Repurposing existing pharmaceuticals will facilitate the treatment of human metapneumovirus (HMPV), as it substantially decreases development costs and timelines by bypassing initial safety testing. Pharmaceuticals such as ribavirin and chloroquine may advance to clinical trials due to their proven safety profiles. A variety of broad-spectrum antiviral medications utilised for treating diverse diseases can be especially beneficial for at-risk groups, including infants and immunocompromised individuals, owing to their limited access to targeted therapy. These patients are safeguarded as certain antivirals target conserved viral pathways (Haraya & Tachibana, 2021).

The results from the clinical applications have been inconsistent. Significant achievements include the application of DAS181, an inhaled sialidase. Administered with ribavirin and IVIG, this treatment significantly decreased HMPV viral load and oxygenation levels in immunocompromised patients, while also increasing recovery times for severe pediatric cases (Choi et al., 2020).

Chloroquine and hydroxychloroquine demonstrated no therapeutic advantage due to restricted lung bioavailability, despite in vitro potential, whereas nitazoxanide showed variable performance in trials, underscoring the difficulties in attaining appropriate respiratory medication concentrations (Saikusa et al., 2017). And nitazoxanide displayed inconsistent efficacy in trials, highlighting challenges in achieving effective respiratory drug concentrations (Albrektsson et al., 1987).

Vaccine Development and Challenges

The lack of a licensed HMPV vaccine, despite comprehensive research, highlights the necessity for additional development. Live-attenuated vaccines (LAVs), especially those utilising gene- and G-deficient strains, exhibit the capacity to elicit neutralising antibodies and T cell responses. Nonetheless, they confront challenges related to excessive attenuation, safety concerns in vulnerable populations, apprehensions over possible reversion to pathogenic strains, and increased virulence (Burhan et al., 2025). Subunit vaccines targeting the prefusion F protein have demonstrated cross-genotype protective efficacy, especially when combined with adjuvants like alum or TLR agonists (Kohli et al., 2024; Yuan, 2012). Multi-epitope mRNA vaccines that include essential viral proteins and immune stimulants (e.g., β-defensin II, Pam2Cys) demonstrate potential for robust immunogenicity (Decool et al., 2022). Challenges persist because of HMPV's genetic variability, swift evolution (e.g., A2b2-111dup), and immune evasion strategies (Wise, 2022). Universal vaccine strategies target conserved epitopes like F protein site III, though immunodominance may vary. Future directions include pan-pneumovirus vaccines leveraging RSV cross-reactivity (Pasquevich et al., 2023) real-time surveillance to guide vaccine updates (Goya et al., 2025).

Non-Pharmaceutical Preventive Strategies

In the absence of vaccinations or targeted antiviral treatments, leveraging strategies employed for COVID-19 and Influenza, Non-Pharmaceutical Interventions (NPIs) are essential for controlling the dissemination of HMPV (Shrivastava & Shrivastava, 2021). Essential measures encompass the utilisation of soap and water, alongside alcohol-based hand hygiene, surface disinfection, and maybe antiseptic mouth rinses to diminish viral shedding (Ge et al., 2020). In high-risk environments, isolating symptomatic patients is essential, especially during the initial five days following symptom onset, owing to the diminished transmission risk in healthcare settings (De Bellis et al., 2024). Public health initiatives such as real-time monitoring, wastewater analysis, and mild interventions like mask regulations amalgamate social functions with viral containment (Neyaz et al., 2024). Non-pharmaceutical interventions (NPIs) vary in effectiveness across age demographics; children benefit from educational and hygiene measures, adults from telecommuting, the elderly from self-isolation and reduced exposure, and at-risk individuals from personal protective equipment (PPE) and specialised treatment areas (Doost-Hoseini et al., 2021). Continuous adherence presents problems, including behavioural weariness, age-related compliance difficulties, and the necessity for customisation (Ismayilova, 2024).

Emerging Antiviral Strategies and Host-Directed Therapies

The development of antiviral medicines is essential for human metapneumovirus (HMPV), as it is now regarded as more perilous than previously believed. Efforts are underway to regulate immune responses and alter the genes governing HMPV infection to inhibit viral replication through precision medicine. This methodology sharply contrasts with dependence on unverified treatments and immunizations. This section emphasises contemporary methodology for addressing HMPV infection and formulating Host-Directed Therapies (HDTs) in conjunction with multidisciplinary strategies for developing infection-targeted therapies.

Novel Antiviral Compounds Targeting Replication and Transcription

Molecular-level antiviral therapy for HMPV is transitioning to encompass both virus and host components. Specific small host-directed compounds, such as HSP70 inhibitors, influence viral replication by inhibiting proteoglycan activity, while antiviral approaches targeting SARS-CoV-2 Mpro protease inhibitors may additionally affect HMPV cysteine proteases (Wu et al., 2024). High-throughput screening approaches accelerate the identification of inhibitors for viral entry and replication. CRISPR-Cas9 gene editing enables the precise inhibition of host genes crucial for viral replication, including HSD17B13 (Guler et al., 2021). Furthermore, the manipulation of host proteostasis pathways such as HSP70 and the ubiquitin-proteasome system influences the effectiveness of viral replication (Ma et al., 2022). Research on GPR75, informed by genome-wide association studies, has guided and directed future therapeutic strategies due to its genetic and evolutionary resistance (Redline et al., 2019).

Advances Aimed at Customising Treatments for HMPV

Strategies utilising genetics, artificial intelligence, and microbiome insights enhance the precision of HMPV management through personalised medication. Genetic factors, including IFITM3 and IL-28B polymorphisms, influence therapy decisions, particularly the dosage of ribavirin. Wearable devices enable the real-time monitoring of oxygen saturation, coughing, and other relevant symptoms, facilitating proactive management of at-risk patients. To enhance global health, particularly in resource-limited nations, equal access to these breakthroughs is essential.

Conclusion

Human metapneumovirus (HMPV) poses a global health risk, particularly to babies, the elderly, and individuals with compromised immune systems. No antivirals or vaccines are available; hence, current therapeutic techniques rely on supportive care. Ribavirin is recognised as ineffective due to its hazardous side effects, although alternative investigational medicines, such as MPV364, monoclonal antibodies, host-directed immunometabolism therapy, and emerging antivirals, demonstrate potential but require further clinical evaluation. Current diagnostic approaches, particularly in resource-limited settings, hinder timely treatment initiation and exhibit biased advantages for vaccine development using mRNA prefusion-stabilised F subunit techniques in conjunction with antigenic diversity. Future emphasis should be on specific viral pathways, adaptable combination antiviral medicines, and innovative vaccine techniques that underscore universal markers. Addressing HMPV requires advancements in real-time genetic surveillance and the widespread accessibility of therapeutic options. Innovative procedures encompass the donation of hydrogen sulfide, nanoparticle drug delivery, and customised treatment strategies to enhance therapeutic efficacy. A cross-disciplinary approach integrating virology, immunology, and global health policies is essential to mitigate the development of HMPV and protect vulnerable populations.

References

Ahmed, R. (2025). Human Metapneumovirus (HMPV): Epidemiology, Pathophysiology, Clinical Management, and Future Prospects in Treatment and Prevention. *RADINKA JOURNAL OF HEALTH SCIENCE*, *2*(3), 312–327.

Albrektsson, T., Brånemark, P. I., Jacobsson, M., & Tjellström, A. (1987). Present clinical applications of osseointegrated percutaneous implants. *Plastic and Reconstructive Surgery*, *79*(5), 721–730.

Burhan, E., Azzumar, F., Sinuraya, F. A. G., Rakasiwi, M. I. D., Akbar, I., Mubarak, F., Rengganis, A. T., Rachmadi, R. A., & Afidjati, H. (2025). Real-world Effectiveness of COVID-19 Vaccine (ChAdOx-1s, CoronaVac, BBIBP-CorV, mRNA-1273, and BNT162b2) in Jakarta: Protocol for Test-negative Design of Healthcare Data. *JMIR Research Protocols*.

Carter, M., Estrada, B., Barik, S., Vidal, R., & Ramsey, K. M. (2006). 204 Epidemiology and Clinical Manifestations of Human Metapneumovirus Infections among Children in Mobile, Alabama. *Journal of Investigative Medicine*, *54*(1), S292.4-S292.

Chatterjee, A., Mavunda, K., & Krilov, L. R. (2021). Current State of Respiratory Syncytial Virus Disease and Management. *Infectious Diseases and Therapy*, *10*(Suppl 1), 5.

Choi, J. W., Withers, S. S., Chang, H., Spanier, J. A., De La Trinidad, V. L., Panesar, H., Fife, B. T., Sciammas, R., Sparger, E. E., Moore, P. F., Kent, M. S., Rebhun, R. B., & McSorley, S. J. (2020). Development of canine PD-1/PD-L1 specific monoclonal antibodies and amplification of canine T cell function. *PLoS ONE*, *15*(7), e0235518.

Chu, R., Gerstein, J., Wu, H., Huang, H., Lou, Y., & Palmer, R. (2020). Development of Rabbit Monoclonal Antibodies for Quantitation of Therapeutic Human Antibodies in Preclinical Non-Human Primate Studies. *Monoclonal Antibodies in Immunodiagnosis and Immunotherapy*, *39*(5), 175–183.

De Bellis, A., Bizzotto, A., Anagnostopoulou, L., Kourentis, L., Marziano, V., Mouchtouri, V., Merler, S., & Guzzetta, G. (2024). Mitigating norovirus spread on cruise ships: A model-based assessment of diagnostic timing and isolation. *MedRxiv*.

Decool, H., Bardiaux, B., Checa Ruano, L., Sperandio, O., Fix, J., Gutsche, I., Richard, C.-A., Bajorek, M., Eléouët, J.-F., & Galloux, M. (2022). Characterisation of the Interaction Domains between the Phosphoprotein and the Nucleoprotein of Human Metapneumovirus. *Journal of Virology*, *96*(2).

Doost-Hoseini, M., Seifi, M., Pakkhesal, M., Saboury, A., Amdjadi, P., & Naghavialhosseini, A. (2021). Evaluation of caries risk reduction following preventive programs in orthodontic patients, using Cariogram computer model: A quasi-experimental trial. *Dental Press Journal of Orthodontics*, *26*(5), e2120218.

Dubey, A., Kumar, M., Tufail, A., & Dwivedi, V. D. (2025). Harnessing Computational Insights to Identify Potent Inhibitors for Human Metapneumovirus (HMPV): A Synergistic Approach with Natural Compounds. *BioRxiv*.

Elemuwa, C. O., Elemuwa, U. G., Akpan, E., & Elemuwa, T. D. (2025). A Mini-Review on the Novel, Emerged, Human Metapneumovirus (HMPV). *International Journal of Advanced Multidisciplinary Research and Studies*, *5*(1), 1106–1109.

Geiser, J., Boivin, G., Huang, S., Constant, S., Kaiser, L., Tapparel, C., & Essaidi-Laziosi, M. (2021). RSV and HMPV Infections in 3D Tissue Cultures: Mechanisms Involved in Virus-Host and Virus-Virus Interactions. *Viruses*, *13*(1), 139.

Goya, S., Nunley, B. E., Longley, P. C., Mathis, J. R., Varela, C. G., Kim, D. Y., Nurik, M., Naccache, S. N., & Greninger, A. L. (2025). Recent human metapneumovirus genomic diversity within expected evolutionary trends. *MedRxiv*.

Guler, R., Ozturk, M., Sabeel, S., Motaung, B., Parihar, S. P., Thienemann, F., & Brombacher, F. (2021). Targeting Molecular Inflammatory Pathways in Granuloma as Host-Directed Therapies for Tuberculosis. *Frontiers in Immunology*, *12*, 733853.

Haraya, K., & Tachibana, T. (2021). Simple Approach to Accurately Predict Pharmacokinetics of Therapeutic Monoclonal Antibodies after Subcutaneous Injection in Humans. *Clinical Pharmacokinetics*, *60*(1), 111–120.

He, J., Qiu, N., Zhou, X., Meng, M., Liu, Z., Li, J., Du, S., Sun, Z., & Wang, H. (2023). Resveratrol analogue, triacetylresveratrol, is a potential immunomodulator of lung adenocarcinoma immunotherapy combination therapies. *Frontiers in Oncology*, *12*, 1007653.

Hengst, M., Häusler, M., Honnef, D., Schelthauer, S., Ritter, K., & Kleines, M. (2008). [Human Bocavirus-infection (HBoV): an important cause of severe viral obstructive bronchitis in children]. *Klinische Padiatrie*, *220*(5), 296–301.

Ismayilova, P. F. (2024). Comparative Study of National Biological Security, with a focus on Azerbaijan: Strategies for Preserving and Controlling the Transmission of Public Health Threats. *Uzhhorod National University Herald. Series: Law*, *2*(82), 70–85.

Khan, A., Khanna, V., & Majumdar, K. (2024). Demographics, Clinical Presentation and Outcome of Metapneumovirus Infection in Adults: A Case Series Analysis at Scarborough General Hospital, United Kingdom. *Cureus*, *16*(11), e73292.

Kinder, J. T., Moncman, C. L., Barrett, C., Jin, H., Kallewaard, N., & Dutch, R. E. (2020). Respiratory Syncytial Virus and Human Metapneumovirus Infections in Three-Dimensional Human Airway Tissues Expose an Interesting Dichotomy in Viral Replication, Spread, and Inhibition by Neutralising Antibodies. *Journal of Virology*, *94*(20).

Kohli, M., Maschio, M., Lee, A., Joshi, K., Carroll, S., Balogh, O., Van de Velde, N., & Beck, E. (2024). The potential clinical impact and cost-effectiveness of the updated COVID-19 mRNA Autumn 2024 vaccines in the United Kingdom. *Journal of Medical Economics*, *27*(1), 1359–1372.

Koizumi, H., Nakahashi-Oda, C., Lyu, W., Yamashita-Kanemaru, Y., Tabuchi, K., Shibuya, K., & Shibuya, A. (2023). Development of Monoclonal Antibodies Specific to Either CD300AR111 or CD300AQ111 or Both. *Monoclonal Antibodies in Immunodiagnosis and Immunotherapy*, *42*(5), 182–185.

Kolli, D., Bao, X., & Casola, A. (2012). Human Metapneumovirus Antagonism of Innate Immune Responses. *Viruses*, *4*(12), 3551.

Kozopas, N. M. (2024). Human Metapneumovirus (HMPV): A Brief Overview of Current Knowledge and Diagnostic Approaches. *Ukrainian Journal of Laboratory Medicine*, *2*(4), 58–63.

Krishnan, A., Kumar, R., Broor, S., Gopal, G., Saha, S., Amarchand, R., Choudekar, A., Purkayastha, D. R., Whitaker, B., Pandey, B., Narayan, V. V., Kabra, S. K., Sreenivas,

V., Widdowson, M. A., Lindstrom, S., Lafond, K. E., & Jain, S. (2019). Epidemiology of viral acute lower respiratory infections in a community-based cohort of rural north Indian children. *Journal of Global Health*, *9*(1), 010433.

Lin, S., Wang, Q., Wang, F., & Shi, H. (2023). Effects of aerosolised inhalation of N-acetylcysteine combined with high flow nasal cannula oxygen therapy on inflammation, oxidative stress, and cognitive function in patients with severe pulmonary infection complicated with respiratory failure. *Tropical Journal of Pharmaceutical Research*, *21*(11), 2467–2472.

Ma, Y., Nakamoto, S., Ao, J., Qiang, N., Kogure, T., Ogawa, K., Nakagawa, M., Fujiwara, K., Iwanaga, T., Kojima, R., Kanzaki, H., Koroki, K., Kobayashi, K., Kanogawa, N., Kiyono, S., Nakamura, M., Kondo, T., Nakagawa, R., Ogasawara, S., … Kato, N. (2022). Antiviral Compounds Screening Targeting HBx Protein of the Hepatitis B Virus. *International Journal of Molecular Sciences*, *23*(19), 12015.

Mäkinen, K., & Hafrén, A. (2014). Intracellular coordination of potyviral RNA functions in infection. *Frontiers in Plant Science*, *5*(MAR), 110.

Malaer, J. D., & Mathew, P. A. (2020). Role of LLT1 and PCNA as Natural Killer Cell Immune Evasion Strategies of HCT 116 Cells. *Anticancer Research*, *40*(12), 6613–6621.

Mattoli, S., & Schmidt, M. (2023). Investigational Use of Mesenchymal Stem/Stromal Cells and Their Secretome as Add-On Therapy in Severe Respiratory Virus Infections: Challenges and Perspectives. *Advances in Therapy*, *40*(6), 2626.

Mishra, B., Mohapatra, D., Tripathy, M., Mamidi, P., & Mohapatra, P. R. (2025). A Re-emerging Respiratory Virus: Human Metapneumovirus (hMPV). *Cureus*, *17*(2), e78354.

Mousa, J. J., Binshtein, E., Human, S., Fong, R. H., Alvarado, G., Doranz, B. J., Moore, M. L., Ohi, M. D., & Crowe, J. E. (2018). Human antibody recognition of antigenic site IV on Pneumovirus fusion proteins. *PLoS Pathogens*, *14*(2), e1006837.

Neyaz, L. A., Alghamdi, H. S., Alghashmari, R. M., Alswat, S. S., Almaghrabi, R. O., Bazaid, F. S., Albarakaty, F. M., Elbanna, K., & Abulreesh, H. H. (2024). A comprehensive review of the current status of culture media for routine standardised isolation of Salmonella and Shigella spp. from contaminated food. *Journal of Umm Al-Qura University for Applied Sciences*.

Ou, L., Chen, S. J., Teng, I. T., Yang, L., Zhang, B., Zhou, T., Biju, A., Cheng, C., Kong, W. P., Morano, N. C., Stancofski, E. S. D., Todd, J. P., Tsybovsky, Y., Wang, S., Zheng, C. Y., Mascola, J. R., Shapiro, L., Woodward, R. A., Buchholz, U. J., & Kwong, P. D. (2023). Structure-based design of a single-chain triple-disulfide-stabilised fusion-glycoprotein trimer that elicits high-titer neutralising responses against human metapneumovirus. *PLOS Pathogens*, *19*(9), e1011584.

Pan, J., Qian, X., Lattmann, S., El Sahili, A., Yeo, T. H., Jia, H., Cressey, T., Ludeke, B., Noton, S., Kalocsay, M., Fearns, R., & Lescar, J. (2019). Structure of the human metapneumovirus polymerase phosphoprotein complex. *Nature*, *577*(7789), 275.

Parameshwari, P., Akondi, B. R., Mallamma, T., & Gowda, J. (2024). Human Metapneumovirus: A Call for Awareness. *Asian Journal of Pharmaceutical Research and Health Care*, *16*(4), 339–343.

Pasquevich, K. A., Coria, L. M., Ceballos, A., Mazzitelli, B., Rodriguez, J. M., Demaría, A., Castro, C. P., Bruno, L., Saposnik, L., Salvatori, M., Varese, A., González, S., González Martínez, V. V., Geffner, J., Álvarez, D., Feleder, E., Halabe, K., Perez Lera, P. E., de Oca, F. M., … Cassataro, J. (2023). Safety, tolerability, and immunogenicity of a new SARS-CoV-2 recombinant Gamma variant RBD-based protein adjuvanted vaccine, used as heterologous booster in healthy adults: a Phase 1 interim report. *MedRxiv*.

Pipitò, L., Mazzola, C. V., Bono, E., Gioè, C., Giammanco, G. M., Bonura, C., & Cascio, A. (2025). A Case of Severe Respiratory Failure Caused by Metapneumovirus and Influenza Virus in a Patient with HIV Infection. *Viruses*, *17*(3), 289.

Pol, S., Corouge, M., & Vallet-Pichard, A. (2016). Daclatasvir–sofosbuvir combination therapy with or without ribavirin for hepatitis C virus infection: from the clinical trials to real life. *Hepatic Medicine : Evidence and Research*, *8*, 21.

Raza, K., Ismailjee, S. B., Crespo, M., Studer, S. M., Sanghavi, S., Paterson, D. L., Kwak, E. J., Rinaldo, C. R., Pilewski, J. M., McCurry, K. R., & Husain, S. (2007). Successful Outcome of Human Metapneumovirus (hMPV) Pneumonia in a Lung Transplant Recipient Treated With Intravenous Ribavirin. *Journal of Heart and Lung Transplantation*, *26*(8), 862–864.

Redline, S., Sands, S. A., Owens, R. L., & Edwards, B. A. (2019). More Than the Sum of the Respiratory Events: Personalised Medicine Approaches for Obstructive Sleep Apnea. *American Journal of Respiratory and Critical Care Medicine*, *200*(6), 691–703.

Saikusa, M., Kawakami, C., Nao, N., Takeda, M., Usuku, S., Sasao, T., Nishimoto, K., & Toyozawa, T. (2017). 180-Nucleotide Duplication in the G Gene of Human metapneumovirus A2b Subgroup Strains Circulating in Yokohama City, Japan, since 2014. *Frontiers in Microbiology*, *8*(MAR), 402.

Satapathy, T., Satapathy, A., Satapathy, A., Yadav, N., Chandrakar, M. C. M., & Chandrakar, K. (2025). Recent outbreaks of Human Metapneumovirus (HMPV): Prevention, Diagnosis and Therapeutic insights. *Journal of Drug Delivery and Therapeutics*, *15*(2), 193–203.

Shrivastava, S., & Shrivastava, P. (2021). Implementing a Combination of Social and Public Health Interventions for the Effective Control of the COVID-19 Pandemic. *Journal of Comprehensive Health*, *9*(1), 38–40.

Snape, M. D., Ghamloush, S. S., Grace, Chen, L., Rakesh Dhar, Mithani, R., Righi, V., Morsy, Louie, Kapoor, A., Girard, B., El Asmar, L., & Shaw, C. A. (2023). 2655. Phase 1 Safety and Immunogenicity Results of Two Investigational mRNA Vaccines, mRNA-1345, a Respiratory Syncytial Virus Vaccine, and mRNA-1653, a Human Metapneumovirus and Parainfluenza Virus Type 3 Combination Vaccine in Seropositive Young Children. *Open Forum Infectious Diseases*, *10*(Suppl 2), ofad500.2266.

Soto, J. A., Gálvez, N. M. S., Benavente, F. M., Pizarro-Ortega, M. S., Lay, M. K., Riedel, C., Bueno, S. M., Gonzalez, P. A., & Kalergis, A. M. (2018). Human Metapneumovirus: Mechanisms and Molecular Targets Used by the Virus to Avoid the Immune System. *Frontiers in Immunology*, *9*(OCT), 2466.

Sousa Paulino, R. de, Borges da Silva, D. B., de Oliveira Santos, K. C., Benega, M. A., & de Paiva*, T. M. (2023). Diversity of Non-Influenza Respiratory Viruses Associated with Influenza-Like Illness during 2009 pre- and pandemic periods in Sao Paulo, Brazil, a Historical Overview. *Journal of Biomedical Research & Environmental Sciences*, *4*(10), 1394–1404.

Tacke, F., Günther, R., Buggisch, P., Klinker, H., Schober, A., John, C., Lutz, T., Pfeiffer-Vornkahl, H., Niederau, C., Cornberg, M., Sarrazin, C., & Mauss, S. (2017). Treatment of HCV genotype 2 with sofosbuvir and ribavirin results in lower sustained virological response rates in real life than expected from clinical trials. *Liver International : Official Journal of the International Association for the Study of the Liver*, *37*(2), 205–211.

Thompson, R. E., Edmonds, K., & Dutch, R. E. (2023). Specific Residues in the C-Terminal Domain of the Human Metapneumovirus Phosphoprotein Are Indispensable for Formation of Viral Replication Centres and Regulation of the Function of the Viral Polymerase Complex. *Journal of Virology*, *97*(5).

Vinci, A., Lee, P. J., & Krilov, L. R. (2018). Human Metapneumovirus Infection. *PaediatricsPaediatrics in Review*, *39*(12), 623–624.

Wei, T., Wang, C., Ma, F., Guo, J., Chen, A., Huang, Y., Xie, Z., & Zheng, L. (2023). Whole genome sequencing and evolution analyses of Human metapneumovirus. *Virus Genes*, *59*(4), 1. -2.

West, K. A., Kumar, S., Scott, M., Emery, J. G., Steidl, U. G., Narayanagari, S.-R., Mitchell, K., Ren, F., Ying, H., Fei, Q., Yang, T., Svensson, E., & Rosen, G. (2023). BOS-371, a monoclonal antibody against IL1RAP: Characterisation in preclinical models of AML. *Journal of Clinical Oncology*, *41*(16_suppl), 7030–7030.

Wise, J. (2022). Moderna will open an mRNA vaccine research and manufacturing centre in the UK. *BMJ (Clinical Research Ed.)*, *377*, o1556.

Wu, Y., Jensen, N., Rossner, M. J., & Wehr, M. C. (2024). Exploiting Cell-Based Assays to Accelerate Drug Development for G Protein-Coupled Receptors. *International Journal of Molecular Sciences*, *25*(10), 5474.

Wyles, D., Pockros, P., Morelli, G., Younes, Z., Svarovskaia, E., Yang, J. C., Pang, P. S., Zhu, Y., McHutchison, J. G., Flamm, S., & Lawitz, E. (2015). Ledipasvir-sofosbuvir plus ribavirin for patients with genotype 1hepatitis C virus previously treated in clinical trials of sofosbuvir regimens. *Hepatology (Baltimore, Md.)*, *61*(6), 1793–1797.

Xiao, X., Tang, A., Cox, K. S., Wen, Z., Callahan, C., Sullivan, N. L., Nahas, D. D., Cosmi, S., Galli, J. D., Minnier, M., Verma, D., Babaoglu, K., Su, H., Bett, A. J., Vora, K. A., Chen, Z., & Zhang, L. (2019). Characterisation of potent RSV neutralising antibodies isolated from human memory B cells and identification of diverse RSV/hMPV cross-neutralising epitopes. *MAbs*, *11*(8), 1415.

Yan-a, W. (2009). Study Overview of Human Metapneumovirus. *Medical Recapitulate*.

Yuan, Q. (2012). Human metapneumovirus: a review of recent progress. *Chinese Journal of Viral Diseases*.

Zhang, H., Ge, C., Fisher, D., Hien, N. T. T., Musabaev, E., Pronyuk, K., Xia, Y., Zhu, Z., Wang, Y., Dang, Y., & Zhao, L. (2025). Antiviral treatment for viral pneumonia: current drugs and natural compounds. *Virology Journal*, *22*(1), 62.

Chapter 8

Advances in Vaccine Development for Human Metapneumovirus (HMPV)

Muskan*
Prabhjot Kaur
Priyanka Kriplani
and Anjali Sharma
Guru Gobind Singh College of Pharmacy, Yamunanagar, Haryana, India

Abstract

Human metapneumovirus, a negative-sense single-stranded virus, belongs to the paramyxoviridae family, which also includes the respiratory syncytial virus and parainfluenza virus. HMPV and RSV are among the leading causes of lower respiratory tract infections in children. HMPV is a significant contributor to illness and death in elderly individuals and immunocompromised populations worldwide. Recurrent infections are common and indicate a significant medical burden. In the absence of efficient treatments, developing a vaccine appears to be a practical means of reducing the strain caused by viral infection. HMPV is classified into two genetic lineages, A and B, each characterised by distinct antigenic properties. These lineages are further divided into subtypes A1 and A2 within lineages A, B1, and B2. Additionally, the A2 subtype is further split into two groups, A2a and A2b. The over 80% protein sequence similarity between subtypes indicates that, while having distinct genetic sequences, different subtypes display a significant degree

* Corresponding Author's Email: muskan20shingari@gmail.com

In: Human Metapneumovirus
Editors: Anjali Sharma, Vishnu Mittal, Devkant Sharma et al.
ISBN: 979-8-90134-063-9

of homology. The selection of epitopes preserved in both lineages can provide future vaccine candidates with protection against a range of HMPV strains. Live attenuated vaccine, mRNA-based vaccine, inactivated vaccine, and viral protein-based vaccine are among the several vaccines that have been developed recently to combat the HMPV virus. For example, Formalin-inactivated influenza vaccine, PIV-3-based HMPV F vaccine, HPIV1-based vaccines, etc. This chapter will discuss current progress and ongoing efforts in the development of a vaccine for HMPV. It is our goal that all of these investigations will someday reduce the medical burden that this clinically significant virus causes.

Keywords: mRNA-based vaccines, inactivated vaccine, respiratory syncytial virus, viral protein-based vaccine, human metapneumovirus, live attenuated vaccine

List of Abbreviations

HMPV	Human Metapneumovirus
RNA	Ribonucleic Acid
RdRp	RNA-dependent RNA polymerase
VLP	Virus-Like Particle
RSV	Respiratory Syncytial Virus
IL	Interleukin
TNF-α	Tumour Necrosis Factor-alpha
IFN-α	Interferon-alpha
COPD	Chronic Obstructive Pulmonary Disease
CTL	Cytotoxic T Lymphocyte
TLR	Toll-Like Receptor
RIG-I	Retinoic Acid-Inducible Gene I
Th1	T-helper Type 1
Th2	T-helper Type 2
BCG	Bacillus Calmette–Guérin
PIV3	Parainfluenza Virus Type 3
F	Fusion protein
G	Glycoprotein
SH	Small Hydrophobic protein
M	Matrix protein
N	Nucleoprotein
P	Phosphoprotein

L	Large (polymerase) protein
M2-1, M2-2	Viral proteins involved in transcription and replication
mRNA	Messenger RNA
CD4+	Cluster of Differentiation 4 Positive T Cell
CD8+	Cluster of Differentiation 8 Positive T Cell
BALB/c	Albino Laboratory-Bred Mice Strain
IgG2a	Immunoglobulin G2a
NCT	National Clinical Trial (Registry Number).

Overview of Human Metapneumovirus

HMPV, a member of the paramyxoviridae family, is a negative-sense, single-stranded RNA virus, closely related to the respiratory syncytial virus and parainfluenza virus. Identified in 2001, HMPV was soon recognised as a common cause of lower respiratory tract infections, particularly in young children, the elderly and individuals with weakened immune systems. The virus is classified into 2 main genetic lineages, A and B, each further divided into sublineages: A1, A2, B1, B2. At present, 5 distinct and long-standing clades of hMPV are known to be circulating. The hMPV antigenome contains 9 open reading frames responsible for viral protein production, arranged in the following order: 3'-N-P-M-F-M2-1-SH-G-5'. According to Porwal et al., (2025), RNA synthesis, which is comprised of two distinct processes—gene transcription and viral replication—requires the large protein L, phosphoprotein P, and nucleoprotein N. Upon entry, the N-encapsidated genome is bound at the leader region by the viral RNA-dependent RNA polymerase (RdRp), which is produced by the combination of the L and P proteins. Once the start and stop signals flanking each viral gene are recognised, the virus sequentially transcribes each gene. During synthesis, mRNAs are polyadenylated and capped. When there is sufficient nucleoprotein to encapsulate newly synthesised antigenomes and genomes, replication most likely begins. Numerous copies of the viral genome can be copied using the positive-sense antigenome that is created when the negative-sense genome is duplicated (Brynes et al., 2025). The M2-2 protein, along with P and L, is essential for the synthesis of viral RNA. It remains uncertain whether HMPV M2-2, similar to RSV M2-2 protein, plays a crucial role in regulating the switch of viral RNA polymerase from transcribing viral genes to replicating the viral genome. The M2-2 protein, small hydrophobic protein SH, glycoprotein G, and phosphoprotein P have all been shown to affect host immunological responses. G, SH, and M-2 are absent from attenuated recombinant hMPVs, either singly or in combination, or avian P is used in place of P. The diagram of Human metapneumovirus (HMPV) is shown in Figure 1. Fusion protein F triggers a robust humoral immune response and is necessary for hMPV entrance. In this chapter, we discuss the recent advances in vaccine development for treating HMPV (Miyakawa et al., 2025).

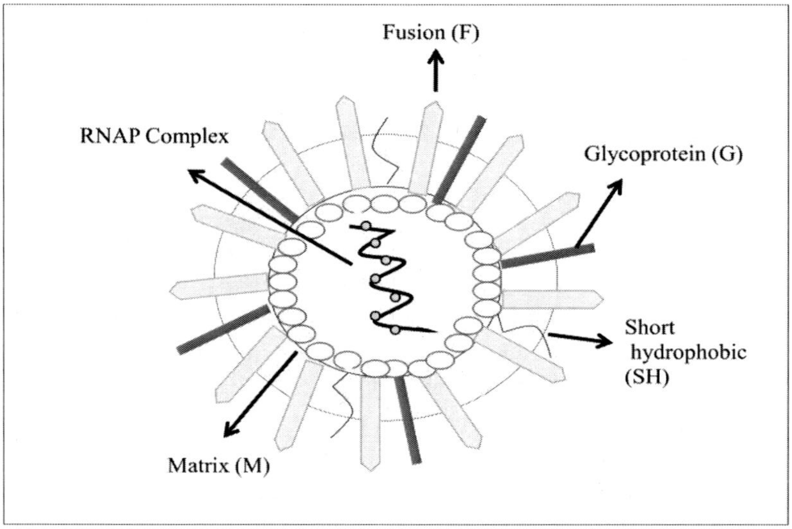

Figure 1. Schematic diagram of Human metapneumovirus.

Epidemiology

hMPV has a seasonal distribution and has been isolated on every continent. In the northern hemisphere, epidemics often occur from January to Mar, and in the southern hemisphere, from June to July. The peak of hMPV seasonal incidence comes in Mar and Apr, after influenza and RSV infection, according to a new study. Another study found that the seasons for hMPV and RSV infections are the same. Since hMPV is a respiratory virus, it is disseminated by infectious airborne droplets. Despite the possibility of re-infection throughout adulthood, seroprevalence studies have shown that a sizable percentage of children (90–100%) had contracted the infection by the time they were 5–10 years old (Chand et al., 2025). Reinfection with hMPV may occur due to a new viral genotype or incomplete immunity from a previous infection. The incubation period ranges from 3- 5 days, with peak viral levels in animal models seen around 4 to 5 days. While hMPV commonly affects children under 2, adults generally experience only mild, flu-like symptoms. Serious side effects, including chronic obstructive pulmonary disease (COPD), can happen in some adult cases, particularly in older people. Adults are more prone than children to have dyspnea. Additionally, hMPV infection has been documented in many immunocompromised patients, including recipients of hematopoietic stem cell transplants, patients with haematological malignancies, and recipients of lung transplants. During a regular respiratory virus season, both hMPV genotypes (A and B) co-circulated, according to two studies, and re-infections with distinct hMPV genotypes happen often (Ji et al., 2024).

Pathogenesis

Persistent hMPV infection results from a weakened and delayed immune response, including sluggish cytotoxic T cell activity and poor viral clearance. The virus hinders T cell activation by targeting and infecting dendritic cells. Consequently, the production of long-term immunity is impeded, and the growth of CD4+ T cells specific to antigens is restricted (Akingbola et al., 2025). It is known that respiratory infections can alter cytokine responses. HMPV stimulated lower levels of cytokines like IL-12, TNF-α, IL-6, and IL-10 compared to influenza and RSV. In animal models, higher levels of IL-2, IL-4, IL-8, IFN-α, and other inflammatory markers are detected in the lungs. This immune response causes inflammation and cellular infiltration around blood vessels and airways. Histological findings show lung tissue damage, hyaline membranes, and macrophages with foamy or hemosiderin content. While HMPV activates the toll-like receptor pathway, its protective role in lung infection remains uncertain. MyD88-deficient animals showed significantly reduced levels of pulmonary inflammation and associated sickness after intranasal infection with hMPV compared to wild-type C57BL/6 mice, per a recent study (Ahmed et al., 2025).

Vaccine Development for HMPV

With no effective treatments available, creating a vaccine appears to be a practical approach to lessen the severity of the viral illness. Two genetic lineages, A and B, have emerged from the human metapneumovirus (HMPV), each with a distinct antigen. According to Wilkhoo et al., (2025), each lineage has two subtypes, A1 and A2, which are further subdivided into A2a and A2b. The genome of the hMPV virus is non-segmented negative-sense RNA, measuring 13 kb. According to Li et al., (2024), this RNA comprises eight genes that collectively code for nine proteins, including the phosphoprotein (P), large protein (L), and nucleoprotein (N), all of which are involved in RNA synthesis. Viral assembly and budding are mediated by the matrix protein (M), while M2 mediates RNA transcription. The G protein mediates attachment, the F protein fuses membranes, and the other three proteins attach to lipid. Although tiny hydrophobic (SH) proteins are believed to regulate the host immune response, little is known about them (Swart et al., 2024). It has been shown that SH proteins can produce viroporin-forming ion ports. In light of this, Table 1 lists the many vaccines created to treat the human metapneumovirus.

Viral Protein-Based Vaccines

The structural proteins of viruses combine to form virus-like particles, or VLPs. They lack the viral genome, which prevents them from reproducing. Even though VLPs are not communicable, B-cell responses are significantly boosted by their capacity to replicate viral structure and exhibit antigens methodically and repetitively. Virus-like particles can be designed to contain only the virus's immunogenic proteins, directing the immune response specifically toward protective antigens. Trinite et al., (2024) found that the human papillomavirus vaccine, a VLP vaccine approved for use in humans, can induce humoral and cellular immune responses. Adjuvants can be directly incorporated into virus-like particles. The cross-protective heterosubtypic immune responses were enhanced by a vaccination that contained influenza virus-like particles and membrane-anchored flagellin. A study reported a VLP vaccine composed of the influenza M1 protein core combined with RSV F or G proteins. In BALB/c mice, intramuscular administration of RSV-F or RSV-G induced IgG2a-dominant antibody responses in both serum and lung fluid.

Mice that had received vaccinations showed significantly reduced lung virus levels after viral challenge. Both types of VLPs elicited strong antibody titers after primer and booster injections. Moreover, VLP vaccination appeared to trigger a CD8+ T cell response, even if the function of T cells in defence was not proven (Van Den Bergh et al., 2022).

Subunit Vaccine

All known paramyxoviruses cause an immune response when fusion proteins are present. The two disulfide-linked polypeptides, F1 and F2, are class I transmembrane glycoproteins that are produced from the inactive precursor, F0, by host proteases. Given the similarity between HMPV and RSV F proteins and the proven safety of RSV F subunits in clinical trials, researchers suggest that an HMPV subunit vaccine could provide protective immunity. Cotton rats immunised with soluble HMPV F protein developed potent neutralising antibodies, but protection in the upper respiratory tract was slightly reduced. Neither a skewed TH2 response nor enhanced alveolitis or eosinophilic infiltrates—indicating worsened disease associated with FI-RSV—were observed in immunocompromised mice (Rush et al., 2022). When F subunit vaccines were administered together with various adjuvants, Syrian golden hamsters developed protective antibody levels against infections brought on by both homologous and heterologous HMPV subgroups. In vitro studies have shown that HMPV M protein enhances dendritic cells' maturation and cytokine release. BALB/c mice vaccinated with both F and M proteins plus alus had reduced lung viral loads and lower TH2/TH1 cytokine ratios compared to those receiving F protein alone. According to Hsieh et al., (2022), this implies that including the M protein in an HMPV vaccination may alter immune responses to a subsequent infection by influencing the cellular immune response. The development of HMPV subunit protein vaccines was hampered by the rapid fall in the neutralising antibody titers that immunisation produced (Huang et al., 2021).

Inactivated Vaccine

Formalin-inactivated influenza vaccines are widely used due to their stability, ease of production, and safety, as they lack replication. In contrast, the formalin-inactivated RSV vaccine led to worsened illness, often linked to a

Th2-skewed immune response, formaldehyde sensitivity, and weak antibody recognition of natural RSV epitopes. Likewise, following a hMPV challenge, mice immunised with formalin-inactivated hMPV similarly displayed vaccine-enhanced lung disease and Th2 response, suggesting that formalin-inactivated hMPV may not be a suitable vaccine candidate (Sun et al., 2023). However, the Th1/Th17 response was higher in vaccinated mice. If hMPV is immunogenic, protective, and has balanced immune responses, nanoemulsion inactivation may be employed; however, further study is needed to determine the safety of nanoemulsion-adjuvanted inactive RSV vaccine candidates (Zhang et al., 2024).

Live Attenuated Vaccines

Live attenuated vaccines come in two varieties: recombinant and non-recombinant. Most non-recombinant live attenuated viruses are generated through natural mutation or deletions during cell passage, sometimes aided by mutagens or cold adaptations. However, these vaccines carry a risk of regaining virulence in vivo, and some attenuated RSV vaccines have shown inadequate safety and effectiveness in clinical trials. Heat-sensitive strains of hMPV have recently been developed, and injected hamsters showed protective immunity (Ogonczyk-Makowska et al., 2024). This indicates that SH has no attenuating impact when deleted and is completely unneeded in vivo (Chupin et al., 2021). rhMPV-ΔM2-2 exhibited comparable immunogenicity and protective efficacy to rhMPV-ΔG; however, it was attenuated more in infected African green monkeys. The avian MPV P protein has been used to replace the P protein in another attenuated recombinant hMPV, called rhMPV-Pavian. Recently, it was approved to use a wild-type recombinant hMPV as a suitable parent virus for the development of live attenuated hMPV vaccine candidates in experimental human infection trials. Despite rhMPV-Pavian's low infectivity in healthy adults, further investigation is required to identify the causes of this low infectivity and whether other attenuated recombinant viruses have similar issues with human infectivity (Dubois et al., 2023).

mRNA-Based Vaccines

The bivalent construct mRNA-1653, which targets the fusion (F) proteins of type 3 (PIV3) and hMPV, is a new development in the field of mRNA vaccines. Healthy individuals between the ages of 18 and 49 participated in Phase 1 clinical trials (NCT03392389) to thoroughly assess this vaccination (Ma et al., 2024). Assessing the vaccine's immunogenic response-stimulating capability, safety, and reactogenicity were the primary objectives of these trials. In a study of healthy individuals who received the mRNA-1653 vaccination, neutralising antibody titers against hMPV (A and B strains) and PIV3 increased dramatically after a single dose. The vaccine was found to be safe and tolerated at dosages ranging from 25 to 300 μg (Snape et al., 2024). The second dose significantly reduced neutralisation titers. Antibody levels are similar across doses; however, the small sample size and demographic homogeneity are acknowledged limitations in extending the data. According to Snape et al., (2023), these findings underscore the need for more clinical studies to validate the vaccine's efficacy and safety in a variety of populations.

Vectored HMPV Vaccines- Epitope Vaccines

Using other respiratory viruses as vectors appears to be a promising strategy for HMPV development. These vectors can efficiently deliver HMPV antigens to target cells, ensuring proper immune presentation and balanced antibody and cellular immune responses. Viral-vectored vaccines allow us to incorporate only the necessary immunogenic regions of a pathogen into a recombinant virus, while removing aspects known to contribute to pathogenicity and host immunity regulation (Parks et al., 2024). The most crucial step is to select the distribution strategy that will best boost the immune system. Viral vectors are now being used to create a range of vaccines against HMPV infection. Additionally, the rational design of the HMPV vaccine has used bacterial vectors. To remove HMPV from mice lungs without inducing pulmonary disease, for example, the P-recombinant Bacillus Calmette–Guérin (BCG) immunisation encouraged the formation of helper and cytotoxic memory T cells (Miranda-Katz et al., 2021). As per Groen et al., (2023), current research should focus on finding the most promising HMPV epitopes in order to develop human HMPV vaccines based on epitopes rationally.

Chimeric Vaccines

A chimeric live vectored PIV3 vaccine expressing the hMPV F and HN genes offered protection in hamsters and African green monkeys. Additionally, following vaccination and challenge, a chimeric vaccine that replaced the AMPV nucleoprotein (N) and phosphoprotein (P) with those of HMPV generated significant amounts of neutralising antibodies. Vaccinations with alphavirus replicons encoding HMPV F protected mice and cotton rats (Ogonczyk-Makowska et al., 2024).

Factors That Should Be Considered in the Development of Future Vaccines against HMPV

While the F protein is key to HMPV immunogenicity, identifying antigens that trigger protective CTL and humoral responses is crucial for vaccine success. Specific CTL peptides from G, SH, M2-2, and N proteins have been shown to enhance Th1 cytokine production and reduce viral load and disease severity in mouse models. Co-immunising the host with peptides containing CTL epitopes could be a practical method to boost the immunogenicity of rhMPV deletion mutants or to extend the immunogenicity of vaccinations based on F proteins (Swart et al., 2024). Given the complete conservation of the epitopes present in the N and M2-2 proteins, it is expected that a CTL epitope vaccine will give protection against both hMPV strains. Finding the viral proteins essential for modifying antiviral signalling is also essential for the development of vaccines. Specific viral proteins, such as G and M2-2, have been found to have a significant role in suppressing the host's innate response to hMPV. Researchers have found that the M2-2 protein has multiple functions. According to Mistry et al., (2025), it has a CTL epitope, targets central adaptors for retinoic acid-inducible gene I (RIG-I) and Toll-like receptors (TLRs), and regulates viral gene transcription and viral RNA replication. Scientists have shown that M2-2 contains unique regulatory domains for the replication of viral genes and genomes. Furthermore, the researchers identified M2-2 motifs that inhibit antiviral signalling (manuscript in process). A live attenuated vaccine candidate based on M2-2 might be developed using all of these M2-2-related facts. The breakdown of viral protein functional domains is often highly desired for vaccine development (Groen et al., 2023).

Table 1. Different vaccines developed for treating human metapneumovirus

Vaccine Used	Product	Human/Animal model used	Observation	Reference
Inactivated vaccine	Heat-inactivated vaccine	Mice	After immunisation, BALB/c mice were given an intranasal challenge to create protective immunity against a similar strain of hMPV.	(Sun et al., 2023)
chimeric vaccine	HMPV antigen on the parainfluenza vaccines	Rhesus and African monkey	African green monkeys were completely protected against a wild-type hMPV challenge by an intranasal vaccination that produced a humoral and cell-mediated immune response unique to hMPV. It was demonstrated that this vaccination adequately attenuated rhesus monkeys.	(Ogonczyk-Makowska et al., 2024)
viral protein Based Vaccine	Virus like particles	Mice	Immunization decreased viral titres in immunized animals' lungs.	(Trinite et al., 2024)
epitope Vaccine	T-lymphocyte Epitope Vaccine	mice	Following a hMPV challenge, vaccination decreased lung pathology, viral load, and Th2-type cytokine production (IL-10, IL-4).	(Parks et al., 2024)
Live attenuated vaccine	ΔM2-2	Mice	Cross-protective immunity against a heterologous strain was established by immunisation and total protection against challenge with a homologous strain.	(Dubois et al., 2023)
	ΔMS-2	hamster	Attenuated and protective against the wild-type hMPV challenge in hamsters	
	ΔM2-2, ΔSH, ΔG	African green monkeys	There was sufficient attenuation of ΔG and ΔM2-2. After being exposed to wild-type hMPV, the lower respiratory tract did not exhibit any noticeable viral shedding.	
Subunit vaccine	HMPV subunit vaccine	Cotton rat	Following an hMPV challenge, immunisation decreased nasal viral shedding in cotton rats; nonetheless, lung pathology was similar to that of control mice.	(Rush et al., 2022)
		hamster	Intra-nasal vaccination with recombinant human PIV-1 expressing the Hmpv f protein demonstrated superior immunogenicity and protection compared to a vaccine expressing the SH and G proteins	
		Cynomolgus macaques	Immunisation produced a strong cellular immune response, a neutralising antibody, and an antibody specific to hMPV F. However, with time, the resultant humoral reaction quickly decreased.	
		Syrian golden hamster	Immunisation produced a strong neutralising antibody response against the homologous virus and significantly lowered viral levels in the nasal turbinates.	

Immune Response to HMPV

RSV can evade innate immunity using the nonstructural proteins NS-1 and NS-2, which disrupt type 1 interferon signalling (Sepulveda-Alfaro et al., 2024). The elimination of viruses also depends on T cells (Sojati et al., 2024). Virus titers were higher in BALB/c mice with both CD4+ and CD8+ T cell depletion after an HMPV exposure. Additionally, compared to individuals without the virus, those with HIV experienced more severe HMPV infections. Even though all people have had HMPV by the age of five, based on the presence of serum antibodies, recurring infections are common throughout life, indicating that protection is not total (Babawale et al., 2024). The most likely reasons for recurring infections are decreased immunity and decreased cross-reactive antibodies. While antibodies to the G protein of RSV, which has many neutralising antigens, are protective, antibodies to the G and SH proteins of HMPV are not (Ruiz-Pozo et al., 2025).

Challenges in Vaccine Development and Future Directions

Compared to COVID-19 vaccinations, HMPV vaccines are less developed. None, however, has advanced past the preclinical stage. The main challenges in developing an HMPV vaccine are limited long-term immunity and immune evasion, though early research suggests strong potential for future respiratory illness prevention. In order to improve long-lasting, highly neutralising postvaccination immunity, vaccine manufacturers are focusing on viral protective epitope immunogenicity, delivery carrier, and improving vaccine formulations (Shapovalova et al., 2025). The HMPV vaccine studies have made significant progress; however, the following issues still need to be addressed. Antigenic variation: Mutation in the HMPV gene can alter antigenic sites, reducing or eliminating protective immunity against circulating strains. While live attenuated vaccines are effective, they may pose risks to immunocompromised individuals, and inactivated vaccines often fail to generate strong immune responses. Durability of immunity: herd immunity requires persistence of immunity throughout time (Costa-Filho et al., 2025). To increase the immunogenicity of HMPV vaccines and ensure that vaccine-induced immunity successfully prevents the virus from spreading, a new delivery system must be developed. According to Satapathy et al., (2025), to provide effective HPMV vaccinations, researchers and vaccine manufacturers should collaborate to develop univalent or multivalent HPMV vaccines that combine HPMV with other respiratory viruses.

Conclusion

Although no licensed vaccines or treatments currently exist for HMPV, promising results from animal studies support the potential of various vaccine candidates and therapies. An ideal vaccine must be safer and more immunogenic than natural infection, as studies in cotton rats showed that F1-HMPV worsened lung disease upon reinfection, making it a less viable option. Vaccinations against subunits seem to provide short-term protection against an initial infection. However, in those who have already been exposed to hMPV, it may bolster the immune system. Additionally, safe and promising subunit vaccinations, especially when given as non-infectious carriers, can provide some protection to risk groups such as the elderly, immunocompromised individuals, and premature infants. The currently available live attenuated hMPV vaccines show promise, particularly for young children and newborns. However, it can be challenging to strike a compromise between a suitable level of immunogenicity and a reasonable degree of attenuation. We are currently investigating the prospect of identifying the primary immune regulatory protein or proteins and related functional patterns in order to generate vaccination candidates with acceptable immunogenicity and attenuation. Numerous vaccination strategies have been studied and assessed in non-human primate and rodent models, taking all relevant considerations into account. None have been tried on humans as of yet, however. According to recent experimental inoculation of adults with recombinant wild-type hMPV, future studies may assess the immunological effectiveness of live attenuated recombinant hMPV in humans.

References

Ahmed, R. (2025). Human Metapneumovirus (HMPV): Epidemiology, Pathophysiology, Clinical Management, and Future Prospects in Treatment and Prevention. *Radinka Journal of Health Science*, *2*(3), 312-327.

Akingbola, A., Adegbesan, A., TundeAlao, S., Adewole, O., Ayikoru, C., Benson, A. E., & Chuku, J. (2025). Human Metapneumovirus: an emerging respiratory pathogen and the urgent need for improved Diagnostics, surveillance, and vaccine development. *Infectious Diseases*, *57*(3), 304-310.

Babawale, P. I., & Guerrero-Plata, A. (2024). Respiratory viral coinfections: insights into Epidemiology, Immune Response, Pathology, and clinical outcomes. *Pathogens*, *13*(4), 316.

Brynes, A. (2025). *Human Metapneumovirus Small Hydrophobic Protein Degrades JAKs to Block Immune Signals* (Doctoral dissertation, University of Pittsburgh).

Chand, S., Karmacharya, R., Magar, S. T., Nongmeikapam, H., Liangkiuwiliu, R., & Talagatoti, D. R. P. (2025). Human Metapneumovirus: An Emerging Respiratory Virus. *National Journal of Community Medicine*, *16*(04), 423-430.

Chupin, C., Pizzorno, A., Traversier, A., Brun, P., Ogonczyk-Makowska, D., Padey, B., & Rosa-Calatrava, M. (2021). Avian cell line DuckCelt®-T17 is an efficient production system for live-attenuated human metapneumovirus vaccine candidate Metavac®. *Vaccines*, *9*(10), 1190.

Costa-Filho, R. C., Saddy, F., Costa, J. L. F., Tavares, L. R., & Castro Faria Neto, H. C. (2025). The silent threat of human metapneumovirus: clinical challenges and diagnostic insights from a severe pneumonia case. *Microorganisms*, *13*(1), 73.

Dubois, J., Ogonczyk-Makowska, D., Vacher, C., Pizzorno, A., Brun, P., Chupin, C., & Rosa-Calatrava, M. (2023). New mucosal bivalent live-attenuated vaccine is protective against Human Metapneumovirus and Respiratory Syncytial Virus.

Groen, K., van Nieuwkoop, S., Meijer, A., van der Veer, B., van Kampen, J. J., Fraaij, P. L., & van den Hoogen, B. G. (2023). Emergence and potential extinction of genetic lineages of human metapneumovirus between 2005 and 2021. *Mbio*, *14*(1), e02280-22.

Hsieh, C. L., Rush, S. A., Palomo, C., Chou, C. W., Pickens, W., Más, V., & McLellan, J. S. (2022). Structure-based design of prefusion-stabilized human metapneumovirus fusion proteins. *Nature communications*, *13*(1), 1299.

Huang, J., Chopra, P., Liu, L., Nagy, T., Murray, J., Tripp, R. A., & Mousa, J. J. (2021). Structure, immunogenicity, and conformation-dependent receptor binding of the postfusion human metapneumovirus F protein. *Journal of Virology*, *95*(18), 10-1128.

Ji, W., Chen, Y., Han, S., Dai, B., Li, K., Li, S., & Jin, Y. (2024). Clinical and epidemiological characteristics of 96 pediatric human metapneumovirus infections in Henan, China after COVID-19 pandemic: a retrospective analysis. *Virology Journal*, *21*(1), 100.

Li, Q., Li, H., Li, Z., & Wang, Y. (2024). Vaccine and therapeutic agents against the respiratory syncytial virus: resolved and unresolved issue. *MedComm*, *5*(12), e70016.

Ma, S., Zhu, F., Xu, Y., Wen, H., Rao, M., Zhang, P., & Pan, P. (2024). Development of a novel multi-epitope mRNA vaccine candidate to combat HMPV virus. *Human Vaccines & Immunotherapeutics*, *20*(1), 2293300.

Miranda-Katz, M., Erickson, J. J., Lan, J., Ecker, A., Zhang, Y., Joyce, S., & Williams, J. V. (2021). Novel HLA-B7-restricted human metapneumovirus epitopes enhance viral clearance in mice and are recognized by human CD8+ T cells. *Scientific reports*, *11*(1), 20769.\

Mistry, L. N., Agarwal, S., Jaiswal, H., Kondkari, S., Mulla, S. A., & Bhandarkar, S. D. (2025). Human Metapneumovirus: Emergence, Impact, and Public Health Significance. *Cureus*, *17*(3).

Miyakawa, R., Zhang, H., Brooks, W. A., Prosperi, C., Baggett, H. C., Feikin, D. R., & Knoll, M. D. (2025). Epidemiology of human metapneumovirus among children with severe or very severe pneumonia in high pneumonia burden settings: the Pneumonia Etiology Research for Child Health (PERCH) study experience. *Clinical Microbiology and Infection*, *31*(3), 441-450.

Ogonczyk-Makowska, D. (2024). *Development of chimeric bivalent vaccines against Respiratory Syncytial Virus and Human Metapneumovirus* (Doctoral dissertation, Université Laval).

Ogonczyk-Makowska, D., Brun, P., Vacher, C., Chupin, C., Droillard, C., Carbonneau, J., & Dubois, J. (2024). Mucosal bivalent live attenuated vaccine protects against human metapneumovirus and respiratory syncytial virus in mice. *NPJ vaccines*, *9*(1), 111.

Parks, O. B. (2024). *The role of age and complement in CD8+ T cell function during human metapneumovirus (HMPV) infection* (Doctoral dissertation, University of Pittsburgh).

Porwal, S., Malviya, R., Sridhar, S. B., Shareef, J., & Wadhwa, T. (2025). Global Impact of hMPV Virus: Transmission, Pathogenesis, Diagnostic and Treatment. *Diagnostic Microbiology and Infectious Disease*, 116809.

Ruiz-Pozo, V. A., Cadena-Ullauri, S., Tamayo-Trujillo, R., Guevara-Ramírez, P., Paz-Cruz, E., Castañeda Cataña, M. A., & Zambrano, A. K. (2025). Interplay between endogenous hormones and immune systems in human metapneumovirus pathogenesis and management. *Frontiers in Pharmacology*, *16*, 1568828.

Rush, S. A. (2022). *Structural and biophysical investigations toward engineering a protein subunit vaccine for human metapneumovirus* (Doctoral dissertation).

Satapathy, T., Satapathy, A., Satapathy, A., Yadav, N., Chandrakar, M., & Chandrakar, K. (2025). Recent outbreaks of Human Metapneumovirus (HMPV): Prevention, Diagnosis and Therapeutic insights. *Journal of Drug Delivery & Therapeutics*, *15*(2).

Sepúlveda-Alfaro, J., Catalán, E. A., Vallejos, O. P., Ramos-Tapia, I., Madrid-Muñoz, C., Mendoza-León, M. J., & Melo-Gonzalez, F. (2024). Human metapneumovirus respiratory infection affects both innate and adaptive intestinal immunity. *Frontiers in Immunology*, *15*, 1330209.

Shapovalova, V. (2025). Human Metapneumovirus: Modern Challenges for Medicine and Pharmaceutics. *SSP Modern Pharmacy and Medicine*, *5*(2), 1-14.

Snape, M. D., Ghamloush, S. S., Chen, G. L., Dhar, R., Mithani, R., Righi, V., & Shaw, C. A. (2023, November). 2655. Phase 1 Safety and Immunogenicity Results of Two Investigational mRNA Vaccines, mRNA-1345, a Respiratory Syncytial Virus Vaccine, and mRNA-1653, a Human Metapneumovirus and Parainfluenza Virus Type 3 Combination Vaccine in Seropositive Young Children. In *Open Forum Infectious Diseases* (Vol. 10, No. Suppl 2, pp. ofad500-2266).

Snape, M. D., Moore, J., Du, J., Reuter, C., Penn, N., Stoszek, S. K., & Shaw, C. A. (2024). Safety and immunogenicity of an mRNA-Based RSV vaccine and an RSV/hMPV combination vaccine in children 5 to 23 months of age. *Preprints. org*, *11*.

Sojati, J., Parks, O. B., Zhang, Y., Walters, S., Lan, J., Eddens, T., & Williams, J. V. (2024). IFN-λ drives distinct lung immune landscape changes and antiviral responses in human metapneumovirus infection. *Mbio*, *15*(5), e00550-24.

Sun, F., Lei, G., Tian, C., Bai, Z., Bai, C., Li, Y., & Yang, P. (2023). Protective efficacy of a novel recombinant influenza virus carrying partial human metapneumovirus F protein epitopes. *Virulence*, (just-accepted), 2284515.

Swart, M., Allen, J., Reed, B., Izquierdo Gil, A., Verspuij, J., Schmit-Tillemans, S., & Brandenburg, B. (2024). Plant Cell Culture-Derived Saponin Adjuvant Enhances Immune Response Against a Stabilized Human Metapneumovirus Pre-Fusion Vaccine Candidate. *Vaccines*, *12*(12), 1435.

Trinité, B., Durr, E., Pons-Grífols, A., O'Donnell, G., Aguilar-Gurrieri, C., Rodriguez, S., & Blanco, J. (2024). VLPs generated by the fusion of RSV-F or hMPV-F glycoprotein to HIV-Gag show improved immunogenicity and neutralizing response in mice. *Vaccine*, *42*(15), 3474-3485.

Van Den Bergh, A., Bailly, B., Guillon, P., von Itzstein, M., & Dirr, L. (2022). Antiviral strategies against human metapneumovirus: Targeting the fusion protein. *Antiviral Research*, *207*, 105405.

Wilkhoo, H. S., Islam, A. W., Wilkhoo, H. S., & Hussain, S. (2025) Clinical Insights and Advancements in Human Metapneumovirus Management and Prognosis, 13(1), e204.

Zhang, Y., Xu, J., Miranda-Katz, M., Sojati, J., Tollefson, S. J., Manni, M. L., & Williams, J. V. (2024). Distinct roles for type I and type III interferons in virulent human metapneumovirus pathogenesis. *PLoS pathogens*, *20*(2), e1011840.

Chapter 9

Environmental and Ecological Factors Influencing Human Metapneumovirus (HMPV) Spread

Kotthapalli Prashanth[1]
Parthasarathi Behera[2]
Jeewon Rajesh[3]
and Sumana Kumar[1,*]

[1]Department of Microbiology, JSS Academy of Higher Education and Research, Mysuru, Karnataka, India
[2]Department of Health Sciences, International Centre for Genetic Engineering and Biotechnology (ICGEB), Aruna Asif Ali Marg, New Delhi, India
[3]Department of Zoology, College of Science, King Saud University, Riyadh, Saudi Arabia

Abstract

Human Metapneumovirus (HMPV) is a prominent respiratory virus with a major impact on the public health system, especially the vulnerable populations. The transmission dynamics and outbreak patterns are shaped by a complex interplay of environmental and ecological factors, including meteorological conditions such as temperature, humidity, wind speed, and sunshine duration. Variations in temperature and precipitation enormously affect outbreak patterns, necessitating adaptive strategies. A crowded environment without proper ventilation facilitates rapid virus spread due to close contact and opportunistic airborne transmission.

* Corresponding Author's Email: sumana.k@jssuni.edu.in

In: Human Metapneumovirus
Editors: Anjali Sharma, Vishnu Mittal, Devkant Sharma et al.
ISBN: 979-8-90134-063-9

Environmental factors such as exposure to air pollutants, including those from cooking fuels and tobacco smoke, can impair lung function and increase the chances of inflammation, making individuals more susceptible to HMPV infection. Contaminated nonporous surfaces like metal and plastic allow viruses to remain viable longer than porous surfaces, enabling transmission. Regular handwashing, avoiding close contact with symptomatic individuals, and maintaining good indoor ventilation are effective mitigation strategies. Research evidence suggests that HMPV may have zoonotic origins, highlighting the importance of including animal reservoirs in surveillance efforts and also with the use of advanced techniques and strategies, including molecular diagnostics and integration of clinical and environmental data, enabling healthcare systems to detect and respond to outbreaks more efficiently. Travel migrations introduce novel variants seeding to new outbreaks in regions previously unexposed leading to increased genetic diversity and the potential for new waves of infection. Advancements in vaccine development and antiviral therapy are fundamental to effective control and management of virus transmission, especially HMPV.

Keywords: human metapneumovirus, ecological factors, environmental influence, airborne transmission, contaminated surfaces

Introduction to HMPV

Human metapneumovirus (HMPV) is a pleomorphic and easily transmissible virus, with particles ranging from 150 nm to 600 nm in size. It causes upper and lower respiratory tract infections and belongs to the family *Pneumoviridae*. HMPV is closely related to the respiratory syncytial virus (RSV). HMPV is now acknowledged as a globally circulating virus responsible for a range of respiratory illnesses, from mild cold-like symptoms to more severe conditions such as bronchiolitis (a lung infection in infants and young children) and pneumonia. HMPV is capable of infecting anyone, regardless of age. However, the chances of experiencing serious illness are notably higher among children younger than five, older adults, especially those aged 65 and above, and immunocompromised individuals or chronic respiratory diseases (Falsey, 2014; Krüger et al., 2025; Schuster & Williams, 2023). HMPV was discovered in 2001 by a Dutch team led by Bernadette G. van den Hoogen, who isolated the virus from nasopharyngeal aspirate samples of children under 5 years of age with unexplained respiratory tract infections in the Netherlands (Van Den Hoogen et al., 2001). Although HMPV was only recently identified, retrospective serological studies and analyses of archived human serum samples indicate that the virus has been circulating in humans for at least fifty years prior to its discovery. The virus was detected in the samples through molecular approaches like randomly arbitrarily primed PCR (RAP-PCR), which eventually enabled genetic sequencing and identification of this previously unrecognised pathogen (Haas et al., 2013; Jesse et al., 2022; Rao et al., 2004). Current research efforts are focused on developing effective vaccines and antiviral treatments, as well as gaining a deeper understanding of the environmental and host factors that influence HMPV transmission and disease severity.

Transmission Dynamics of HMPV

The transmission dynamics of HMPV are influenced by environmental factors along with host-related factors such as age, immune responses, and related health conditions, which affect viral stability and host susceptibility. The incubation period of HMPV is three-six to six days, with most infections resolving within two to five days, though severe cases occur. The virus survives on surfaces for hours, increasing transmission risk through contaminated objects (Akingbola et al., 2025; Mistry et al., 2025; Satapathy et al., 2025). Socioeconomic conditions also impact the spread and severity of HMPV, especially in crowded or resource-limited environments. The identification of this virus has advanced the understanding of respiratory infections and highlighted the need for surveillance (Mistry et al., 2025).

Prevention

HMPV typically circulates during late winter and spring (February-May) in temperate regions. The virus exhibits peak contagiousness during the initial days of illness, coinciding with the height of symptom manifestation. Preventive strategies encompass handwashing with soap for a duration of at least twenty seconds, avoiding contact with individuals exhibiting illness, and disinfecting frequently touched surfaces. It is crucial to cover the mouth and nose when coughing or sneezing and to remain at home when symptomatic to mitigate virus transmission. The use of alcohol-based sanitisers is essential when soap is unavailable. When coughing, individuals should cover their mouth with a tissue or elbow and wash their hands following tissue disposal.

Wearing masks in crowded environments is recommended to reduce droplet spread. Limiting exposure to crowded areas during outbreaks is advisable. Increasing awareness of HMPV symptoms and encouraging early reporting are important. Although a vaccine specific to HMPV is not currently available, staying updated with other respiratory vaccines, such as those for influenza and pneumococcal diseases, can help reduce the overall burden of respiratory illnesses (Akingbola et al., 2025; Mistry et al., 2025; Satapathy et al., 2025). Adopting a healthy lifestyle which encompasses balanced nutrition, regular exercise, and sufficient sleep plays an important role in supporting immune function. Shared, environments such as offices, schools, and public places also involved in airborne transmission, in which symptomatic individuals should be incentivised with sick leave policies to reduce the transmission and should be made aware of hygiene practices such as hand washing and monitored accordingly (Abe & Abe, 2019; Adedokun et al., 2025; Powell et al., 2022; Principi & Esposito, 2014; Shao et al., 2021). Pathways of Environmental and Ecological Influence on HMPV Spread are shown in Figure 1.

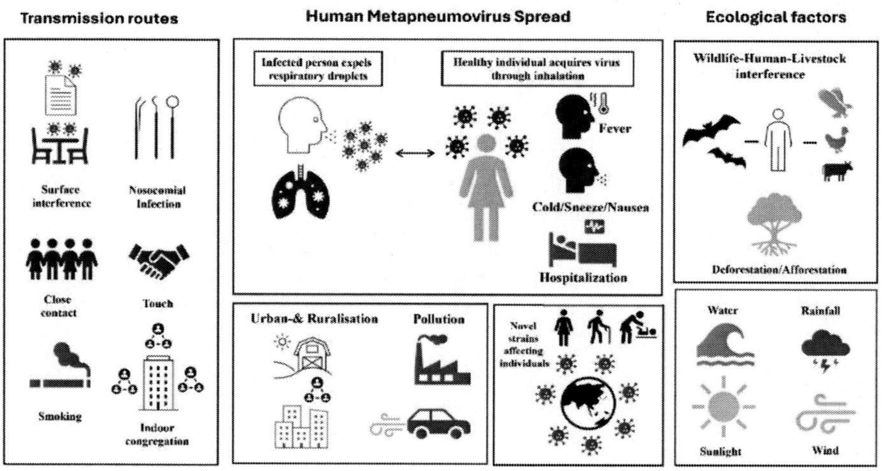

Figure 1. Pathways of environmental and ecological influence on HMPV spread.

Environmental Determinants of HMPV Transmission

Environmental factors play a significant role, and addressing related factors that may exacerbate HMPV outbreaks is vital, which can be achieved by improving access to healthcare, enhancing surveillance, and utilising data analytic approaches to enable timely detection and intervention. HMPV stability changes with temperature and surface type, persisting longer at lower temperatures, while higher temperature reduces viral stability and transmission risk.

Surface Survival Characteristics

Surface-mediated transmission is one of the environmental factors that is involved in indirect viral spread, wherein the virus is deposited on surfaces by an infected person and subsequently transferred to others through contact. Nonporous surfaces such as plastic, stainless steel, and hospital-based equipment are capable of retaining infectious viruses for 24 to 48 hours at room temperature with moderate humidity and persisting for up to seven days; however, the infectivity diminishes rapidly once the virus has dried. Metal and glass surfaces in hospitals pose transmission risks, highlighting the importance of surface hygiene for infection control. On the other hand, on porous surfaces such as paper, fabric, and tissue, the virus quickly loses its stability within hours due to absorption and quick drying (Dancer, 2014; Geiser et al., 2021; Olopade et al., 2025; Rajeswar Dutt et al., 2025; Tollefson et al., 2010).

Seasonality and Climate

HMPV infections peak during late winter and early spring due to increased indoor congregation. Climate change affects viral epidemiology, altering outbreak patterns through environmental and ecological behaviours. Rising temperatures and humidity levels create favourable conditions for the transmission of the virus. The role of climate risk integration in public health planning is crucial, as it can modify HMPV transmission through meteorological factors (Quintero-Salgado et al., 2024). Climate change is disrupting seasonal cycles, altering the viral transmission periods, as this disruption may lead to off-season outbreaks, with infections occurring outside their typical peak seasons, thereby increasing health risks. As climate change induces unpredictable weather conditions, the regularity of HMPV seasonal outbreaks may become less predictable, potentially occurring in new locations with regional variations on local climate changes (Balekundri & Ahire, 2025).

Rainfall Patterns and Seasonal Variations

Rainfall and HMPV transmission remained unresolved, though weather may affect transmission. Rainfall mainly impacts HMPV in tropical and subtropical regions. Principal component analyses (PCAs) uncovered and wind speed, which wind speed accounts for infection rate variance, highlighting climate-virus interactions. In milder winters, there is evidence of decreased viral shedding while extreme weather disrupts transmission (Lim et al., 2020). In climate-sensitive areas, rainfall and humidity trends affect HMPV stability, which makes public health measures essential for managing transmission dynamics (Darniot et al., 2018; Price et al., 2019). In China, HMPV cases increase during the winter and early spring months (November-April), coinciding with low temperatures and reduced rainfall (Al-Tawfiq & Memish, 2025). In contrast, in Malaysia, elevated relative humidity and rainfall may correlate with prevalence of HMPV (Chow et al., 2016; Yew et al., 2019).

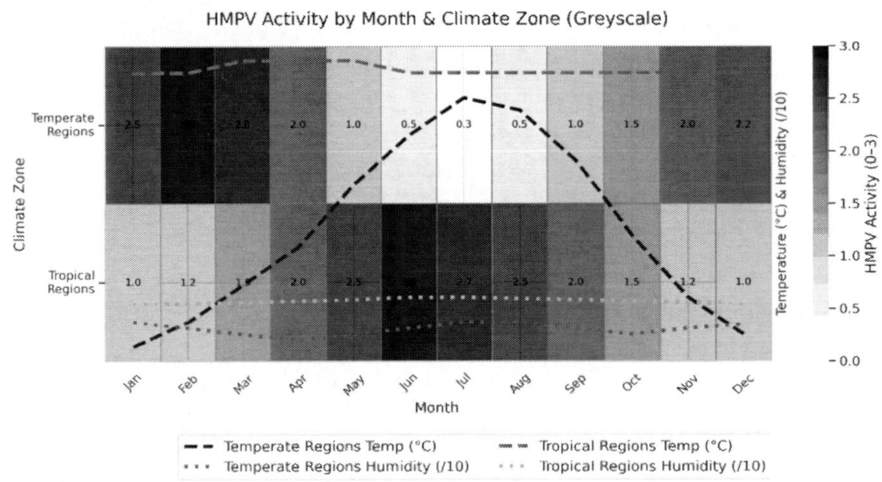

Figure 2. HMPV Activity in Temperate and Tropical Regions with Climatic Overlays: The heatmap illustrates the monthly variations in relative HMPV activity (on a scale of 0–3) across two primary climate zones—Temperate and Tropical regions. Higher HMPV activity is indicated by warmer colours (yellow), while lower activity is represented by cooler tones (purple). Overlaid line plots show average monthly temperature and scaled relative humidity. (Dashed lines represent mean monthly temperature in °C (blue for temperate, green for tropical regions. Dotted lines represent mean monthly humidity divided by 10 for visual scale fitting (orange for temperate, red for tropical regions). Black stars indicate peak HMPV transmission periods in each climate zone.

Influence of Weather (Temperature, Wind Speed, Precipitation, and Humidity) on HMPV Transmission

Temperature and humidity are critical factors influencing the stability and infectivity of HMPV. The virus exhibits greater stability at lower temperatures, whereas elevated temperatures, such as 37°C, significantly diminish its infectivity. At ambient or room temperatures (20-25°C), the virus can persist for up to seven days in liquid suspensions and for 24-48 hours on nonporous surfaces. At 4°C, the virus remains stable for prolonged durations in both liquid and dried forms. Conversely, at 37°C, viral degradation occurs within hours, although the virus can withstand repeated freezing at -80°C without substantial loss of viability. Infectious virus can persist for several hours at room temperature and for extended periods at 4°C, while exposure to 37°C results in a rapid decline in infectivity. Empirical studies indicate that lower relative humidity (20-35%) facilitates airborne transmission, whereas higher humidity levels can mitigate it. Nonetheless, moderate to high humidity may enhance surface stability and influence droplet dynamics. Continuous recording of temperature, humidity and wind speed provided data for statistical modelling and prediction of HMPV outbreaks (Vidal et al., 2019; Ye et al., 2023). Multivariate regression analyses showed temperature as the primary predictor of HMPV incidence, consistent with respiratory viruses due to indoor crowding and virus survival in cold environments (Wang et al., 2012). In Europe and North America, HMPV circulates from winter through spring, with the highest activity from January to March (Cattoir et al., 2019; Jobe et al., 2025; Moe et al., 2017). In Japan and South Korea, HMPV activity peaks later than in Europe and North America, with the peak season in April and May, likely due to both climatic and social factors (Cho et al., 2023; Ju et al., 2006; Kaida et al., 2006; Nidaira et al., 2012; Sasaki et al., 2005). Understanding seasonality requires integrating environmental and biological factors across regions. Monthly temperature, humidity values, and seasonal data were derived from global climate datasets, including the Global Precipitation Climatology Centre (GPCC), the Global Precipitation Climatology Project (GPCP), and national meteorological agencies (Figure 2).

Temperature, wind speed and moderate humidity (around 55%) independently correlate with increased HMPV activity, clustering at specific temperature intervals (8°C-22°C) and diurnal changes of 6°C-14°C, suggesting that moderate humidity helps in viral stability, while temperature fluctuations may enhance survival or alter susceptibility (Chesa Andini Saputra, 2025; Varela-Lasheras et al., 2023). Humidity and photoperiod influence HMPV and respiratory virus epidemiology, though less than temperature and precipitation. Sunshine duration and atmospheric pressure have been found to correlate with HMPV activity. Increased sunshine duration is independently associated with higher HMPV positivity, potentially by influencing indoor-outdoor movement and ventilation patterns. Reduced winter daylight and sunlight exposure can lower vitamin D levels, weakening immunity (García-Arroyo et al., 2022; He et al., 2023). Studies found weak links between HMPV cases and humidity or sunshine duration. The combination of low humidity, cold temperatures and limited sunlight increases susceptibility to respiratory infections. These meteorological factors have complex impacts best understood through region-specific analysis. However, environmental conditions alone do not determine HMPV spread - human behaviour and social interactions in public spaces equally contribute to viral transmission (Li et al., 2019; Zhang et al., 2013).

Airflow, Air Quality and Ventilation Strategies

Enhancing air circulation serves to dilute viral particles present in the atmosphere, thereby reducing the likelihood of inhalation by susceptible individuals. Improved ventilation diminishes the risk of transmission by dispersing viral particles, whereas insufficient ventilation increases the risk of infection. It is advisable to open windows and doors to facilitate the circulation of fresh air, particularly in crowded or poorly ventilated environments (Ai & Melikov, 2018; Alqarni et al., 2024; Bathula et al., 2021; Ferrari et al., 2022; Nair et al., 2022). The utilisation of mechanical ventilation systems (HVAC) is recommended to ensure comprehensive air exchange within indoor settings. Air purification system with HEPA filters significantly reduces viral concentration where natural ventilation is constrained (Absar Alam et al., 2023; Dubey et al., 2021). HMPV establishes focal lung lesions and persists within the respiratory tract, particularly under conditions of poor ventilation or elevated pollution levels. Exposure to tobacco smoke increases susceptibility to HMPV infection by compromising airway defence mechanisms in both active smokers and individuals exposed to environmental smoke. Tobacco smoke induces airway inflammation and impairs mucociliary clearance, thereby altering immune cell function and facilitating the proliferation of pathogens such as HMPV within the airways (Adivitiya et al., 2021; Duffney et al., 2020; Strzelak et al., 2018; Wang et al., 2023). Additionally, it suppresses antiviral pathways and the expression of interferon-inducible genes, which are essential for viral control. Urban populations in high-pollution areas may face elevated HMPV risks due to compounded environmental stressors. Improving ventilation reduces airborne HMPV transmission, while mitigating pollution exposure preserves integrity and immune function (Cardoso et al., 2004; Ferrari et al., 2022; Islam et al., 2021; Pica & Bouvier, 2012).

Geographic Variations Affecting Transmission

HMPV is found worldwide, with all major continents reporting cases. Different genotypes (notably A and B, with sublineages such as A2b, A2c, B1, and B2) circulate in various regions, and new genetic variants continue to emerge and spread across countries. Regional differences in genotype distribution and surveillance introduce uncertainty, requiring coordinated data collection and meta-analytic methods for consistent findings. Recent studies have documented the predominance and geographic spread of A2c variants with gene duplications in China, Spain, Japan, and Croatia. Asia, particularly China and Japan, has been highlighted as a new epicentre for HMPV transmission and the emergence of novel variants since 2005, with evidence of frequent cross-border transmission between these regions. Phylogeographic analyses showed HMPV distribution shifts over time, influenced by population movement and viral evolution (Oketch et al., 2021).

Behavioural Factors Affecting Transmission

Environments characterised by frequent and close interactions, such as schools, daycare centres, and family households, serve as significant transmission hubs due to increased opportunities for person-to-person spread. High household density and crowded settings with poor ventilation facilitate viral spread. Individuals attending public places while symptomatic contribute to community transmission, making self-isolation essential. Children under 14 are more susceptible to HMPV due to close contact and inconsistent hygiene. Adults, as index cases, risk spreading HMPV through household interactions. Socio-environmental factors, including family structure and living conditions, also play a critical role in the epidemiology of HMPV (Caracciolo et al., 2008). With industrialisation, much of human life is spent indoors, insulated from outdoor seasonal climate fluctuations. These closed, airtight living conditions create constant indoor environments, diminishing the direct influence of outdoor seasonal changes on infection risk. Consequently, the majority of respiratory virus transmission relies more on person-to-person contact during workdays or at home rather than adverse weather conditions, making it a major factor in the seasonality of HMPV infection (Mucha et al., 2024; Niza et al., 2024).

Role of Urbanisation and Population Density

Urbanisation creates densely populated environments where close proximity increases direct and indirect contact between individuals, facilitating HMPV transmission. Urban areas foster human-animal interfaces that enable disease transmission. Although HMPV is a human pathogen, urbanisation dynamics like increased movement and crowding can amplify its spread. Reducing crowd density effectively lowers transmission risk by limiting contact with infected individuals and contaminated surfaces. Urbanisation often brings about socioeconomic changes, including the growth of informal settlements where population density is highest and access to healthcare and sanitation may be limited. Environmental stressors common in urban settings, such as pollution and poor ventilation, can also impair immune responses and facilitate the persistence and transmission of respiratory pathogens (Neiderud, 2015; Pickett et al., 2011).

Socioeconomic Influences on Transmission Dynamics

Socioeconomic factors, including household structure and healthcare access, influence HMPV spread within communities, and lower socioeconomic status often leads to crowded living conditions and reduced preventive measures, contributing to elevated transmission rates. Delayed diagnosis can lead to prolonged viral shedding and increased community spread. In densely populated areas with multi-generational households, transmission rates can reach 12.2%. Though direct links between socioeconomic status and HMPV transmission are less quantified, indirect effects through limited healthcare access and crowded conditions remain significant (Al Hajjar et al., 2011; Bell et al., 2024; Koetz et al., 2006).

Virological and Clinical Surveillance for HMPV Prediction

HMPV infection presents with cough, runny nose, sore throat, nasal congestion, and fever. Severe cases may involve wheezing, bronchiolitis or pneumonia, requiring hospitalisation and oxygen therapy. HMPV surveillance includes virological and clinical monitoring through systems like the National Respiratory and Enteric Virus Surveillance System (NREVSS). Surveillance is essential for detecting outbreaks and uses molecular techniques, including nucleic acid amplification tests (NAAT), reverse transcriptase-polymerase chain reaction (RT-PCR), on respiratory samples from suspected cases and epidemiological data in identifying seasonal patterns (Dani et al., 1999). Real-time data collection enables timely public health responses during high-risk periods. Weekly positive cases are recorded for tracking trends. HMPV infections are typically mild, though recent hospital admissions have increased due to multiple respiratory viruses. While COVID-19 disrupted HMPV seasonality, patterns are returning to pre-pandemic levels. Healthcare settings require droplet precautions and hand hygiene, as no vaccine exists. Health authorities monitor trends for public health responses (Deval et al., 2024; Feng et al., 2024; Fox, 2007; Williams et al., 2002).

Ecological Factors Influencing HMPV Transmission

The evolution of novel strains of HMPV is shaped by a complex interplay of ecological and evolutionary forces. Key ecological factors include host immune pressure, transmission dynamics and population structure, mutation and recombination, environmental and socioeconomic factors, and zoonotic and cross-species transmission. Immune evasion is a major driver of HMPV evolution. The genetic diversity, particularly in the G gene, allows the virus to escape host antibodies, leading to recurrent infections and the emergence of new strains. Positive selection at certain amino acid sites, especially in surface glycoproteins (G and F), suggests adaptation to evade immune responses (Parida et al., 2023; Piñana et al., 2020). Despite the advances in virology and epidemiology, the role of ecological factors and regional seasonality in shaping HMPV outbreaks remains elusive. HMPV outbreaks rarely coincide with influenza or RSV due to viral interference through host responses or receptor competition, resulting from overlapping cellular receptors, interferon responses or protective antibodies (Aune et al., 2021; Caracciolo et al., 2008;

Mahalingam et al., 2006; Papenburg & Boivin, 2010; Wolf et al., 2006; X et al., 2025). Extensive viral gene flow across geographical regions and seasons occurs due to human movement and transmission patterns, facilitating the spread and mixing of different strains. Some strains demonstrate wider geographical spread, likely due to their fitness, which may be influenced by host population immunity and transmission opportunities. High mutation rates, typical of RNA viruses, generate genetic diversity. Most mutations are removed by purifying selection, but some beneficial mutations are retained, especially those conferring immune escape or increased fitness. Recombination between and within HMPV lineages contributes to the emergence of novel strains by shuffling genetic material, particularly in the F, SH, and G genes. Elucidating these relationships is crucial for predicting the outbreak patterns and subsequently implementing timely control measures (Devanathan et al., 2025; Duffy, 2018; Hughes & Hughes, 2007; Juhasz & Easton, 1994; Piñana et al., 2023).

Animal Reservoir and Zoonotic Potential

Although HMPV is primarily known as a pathogen infecting humans, research into related viruses has raised important questions about its potential animal reservoirs. For instance, avian metapneumovirus (AMV) is a well-studied respiratory pathogen in poultry, and genetic analyses have revealed distinctive homology between AMPV and HMPV. This homology indicates a shared evolutionary lineage where its ancestors may have crossed species barriers in the past (Mase et al., 2003). Studies have shown small laboratory animals were used to study virus-host interactions (Schildgen et al., 2007). In addition, retrospective analyses of other respiratory viruses, such as coronaviruses and influenza viruses, have shown that animal reservoirs plausibly serve as the spillover source for new human infections. Though HMPV is primarily human-specific, its genetic homology with avian metapneumovirus suggests theoretical zoonotic risks. Surveillance at wildlife-livestock interfaces is prudent but still remains unproven. However, effective monitoring requires global coordination beyond a few developed countries to address surveillance gaps worldwide (Hassell et al., 2021; Wiethoelter et al., 2015).

Wildlife-Livestock-Human Interface

The interface among wildlife-livestock-humans is increasingly recognised as a critical zone for the emergence and spillover of novel respiratory viruses. This dynamic interface facilitates the movement of pathogens across species barriers, often resulting in new public threats. The transmission of avian influenza, likely from wild birds to poultry and occasionally to humans, underscores the role of direct or indirect contact in facilitating interspecies pathogen transfer. Such events highlight how both direct interactions (handling and slaughtering) and indirect exposure (contaminated water and shared environments) can enable interspecies pathogen transfer. Although there is currently no direct evidence of HMPV transmission between animals and humans, the experience with zoonotic outbreaks of other viruses highlights the necessity for vigilance (Hassell et al., 2017). Deforestation, urban expansion, and agricultural development disrupt natural habitats, increasing contact rates between wildlife-livestock-humans. High-density farming operations create conditions conducive to viral amplification and mutation, increasing the likelihood of spillover events. Expansion into previously undisturbed ecosystems brings people into closer proximity with wildlife reservoirs of novel pathogens. Strengthening biosecurity measures and monitoring these interfaces—particularly in regions with high biodiversity and dense human populations—are essential steps to prevent the emergence of new zoonotic respiratory infections (Daszak et al., 2000; McFarlane et al., 2013; McMichael, 2004; Patz et al., 2004).

Ecosystem Disruptions

Anthropogenic disruptions in ecosystems significantly affect viral transmission and emergence. Deforestation, urbanisation, and habitat destruction increase zoonotic disease spillover risk by disrupting the wildlife-domestic animal-human equilibrium. Climate change-induced habitat loss forces animal migration to new areas, increasing exposure to novel hosts and viruses. The United Nations Environment Programme reports that 60% of human infectious diseases are zoonotic, and 75% of emerging infectious diseases originate from animals with novel pathogens, highlighting the importance of ecological balance (Rahman et al., 2020; Sun et al., 2024). Rapid urbanisation, driven by population growth and economic development, occurs without adequate environmental safeguards, disrupting human-wildlife equilibrium and increasing zoonotic spillover risks. Habitat fragmentation can trigger disease outbreaks in wildlife, and while isolated patches may limit transmission, severe outbreaks often occur. The loss of ecological niches and predators allows pathogen carriers to proliferate, increasing spillover risk and viral adaptation. As climate change reshapes landscapes, these disruptions increase novel pathogen emergence risk and complicate disease management. Environmental degradation also creates social impacts that predispose populations to infections (Combs et al., 2022; Marrana, 2022).

Conclusion

The HMPV transmission is associated with environmental factors, ecological and behavioural patterns. Understanding these factors allows for the development of more effective control strategies for vulnerable populations. Molecular diagnostics have enhanced the identification of the virus and improved the overall understanding of its epidemiology. By integrating enhanced surveillance strategies with environmental data, chances of predicting outbreaks drastically increase. Although there is no approved vaccine yet, promising candidates, including live-attenuated, subunit, and virus-like particle vaccines, are currently in trials. Vaccine strategies incorporating novel platforms like mRNA and nanoparticle delivery to address challenges related to antigenic variability and immunity. Ongoing research into diagnostics, vaccines, and therapeutics, coupled with global surveillance, is essential in reducing the burden of HMPV. Additionally, lessons learned from responses to RSV, influenza, and COVID-19 should inform HMPV preparedness programs to address emerging challenges.

References

Abe, M., & Abe, H. (2019). Lifestyle medicine – An evidence based approach to nutrition, sleep, physical activity, and stress management on health and chronic illness. *Personalized Medicine Universe*, 8, 3–9.

Absar Alam, M., Kumar, R., Yadav, A. S., Arya, R. K., & Singh, V. P. (2023). Recent developments trends in HVAC (heating, ventilation, and air-conditioning) systems: A comprehensive review. *Materials Today: Proceedings*.

Adedokun, K. A., Adekola, S. A., Tajudeen, A., Bello-Ibiyemi, A. A., Babandina, M. M., Magwe, E. A., & Bello, A. (2025). Rising global threat of human metapneumovirus (hMPV in 2024/2025): pathogenesis, immune dynamics, vulnerabilities in immunocompromised individuals, and lessons from past pandemics. *Journal of Rare Diseases* 2025 4:1, 4(1), 1–20.

Adivitiya, Kaushik, M. S., Chakraborty, S., Veleri, S., & Kateriya, S. (2021). Mucociliary Respiratory Epithelium Integrity in Molecular Defense and Susceptibility to Pulmonary Viral Infections. *Biology* 2021, Vol. 10, Page 95, 10(2), 95.

Ai, Z. T., & Melikov, A. K. (2018). Airborne spread of expiratory droplet nuclei between the occupants of indoor environments: A review. *Indoor Air*, 28(4), 500–524.

Akingbola, A., Adegbesan, A., TundeAlao, S., Adewole, O., Ayikoru, C., Benson, A. E., Shekoni, M., & Chuku, J. (2025). Human Metapneumovirus: an emerging respiratory pathogen and the urgent need for improved Diagnostics, surveillance, and vaccine development. *Infectious Diseases*.

Al Hajjar, S., Al Thawadi, S., Al Seraihi, A., Al Muhsen, S., & Imambaccus, H. (2011). Human metapneumovirus and human coronavirus infection and pathogenicity in Saudi children hospitalized with acute respiratory illness. *Annals of Saudi Medicine*, 31(5), 523–527.

Alqarni, Z., Rezgui, Y., Petri, I., & Ghoroghi, A. (2024). Viral infection transmission and indoor air quality: A systematic review. *Science of The Total Environment*, 923, 171308.

Al-Tawfiq, J. A., & Memish, Z. A. (2025). The surge of human metapneumovirus (hMPV) cases in China and global implications. *New Microbes and New Infections*, 63, 101563.

Aune, K. T., Davis, M. F., & Smith, G. S. (2021). Extreme Precipitation Events and Infectious Disease Risk: A Scoping Review and Framework for Infectious Respiratory Viruses. *International Journal of Environmental Research and Public Health* 2022, Vol. 19, Page 165, 19(1), 165.

Balekundri, A., & Ahire, E. D. (2025). The growing concern of human metapneumovirus. *Community Acquired Infection*, 12, 2025.

Bathula, S., Anand, S., Thajudeen, T., Mayya, Y. S., Chaudhury, P., & Shashank, C. (2021). Survival of expiratory aerosols in a room: Study using a bi-compartment and bi-component indoor air model. *Aerosol and Air Quality Research*, 21(5).

Bell, C., He, C., Norton, D., Goss, M., Chen, G., & Temte, J. (2024). Household transmission of human metapneumovirus and seasonal coronavirus. Epidemiology and Infection, 152. Caracciolo, S., Minini, C., Colombrita, D., Rossi, D., Miglietti, N., Vettore, E., Caruso, A., & Fiorentini, S. (2008). Human metapneumovirus infection in young children hospitalized with acute respiratory tract disease: virologic and clinical features. *Pediatric Infectious Disease Journal*, 27(5), 406–412.

Cardoso, M. R. A., Cousens, S. N., De Góes Siqueira, L. F., Alves, F. M., & D'Angelo, L. A. V. (2004). Crowding: risk factor or protective factor for lower respiratory disease in young children? *BMC Public Health*, 4, 19.

Cattoir, L., Vankeerberghen, A., Boel, A., Van Vaerenbergh, K., & De Beenhouwer, H. (2019). Epidemiology of RSV and hMPV in Belgium: a 10-year follow-up. *Acta Clinica Belgica*, 74(4), 229–235.

Chesa Andini Saputra, A. (2025, January). *Weather, High Mobility Are Factors Contributing to HMPV Transmissions.* https://jakartaglobe.id/news/weather-high-mobility-are-factors-contributing-to-hmpv-transmissions.

Cho, S. J., Kim, S. H., Lee, H., Lee, Y. U., Mun, J., Park, S., Park, J., Park, J. S., Lee, K., Lee, C. M., Seo, J., Kim, Y., & Chung, Y. S. (2023). Re-Emergence of HMPV in Gwangju, South Korea, after the COVID-19 Pandemic. *Pathogens*, 12(10), 1218.

Chow, W. Z., Chan, Y. F., Oong, X. Y., Ng, L. J., Nor'E, S. S., Ng, K. T., Chan, K. G., Hanafi, N. S., Pang, Y. K., Kamarulzaman, A., & Tee, K. K. (2016). Genetic diversity, seasonality and transmission network of human metapneumovirus: identification of a unique sub-lineage of the fusion and attachment genes. *Scientific Reports*, 6, 27730.

Combs, M. A., Kache, P. A., VanAcker, M. C., Gregory, N., Plimpton, L. D., Tufts, D. M., Fernandez, M. P., & Diuk-Wasser, M. A. (2022). Socio-ecological drivers of multiple zoonotic hazards in highly urbanized cities. *Global Change Biology*, 28(5), 1705–1724.

Dancer, S. J. (2014). Controlling Hospital-Acquired Infection: Focus on the Role of the Environment and New Technologies for Decontamination. *Clinical Microbiology Reviews*, 27(4), 665.

Dani, M. A. C., Arns, C. W., & Durigon, E. L. (1999). Molecular characterization of Brazilian avian pneumovirus isolates using reverse transcription-polymerase chain reaction, restriction endonuclease analysis and sequencing of a G gene fragment. *Avian Pathology*, 28(5), 473–476.

Darniot, M., Pitoiset, C., Millière, L., Aho-Glélé, L. S., Florentin, E., Bour, J. B., & Manoha, C. (2018). Different meteorological parameters influence metapneumovirus and respiratory syncytial virus activity. *Journal of Clinical Virology*, 104, 77–82.

Daszak, P., Cunningham, A. A., & Hyatt, A. D. (2000). Emerging infectious diseases of wildlife - Threats to biodiversity and human health. *Science*, 287(5452), 443–449.

Deval, H., Kumar, N., Srivastava, M., Potdar, V., Mehta, A., Verma, A., Singh, R., Kavathekar, A., Kant, R., & Murhekar, M. (2024). Human metapneumovirus (hMPV): an associated etiology of severe acute respiratory infection in children of Eastern Uttar Pradesh, India. *Access Microbiology*, 6(9), 000829.v4.

Devanathan, N., Philomenadin, F. S., Panachikuth, G., Jayagandan, S., Ramamurthy, N., Ratchagadasse, V. R., Chandrasekaran, V., & Dhodapkar, R. (2025). Emerging lineages A2.2.1 and A2.2.2 of human metapneumovirus (hMPV) in pediatric respiratory infections: Insights from India. *IJID Regions*, 14, 100486.

Dubey, S., Rohra, H., & Taneja, A. (2021). Assessing effectiveness of air purifiers (HEPA) for controlling indoor particulate pollution. *Heliyon*, 7(9), e07976.

Duffney, P. F., Embong, A. K., McGuire, C. C., Thatcher, T. H., Phipps, R. P., & Sime, P. J. (2020). Cigarette smoke increases susceptibility to infection in lung epithelial cells by upregulating caveolin-dependent endocytosis. *PLOS ONE*, 15(5), e0232102.

Duffy, S. (2018). Why are RNA virus mutation rates so damn high? *PLOS Biology*, 16(8), e3000003. https://doi.org/10.1371/JOURNAL.PBIO.3000003

Falsey, A. R. (2014). Human Metapneumovirus. *Mandell, Douglas, and Bennett's Principles and Practice of Infectious Diseases*, 2, 1961-1966.e2. https://doi.org/10.1016/B978-1-4557-4801-3.00161-2.

Feng, Y., He, T., Zhang, B., Yuan, H., & Zhou, Y. (2024). Epidemiology and diagnosis technologies of human metapneumovirus in China: a mini review. *Virology Journal,* 21(1), 1–11.

Ferrari, S., Blázquez, T., Cardelli, R., Puglisi, G., Suárez, R., & Mazzarella, L. (2022). Ventilation strategies to reduce airborne transmission of viruses in classrooms: A systematic review of scientific literature. *Building and Environment*, 222, 109366.

Fox, J. D. (2007). Respiratory virus surveillance and outbreak investigation. *Journal of Clinical Virology*, 40(SUPPL. 1), S24.

García-Arroyo, L., Prim, N., Del Cuerpo, M., Marín, P., Roig, M. C., Esteban, M., Labeaga, R., Martí, N., Berengua, C., Gich, I., Navarro, F., & Rabella, N. (2022). Prevalence and seasonality of viral respiratory infections in a temperate climate region: A 24-year study (1997–2020). *Influenza and Other Respiratory Viruses*, 16(4), 756–766.

Geiser, J., Boivin, G., Huang, S., Constant, S., Kaiser, L., Tapparel, C., & Essaidi-Laziosi, M. (2021). RSV and HMPV Infections in 3D Tissue Cultures: Mechanisms Involved in Virus-Host and Virus-Virus Interactions. *Viruses* 2021, Vol. 13, Page 139, 13(1), 139.

Haas, L. E. M., Thijsen, S. F. T., van Elden, L., & Heemstra, K. A. (2013). Human metapneumovirus in adults. *Viruses*, 5(1), 87–110.

Hassell, J. M., Begon, M., Ward, M. J., & Fèvre, E. M. (2017). Urbanization and Disease Emergence: Dynamics at the Wildlife–Livestock–Human Interface. *Trends in Ecology & Evolution*, 32(1), 55.

Hassell, J. M., Bettridge, J. M., Ward, M. J., Ogendo, A., Imboma, T., Muloi, D., Fava, F., Robinson, T. P., Begon, M., & Fèvre, E. M. (2021). Socio-ecological drivers of vertebrate biodiversity and human-animal interfaces across an urban landscape. *Global Change Biology*, 27(4), 781–792.

He, Y., Liu, W. J., Jia, N., Richardson, S., & Huang, C. (2023). Viral respiratory infections in a rapidly changing climate: the need to prepare for the next pandemic. *EBioMedicine*, 93, 104593.

Hughes, A. L., & Hughes, M. A. K. (2007). More Effective Purifying Selection on RNA Viruses than in DNA Viruses. *Gene*, 404(1–2), 117.

Islam, M., Sultana, Z. Z., Iqbal, A., Ali, M., & Hossain, A. (2021). Effect of in-house crowding on childhood hospital admissions for acute respiratory infection: A matched case–control study in Bangladesh. *International Journal of Infectious Diseases*, 105, 639–645.

Jesse, S. T., Ludlow, M., & Osterhaus, A. D. M. E. (2022). Zoonotic Origins of Human Metapneumovirus: A Journey from Birds to Humans. *Viruses*, 14(4), 677.

Jobe, N. B., Rose, E., Winn, A. K., Goldstein, L., Schneider, Z. D., & Silk, B. J. (2025). Human Metapneumovirus Seasonality and Co-Circulation with Respiratory Syncytial Virus — United States, 2014–2024. MMWR. *Morbidity and Mortality Weekly Report*, 74(11), 182–187.

Ju, Y. C., Tae, H. H., Byung, E. K., Chang, K. K., Sang, W. K., & Hwang, E. S. (2006). Human metapneumovirus infection in hospitalized children with acute respiratory disease in Korea. *Journal of Korean Medical Science*, 21(5), 838–842.

Juhasz, K., & Easton, A. J. (1994). Extensive sequence variation in the attachment (G) protein gene of avian pneumovirus: Evidence for two distinct subgroups. *Journal of General Virology*, 75(11), 2873–2880.

Kaida, A., Iritani, N., Kubo, H., Shiomi, M., Kohdera, U., & Murakami, T. (2006). Seasonal distribution and phylogenetic analysis of human metapneumovirus among children in Osaka City, Japan. *Journal of Clinical Virology*, 35(4), 394–399.

Koetz, A., Nilsson, P., Lindén, M., van der Hoek, L., & Ripa, T. (2006). Detection of human coronavirus NL63, human metapneumovirus and respiratory syncytial virus in children with respiratory tract infections in south-west Sweden. *Clinical Microbiology and Infection*, 12(11), 1089–1096.

Krüger, N., Laufer, S. A., & Pillaiyar, T. (2025). An overview of progress in human metapneumovirus (hMPV) research: Structure, function, and therapeutic opportunities. *Drug Discovery Today*, 30(5), 104364.

Li, Y., Reeves, R. M., Wang, X., Bassat, Q., Brooks, W. A., Cohen, C., Moore, D. P., Nunes, M., Rath, B., Campbell, H., Nair, H., Acacio, S., Alonso, W. J., Antonio, M., Ayora Talavera, G., Badarch, D., Baillie, V. L., Barrera-Badillo, G., Bigogo, G., … Zar, H. J. (2019). Global patterns in monthly activity of influenza virus, respiratory syncytial virus, parainfluenza virus, and metapneumovirus: a systematic analysis. *The Lancet Global Health*, 7(8), e1031–e1045.

Lim, Y. K., Kweon, O. J., Kim, H. R., Kim, T. H., & Lee, M. K. (2020). Clinical Features, Epidemiology, and Climatic Impact of Genotype-specific Human Metapneumovirus Infections: Long-term Surveillance of Hospitalized Patients in South Korea. *Clinical Infectious Diseases*, 70(12), 2683–2694.

Mahalingam, S., Schwarze, J., Zaid, A., Nissen, M., Sloots, T., Tauro, S., Storer, J., Alvarez, R., & Tripp, R. A. (2006). Perspective on the host response to human metapneumovirus infection: What can we learn from respiratory syncytial virus infections? *Microbes and Infection*, 8(1), 285–293.

Marrana, M. (2022). Epidemiology of disease through the interactions between humans, domestic animals, and wildlife. *One Health: Integrated Approach to 21st Century Challenges to Health*, 73–111.

Mase, M., Yamaguchi, S., Tsukamoto, K., Imada, T., Imai, K., & Nakamura, K. (2003). *Presence of Avian Pneumovirus Subtypes A and B in Japan.*

McFarlane, R. A., Sleigh, A. C., & McMichael, A. J. (2013). Land-use change and emerging infectious disease on an island continent. *International Journal of Environmental Research and Public Health*, 10(7), 2699–2719.

McMichael, A. J. (2004). Environmental and social influences on emerging infectious diseases: Past, present and future. *Philosophical Transactions of the Royal Society B: Biological Sciences*, 359(1447), 1049–1058.

Mistry, L. N., Agarwal, S., Jaiswal, H., Kondkari, S., Mulla, S. A., & Bhandarkar, S. D. (2025). Human Metapneumovirus: Emergence, Impact, and Public Health Significance. *Cureus*, 17(3), e80964.

Moe, N., Stenseng, I. H., Krokstad, S., Christensen, A., Skanke, L. H., Risnes, K. R., Nordbø, S. A., & Døllner, H. (2017). The Burden of Human Metapneumovirus and Respiratory Syncytial Virus Infections in Hospitalized Norwegian Children. *The Journal of Infectious Diseases*, 216(1), 110.

Mucha, W., Mainka, A., & Brągoszewska, E. (2024). Impact of ventilation system retrofitting on indoor air quality in a single-family building. *Building and Environment*, 262, 111830.

Nair, A. N., Anand, P., George, A., & Mondal, N. (2022). A review of strategies and their effectiveness in reducing indoor airborne transmission and improving indoor air quality. *Environmental Research*, 213, 113579.

Neiderud, C. J. (2015). How urbanization affects the epidemiology of emerging infectious diseases. *Infection Ecology & Epidemiology*, 5(1).

Nidaira, M., Taira, K., Hamabata, H., Kawaki, T., Gushi, K., Mahoe, Y., Maeshiro, N., Azama, Y., Okano, S., Kyan, H., Kudaka, J., Tsukagoshi, H., Noda, M., & Kimura, H. (2012). Molecular Epidemiology of Human Metapneumovirus from 2009 to 2011 in Okinawa, Japan. *Japanese Journal of Infectious Diseases*, 65(4), 337–340.

Niza, I. L., Bueno, A. M., Gameiro da Silva, M., & Broday, E. E. (2024). Air quality and ventilation: Exploring solutions for healthy and sustainable urban environments in times of climate change. *Results in Engineering*, 24, 103157.

Oketch, J. W., Kamau, E., Otieno, J. R., Mwema, A., Lewa, C., Isoe, E., Nokes, D. J., & Agoti, C. N. (2021). Comparative analysis of spatial-temporal patterns of human metapneumovirus and respiratory syncytial virus in Africa using genetic data, 2011–2014. *Virology Journal*, 18(1).

Olopade, B. K., Rahman, M. F., Khyum, M. M. O., & Ramkumar, S. (2025). Persistence and control of viruses on fomites and environmental matrices. *Future Virology*.

Papenburg, J., & Boivin, G. (2010). The distinguishing features of human metapneumovirus and respiratory syncytial virus. *Reviews in Medical Virology*, 20(4), 245–260.

Parida, P., Sudheesh, N., Sanjay, E. R., Jagadesh, A., Marate, S., & Govindakaranavar, A. (2023). The emergence of human metapneumovirus G gene duplication in hospitalized patients with respiratory tract infection, India, 2016–2018. *Molecular Biology Reports*, 50(2), 1109–1116.

Patz, J. A., Daszak, P., Tabor, G. M., Aguirre, A. A., Pearl, M., Epstein, J., Wolfe, N. D., Kilpatrick, A. M., Foufopoulos, J., Molyneux, D., Bradley, D. J., Amerasinghe, F. P., Ashford, R. W., Barthelemy, D., Bos, R., Bradley, D. J., Buck, A., Butler, C., Chivian, E. S., … Zakarov, V. (2004). Unhealthy landscapes: Policy recommendations on land use change and infectious disease emergence. *Environmental Health Perspectives*, 112(10), 1092–1098.

Pica, N., & Bouvier, N. M. (2012). Environmental factors affecting the transmission of respiratory viruses. *Current Opinion in Virology*, 2(1), 90–95.

Pickett, S. T. A., Cadenasso, M. L., Grove, J. M., Boone, C. G., Groffman, P. M., Irwin, E., Kaushal, S. S., Marshall, V., McGrath, B. P., Nilon, C. H., Pouyat, R. V., Szlavecz, K., Troy, A., & Warren, P. (2011). Urban ecological systems: Scientific foundations and a decade of progress. *Journal of Environmental Management*, 92(3), 331–362.

Piñana, M., González-Sánchez, A., Andrés, C., Abanto, M., Vila, J., Esperalba, J., Moral, N., Espartosa, E., Saubi, N., Creus, A., Codina, M. G., Folgueira, D., Martinez-Urtaza, J., Pumarola, T., & Antón, A. (2023). The emergence, impact, and evolution of human metapneumovirus variants from 2014 to 2021 in Spain. *Journal of Infection*, 87(2), 103–110.

Piñana, M., Vila, J., Maldonado, C., Galano-Frutos, J. J., Valls, M., Sancho, J., Nuvials, F. X., Andrés, C., Martín-Gómez, M. T., Esperalba, J., Codina, M. G., Pumarola, T., & Antón, A. (2020). Insights into immune evasion of human metapneumovirus: novel 180- and 111-nucleotide duplications within viral G gene throughout 2014-2017 seasons in Barcelona, Spain. *Journal of Clinical Virology*, 132.

Powell, E., Sumner, E., Shaw, A. G., Calvez, R., Fink, C. G., & Kroll, J. S. (2022). The temporal pattern and lifestyle associations of respiratory virus infection in a cohort study spanning the first two years of life. *BMC Pediatrics*, 22(1), 1–10.

Price, R. H. M., Graham, C., & Ramalingam, S. (2019). Association between viral seasonality and meteorological factors. *Scientific Reports*, 9(1), 1–11.

Principi, N., & Esposito, S. (2014). Paediatric human metapneumovirus infection: Epidemiology, prevention and therapy. *Journal of Clinical Virology*, 59(3), 141–147.

Quintero-Salgado, E., Briseno-Ramírez, J., Vega-Cornejo, G., Damian-Negrete, R., Rosales-Chavez, G., & De Arcos-Jiménez, J. C. (2024). Seasonal Shifts in Influenza, Respiratory Syncytial Virus, and Other Respiratory Viruses After the COVID-19 Pandemic: An Eight-Year Retrospective Study in Jalisco, Mexico. *Viruses*, 16(12), 1892.

Rahman, M. T., Sobur, M. A., Islam, M. S., Ievy, S., Hossain, M. J., Zowalaty, M. E. E., Rahman, A. M. M. T., & Ashour, H. M. (2020). Zoonotic Diseases: Etiology, Impact, and Control. *Microorganisms*, 8(9), 1405.

Rajeswar Dutt, K., Kumar Yadav, M., Singh, A., Kumar Mahto, I., Rawani, S., Singh, G., Kumar, S., Kashyap, S., Goray, J., Kumar Singh, P., & Roy, A. (2025). The Hidden Menace: Human Metapneumovirus Infection (hMPV): A Review of Clinical Manifestations, Diagnosis, And Management Strategies. *International Journal of Scientific Research and Technology*, 2(2).

Rao, B. L., Gandhe, S. S., Pawar, S. D., Arankalle, V. A., Shah, S. C., & Kinikar, A. A. (2004). First Detection of Human Metapneumovirus in Children with Acute Respiratory Infection in India: a Preliminary Report. *Journal of Clinical Microbiology*, 42(12), 5961.

Sasaki, A., Suzuki, H., Saito, R., Sato, M., Sato, I., Sano, Y., & Uchiyama, M. (2005). Prevalence of human metapneumovirus and influenza virus infections among Japanese children during two successive winters. *Pediatric Infectious Disease Journal*, 24(10), 905–908.

Satapathy, T., Satapathy, A., Satapathy, A., Yadav, N., Manisha Chandrakar, M. C., & Chandrakar, K. (2025). Recent outbreaks of Human Metapneumovirus (HMPV): Prevention, Diagnosis and Therapeutic insights. *Journal of Drug Delivery and Therapeutics*, 15(2), 193.

Schildgen, O., Simon, A., & Williams, J. (2007). Animal models for human Metapneumovirus (HMPV) infections. *Veterinary Research*, 38(1), 117–126.

Schuster, J. E., & Williams, J. V. (2023). Human Metapneumovirus. *Antibodies for Infectious Diseases*, 237–247.

Shao, T., Verma, H. K., Pande, B., Costanzo, V., Ye, W., Cai, Y., & Bhaskar, L. V. K. S. (2021). Physical Activity and Nutritional Influence on Immune Function: An Important Strategy to Improve Immunity and Health Status. *Frontiers in Physiology*, 12, 751374.

Strzelak, A., Ratajczak, A., Adamiec, A., & Feleszko, W. (2018). Tobacco Smoke Induces and Alters Immune Responses in the Lung Triggering Inflammation, Allergy, Asthma and Other Lung Diseases: A Mechanistic Review. *International Journal of Environmental Research and Public Health*, 15(5), 1033.

Sun, Z. S., Wan, E. Y., Agbana, Y. L., Zhao, H. Q., Yin, J. X., Jiang, T. G., Li, Q., Fei, S. W., Wu, L. B., Li, X. C., Zhang, Q. Y., Liu, J. S., Gu, S. Y., Guo, Z. Y., Xue, J. B., Han, L. F., Zhang, X. X., Xia, S., Welburn, S. C., … Kassegne, K. (2024). Global One Health index for zoonoses: A performance assessment in 160 countries and territories. *IScience*, 27(4), 109297.

Tollefson, S. J., Cox, R. G., & Williams, J. V. (2010). Studies of culture conditions and environmental stability of human metapneumovirus. *Virus Research*, 151(1), 54–59.

Van Den Hoogen, B. G., De Jong, J. C., Groen, J., Kuiken, T., De Groot, R., Fouchier, R. A. M., & Osterhaus, A. D. M. E. (2001). A newly discovered human pneumovirus isolated from young children with respiratory tract disease. *Nature Medicine*, 7(6), 719–724.

Varela-Lasheras, I., Perfeito, L., Mesquita, S., & Gonçalves-Sá, J. (2023). The effects of weather and mobility on respiratory viruses dynamics before and during the COVID-19 pandemic in the USA and Canada. *PLOS Digital Health*, 2(12), e0000405.

Vidal, L. R. R., Pereira, L. A., Debur, M. C., Raboni, S. M., Nogueira, M. B., Cavalli, B., & Almeida, S. M. (2019). A influência da temperatura e índice pluviométrico nas infecções virais humanas. *Brazilian Journal of Health and Pharmacy*, 1(1), 12–20.

Wang, Y., Chen, Z., Yan, Y. D., Guo, H., Chu, C., Liu, J., Ding, Y., Shao, X., Xu, J., & Ji, W. (2012). Seasonal distribution and epidemiological characteristics of human metapneumovirus infections in pediatric inpatients in Southeast China. *Archives of Virology*, 158(2), 417.

Wang, Y., Ninaber, D. K., Faiz, A., van der Linden, A. C., van Schadewijk, A., Lutter, R., Hiemstra, P. S., van der Does, A. M., & Ravi, A. (2023). Acute cigarette smoke exposure leads to higher viral infection in human bronchial epithelial cultures by altering interferon, glycolysis and GDF15-related pathways. *Respiratory Research,* 24(1), 1–16.

Wiethoelter, A. K., Beltrán-Alcrudo, D., Kock, R., & Mor, S. M. (2015). Global trends in infectious diseases at the wildlife-livestock interface. Proceedings of the National *Academy of Sciences of the United States of America*, 112(31), 9662–9667.

Williams, B. G., Gouws, E., Boschi-Pinto, C., Bryce, J., & Dye, C. (2002). Estimates of world-wide distribution of child deaths from acute respiratory infections. *Lancet Infectious Diseases*, 2(1), 25–32.

Wolf, D. G., Greenberg, D., Kalkstein, D., Shemer-Avni, Y., Givon-Lavi, N., Saleh, N., Goldberg, M. D., & Dagan, R. (2006). Comparison of human metapneumovirus, respiratory syncytial virus and influenza A virus lower respiratory tract infections in hospitalized young children. *Pediatric Infectious Disease Journal*, 25(4), 320–324.

X, S., R, Z., J, Z., Y, L., K, G., Q, Z., X, G., N, Z., H, X., H, W., C, Y., Z, Z., & B, Z. (2025). Global meta-analysis of short-term associations between ambient temperature and pathogen-specific respiratory infections, 2004 to 2023. *Euro Surveillance : Bulletin Europeen Sur Les Maladies Transmissibles = European Communicable Disease Bulletin*, 30(11).

Ye, H., Zhang, S., Zhang, K., Li, Y., Chen, D., Tan, Y., Liang, L., Liu, M., Liang, J., An, S., Wu, J., Zhu, X., Li, M., & He, Z. (2023). Epidemiology, genetic characteristics, and association with meteorological factors of human metapneumovirus infection in children in southern China: A 10-year retrospective study. *International Journal of Infectious Diseases*, 137, 40–47.

Yew, S. M., Tan, K. L., Yeo, S. K., Ng, K. P., & Kuan, C. S. (2019). Molecular epidemiology of respiratory viruses among Malaysian Young children with a confirmed respiratory infection during 2014–2015. *Journal of Thoracic Disease,* 11(11), 4626.

Zhang, X. L., Shao, X. J., Wang, J., & Guo, W. L. (2013). Temporal characteristics of respiratory syncytial virus infection in children and its correlation with climatic factors at a public pediatric hospital in Suzhou. *Journal of Clinical Virology*, 58(4), 666–670.

Chapter 10

Human Metapneumovirus (HMPV) Genotypes and Their Clinical Significance

Priya Sahani[1]
Anupama Ojha[2]
and Sarad Kumar Mishra[1,*]
[1]Department of Biotechnology, Deen Dayal Upadhyaya Gorakhpur University, Gorakhpur, Uttar Pradesh, India
[2]Department of Biochemistry, Shri Gorakshnath Medical College Hospital and Research Centre, Mahayogi Gorakhnath University, Gorakhpur, Sonbarsa, Gorakhpur, India

Abstract

Human metapneumovirus (HMPV) is a worldwide-distributed respiratory virus causing a large number of acute respiratory infections, especially in children, people, older adults, and individuals with compromised immune systems. Human metapneumovirus (HPMV) is an important cause of viral pneumonia, which can be fatal when infection is severe and reaches the lungs. HMPV belongs to the Paramyxoviridae family, and the structure of HMPV is genetically heterogeneous, which can be divided into two main genotypes, A and B. These two genotypes contain sublineages (A1, A2, B1, and B2). And those play significant roles in Viral pathogenicity, transmissibility, and various immune evasiveness are all decided by this genetic diversity can be exhibited in the human body. Epidemiologic investigations have demonstrated that HMPV genotypes possess individual seasonal patterns and geographic distribution, in that various genotype predominance is observed in

* Corresponding Author's Email: sarad.biotech@ddugu.ac.in

In: Human Metapneumovirus
Editors: Anjali Sharma, Vishnu Mittal, Devkant Sharma et al.
ISBN: 979-8-90134-063-9

different epidemic seasons. Genotype A is characterised by more severe respiratory distress, especially in children and immunocompromised adults, due to the enhanced inflammatory reaction. The type of Genotype B is also characterised by moderate and linked with higher infections over constant periods, which indicates differences in viral replication and immune evasion. Advances in molecular technology for diagnostics, e.g., real-time PCR and sequencing, have made detection of HMPV genotypes feasible for application in epidemiological surveillance. Advancements in molecular diagnostic technology hey are processed by including real-time PCR and sequencing, have allowed for accurate detection of the HMPV genotypes to monitor viral spread. Elucidation of the clinical relevance of HMPV genotypes will help improve patient care and guide vaccine development. Also, the genotype of HMPV in the field of research is imperative in the establishment of effective prevention and treatment programs, particularly among those at high risk.

Keywords: human metapneumovirus, immunological response, genotypes, epidemiology, clinical relevance, and molecular diagnostics

List of Abbreviations

HMPV	Human Metapneumovirus
RTI	Respiratory Tract Infection
COPD	Chronic Obstructive Pulmonary Disease
PCR	Polymerase Chain Reaction
TLRs	Toll-Like Receptors
RIG-I	Retinoic Acid-Inducible Gene I
PRRs	Pattern Recognition Receptors
RNA	Ribonucleic Acid
DNA	Deoxyribonucleic Acid
F protein	Fusion protein
G protein	Glycoprotein
N protein	Nucleoprotein
P protein	Phosphoprotein
M protein	Matrix protein
SH	Small Hydrophobic protein
L protein	Large Polymerase protein
M2-1, M2-2	Matrix-associated regulatory proteins
NF-κB	Nuclear Factor Kappa B
MAVS	Mitochondrial Antiviral Signalling Protein

SCT	Stem Cell Transplant
RSV	Respiratory Syncytial Virus.

Introduction

The cause of respiratory tract infections in children, the elderly, and those with compromised immune systems is frequently the human metapneumovirus (HMPV), which causes a viral pneumonia infection. This infection can be life-threatening if it spreads to the lower respiratory tract. HMPV, which belongs to the family Paramyxoviridae, is genetically varied and is classified into two broad genotypes, A and B, each split into subgroups A1, A2, B1, and B2. The genetic structure of the HMPV virus includes various types of structures which has different particular functions at the genetic level. This genetic difference has a dramatic impact on the virus's virulence for disease, transmission between hosts, and evasiveness from the immune system. Epidemiological studies of HMPV have identified specific genotypes in seasonal and geographical areas, with other strains being predominant in different epidemics. Genotype A is commonly linked to more severe respiratory illness because it is the most severe infection on the respiratory organ, particularly in children and the immunocompromised, potentially by an overexaggeration of the inflammatory reaction.

In contrast, Genotype B tends to result in mild but prolonged infection, suggesting heterogeneity in viral replication ability and interaction with the immune system. The backbone of management is supportive care methods, mainly the vaccines, such as extra oxygen, antipyretics, and intravenous fluids for hydration if required (Vinci et al., 2018). The most common method by which the human metapneumovirus (HMPV) is spread is by respiratory droplets emitted from an individual's body when they sneeze or cough. The virus may also be transmitted by close, personal contact, like shaking hands or touching contaminated surfaces. One is at risk of getting infected if they touch their mouth, nose, or eyes after touching such contaminated surfaces. The most critical significance of measures of preventing infection, such as proper hand washing and regular surface disinfection, is underlined by the severity of this method of transmission in healthcare (CDC, 2024).

Taxonomy and Genetic Diversity of HMPV

Genetic differences between host factors play a significant role in determining the susceptibility to infection by the Human Metapneumovirus (HMPV) in an individual population of children. Various immune factors help fight against disease. One of the most significant components in the identification and response to viral infection is the pattern recognition receptors (PRRs), including Toll-like receptors (TLRs) and the RIG-I pathway.

They identify the activities of a viral pathogen and activate the immune system. The HMPV virus possesses the receptors. These receptors play the role of identifying viral pathogens and provoking an immune reaction. Genetic variations within the encoding genes of the receptors may have a striking influence on whether or not the host can mount an appropriate immune response against HMPV (Zhang et al., 2014). HMPV virus shares the same genetic polymorphisms in specific Toll-like receptors (TLRs), such as TLR3, that have been implicated in variation in susceptibility to respiratory infections, including Human Metapneumovirus (HMPV) ones. The differences in genes can influence the immune response and metabolic activities; hence, either enhanced or reduced inflammatory responses may result, affecting the severity of infection and other metabolic disturbances in the body. Understanding these genetic determinants is key to identifying the population and the children that is most likely to be at higher risk for severe HMPV infections. It may be invaluable in the creation of specific treatment protocols or vaccines aimed at improving clinical outcomes in such high-risk populations (Liu et al, 2018).

Classification under the Paramyxoviridae Family

The taxonomic classification of this HMPV virus has an integral part in its structure that is a lipid envelope, single-stranded, negative-sense, non-segmented RNA virus that has been categorised from the Paramyxoviridae family, and its genus is Metapneumovirus and its Pneumoviridae family in 2016. It is propagated by different types of respiratory droplets that are infectious and disturb the metabolic activities. Severe HMPV infection has been linked with immunocompromised status, premature birth, and underlying chronic cardiac, pulmonary, or neurological disorders (Uche et al., 2018).

Table 1. Conserved regions and functions of key genes and proteins HMPV

Gene	Protein	Function	Highly Conserved Regions	Conserved Nucleotides (nt)	Conserved Amino Acids (aa)	References
N Gene	Nucleoprotein (N)	Encapsulates viral RNA, forming a ribonucleoprotein complex for replication.	RNA-binding and oligomerisation domains	High conservation in the coding region	Conserved RNA-binding motifs	van et al., 2004
P Gene	Phosphoprotein (P)	Co-factor for the RNA polymerase complex; interacts with N and L proteins.	N-terminal domain and oligomerisation sites	Key nt sequences for polymerase interaction	Conserved phosphoprotein regions	Biacchesi et al., 2005
M Gene	Matrix protein (M)	Facilitates viral assembly and budding.	M2-1 zinc-binding domain; M2-2 regulatory sites	Regulatory nt sequences	Conserved zinc-binding motifs	Luytjes et al., 1989
F Gene	Fusion protein (F)	Mediates membrane fusion and viral entry into host cells	Perfusion and post-fusion forms, heptad repeats	Conserved fusion domains	Heptad repeats and fusion peptide motifs	Chang et al., 2012
M2 Gene	M2-1, M2-2 Proteins	Regulates transcription elongation and replication processes.	M2-1 zinc-binding domain; M2-2 regulatory sites	Regulatory nt sequences	Conserved zinc-binding motifs	Schmidt et al., 2009
SH Gene	Small hydrophobic protein	Function unclear; may play a role in immune evasion.	Transmembrane domains	Transmembrane nt regions	Conserved hydrophobic residues	van et al., 2004
G Gene	Glycoprotein (G)	Enhances viral attachment to host cells, modulates immune responses.	Receptor-binding domain	Conserved receptor-interaction nt	Immune-modulating regions	Melero et al., 2007 (assumed)
L Gene	Large Polymerase Protein (L)	Catalytic core of the RNA polymerase complex.	Polymerase active site motifs	Polymerase catalytic nt	Highly conserved polymerase aa motifs	Collins et al., 2009

Genetic Structure of Human Metapneumovirus

The human metapneumovirus is an enveloped virus whose negative-sense RNA genome has a length of about 13 kilobases. It is a member of the Pneumoviridae subfamily of paramyxoviruses. The eight genes code for proteins in this virus include the different structures Nucleocapsid (N), phosphoprotein (P), matrix (M), fusion (F), second matrix (M2), small hydrophobic (SH), attachment (G), and RNA-dependent RNA polymerase (L) that constitute the components of the genome. They are grouped in an order: 3′-N-P-M-F-M2-SH-G-L-5′ (Biacchesi et al., 2006).

The RNA core of HMPV is contained in a lipid envelope and is surrounded by a matrix (M) protein. Three glycoproteins (F), small hydrophobic (SH), and attachment (G) protrude as spikes of about 13–17 nm long, which are in the membrane. These various types of central nucleic acids in the virus aggregate to form a nucleocapsid of around 17 nm diameter and are accompanied by proteins like P, N, L, M2-1, and M2-2. The G and F proteins facilitate the fusion of various parts of the virus with the heparin sulfate receptors on the host cell surface. After fusion, the viral nucleocapsid is released into the cytoplasm of the host cell, where it replicates. The new viral genome gets assembled to create new nucleocapsids composed of the P proteins, N proteins, L proteins, and M2 proteins. These new virions proceed to the host cell membrane, from where they bud off, carrying F, SH, and G proteins as part of their envelope (Feuillet et al., 2012).

A and B Major Genotypes and Their Sub-Lineages A1, A2, B1, B2

Based on the genetic traits of HMPV, its virulence, and severe infections, it has six lineages (A1, A2a, A2b, A2c, B1, and B2) that are distinguished (Nao et al., 2020).

Table 2. Genetic characteristics of HMPV lineages

Lineage	Subgroups	Distinguishing Features	References
A	A1, A2	Higher virulence is frequent in severe infections	(Biacchesi et al., 2003)
B	B1, B2	Less virulent, more prevalent in mild cases	(Williams et al., 2006)

Evolutionary Factors and Genetic Changes through Time

In the HMPV virus, new sub-lineages such as A2c arose due to continuous genetic drift of the human metapneumovirus, especially in the F and G genes. Such genetic variability might influence immune recognition and pathogenicity of this infection, in addition to antigenic diversity. As with RSV patterns, genotype shift (e.g., A2 to B2) also occurs in a different type of alternating fashion every two to three years. Point mutations and recombination characterise HMPV evolution. Knowledge of viral evolution and an informed vaccine development process requires ongoing monitoring (Piyaratna et al., 2011).

Epidemiology and Seasonal Distribution of HMPV Genotypes

The dangerous respiratory virus, Human metapneumovirus, was first discovered in 2001, primarily affecting small children, the elderly, and people with compromised immune and metabolic systems. Around the world, HMPV is responsible for about 5–15% of pediatric acute respiratory illnesses (Panda et al., 2023). HMPV has a seasonally distinct type of occurrence and has been isolated on all continents. The spatio-temporal distribution of the HMPV genotypes possesses varied divisions. Spring and winter are the times through which outbreaks are known to occur, January to March of the northern hemisphere and June to July of the southern hemisphere (Pilger et al., 2011). Based on a recent study, RSV and influenza seasons are followed by March and April, when the height of HMPV seasonal cases is reached (Kahn et al., 2006). Based on another study, seasons for RSV and HMPV infections overlap (Chan et al.,2007). According to seroprevalence studies, a significant proportion of children (90–100%) have contracted the virus by the time they are 5–10 years old; however, re-infection can happen at any point during adulthood (Van et al., 2001).

This could be the result of infection by a new viral genotype or the loss of the immune system; insufficient immunity can develop during the initial infection. Although it varies from person to person, the incubation period typically lasts three to five days. Peak virus titers are observed in cotton rats and BALB/c mice between days 4 and 5 of animal research (Hamelin et al., 2005). Children under the age of two are particularly susceptible to HMPV, which is prevalent in the pediatric population. Adults infected with HMPV typically only exhibit mild flu-like symptoms. However, serious side effects, including chronic obstructive pulmonary disease (COPD), can happen in some adult cases, particularly in older persons. 29 Adults are more prone than children to have dyspnea (Falsey et al., 2003). Additionally, MPV infection has been documented in several immunocompromised patients, including recipients of hematopoietic stem cell transplants, patients with haematological malignancies, and recipients of lung transplants (Dokos et al.,2013). Premature birth, youth, a history of nosocomial infections, and underlying chronic pulmonary, cardiac, or neurological conditions are risk factors for severe HMPV infection (Principi et al., 2014).

Pathogenesis and Immune Evasion Mechanisms

The HMPV fusion (F) surface glycoprotein interacts with heparan sulfate proteoglycans (HSPGs) on human airway epithelial cells, serving as the primary glycoprotein receptor to initiate the infection process (Dick et al., 2012). Heparan sulfate proteoglycans (HSPGs) are essential extracellular matrix constituents, consisting of heparan sulfate (HS) chains made up of repeating and important parts of N-acetyl glucosamine (GlcNAc) linked to iduronic acid (IdoA) or glucuronic acid (GlcA), which are attached to a core protein anchored to the cell membrane. Moreover, human cell surfaces also bear a complex mixture of terminal glycan structures that viruses can use for their adhesion (Cummings et al., 2019). The human lung glycans have a mixture of bi-, tri-, and tetra-antennary complex N-glycans that typically have two to four N-acetyllactosamine (LacNAc, Galβ1-4GlcNAc) moieties. They may also have core fucosylation and are often salivated on the terminal residues. In addition, the O-glycans, glycosphingolipids, and mucins of the lung have similar extensions that involve (Neu5Acα2-3/6) Galβ1-4GlcNAc sequences, and the respiratory infections also involve these sequences. (Jia et al., 2020). In addition to having fewer linear poly-LacNAc extensions, the nasopharynx segment has a similar diversity of complex N-glycans. The nasopharynx has a comparable diversity of complex N-glycans but with fewer linear poly-LacNAc extensions. The significant variability of glycans, in chain lengths as well as in core structures, fosters a highly diverse glycan environment in the respiratory tract and upper and lower segments, which may be potential glycoreceptors for HMPV.

The nasopharynx contains an analogous range of complex N-glycans, with fewer linear poly-LacNAc extensions. The large diversity of glycans, varying in chain lengths and core structures, promotes a very diverse glycan environment in the respiratory tract and upper and lower regions, which could be possible glycoreceptors for HMPV. The production of type I interferons (IFN-I) is triggered when different recognition receptors, such as Toll-like receptors (TLRs) and RIG-I-like receptors (RLRs), detect viral components such as DNA, RNA, and proteins. This signaling activates important kinases including TBK1 and IKKε, and this in turn encourages the activation of transcription factors IRF3 and IRF7 is activated by the transcription factors These elements are essential for stimulating the synthesis of the interferons IFN-α and IFN-β. Specific proteins have been linked to vulnerability to viral infections; some of them have been emphasised in mouse model research, while others have been the subject of human studies. Gene names follow traditional human gene nomenclature, whereas viral RNA, viral DNA, and cellular DNA are represented by blue, yellow, and green helices, respectively. (Walther et al., 2013).

Clinical Manifestations of HMPV Infections

HMPV typically has a non-specific clinical presentation overlapping with other respiratory viruses. The different types of symptoms are fever, cough, nasal congestion, wheezing, dyspnea, and pharyngitis. Severe acute respiratory failure necessitating mechanical support can present in exceptional cases, particularly in infants and those with comorbidities (Nicholson et al., 2020). With a peak incidence at 6–12 months of age, HMPV accounts for about 6–10% of RTI-related hospitalisations in children less than 5 years old (Williams et al., 2023). The most frequent reasons for hospitalisation are pneumonia and bronchiolitis (Matsuda et al., 2013). For HMPV positive results, fever persists for 10 days, reaching the highest value during illness (Van et al., 2003). Fever is a rare symptom of re-infection with HMPV in young adults who have only mild cold and influenza-like disease. However, re-infection in older adults can cause profound symptoms (e.g., pneumonitis) and even death (Falsey et al., 2003). In many studies, small children have varying lower respiratory tract infections, which are attributed to HMPV. Wheezing has been reported as a standard clinical symptom. Both adults and young children who have HMPV infections may experience exacerbations of their asthma (Williams et al., 2005). Patients with COPD are more likely to contract HMPV, and HMPV enhances COPD (Perotin et al., 2013). Additionally, some findings have indicated that a variety of disorders affecting the central nervous system, from severe encephalitis to febrile seizures, may be linked to HMPV infection in children (Arnold et al., 2009).

Diagnostic Strategies and Genotypic Identification

In order to restrict the epidemic and provide patients with timely medical care, effective disease control measures will be developed with the help of early diagnosis of HMPV infection. Since HMPV and RSV have largely conserved F protein amino acid sequences (Kim et al, 2016), few serological methods have been developed to detect antibodies specific to HMPV (Ishiguro et al., 2021). Numerous nucleic acid-based molecular HMPV detection technologies are already on the market, significantly reducing the difficulty of diagnosing HMPV in a variety of diagnostic settings. (Cong et al., 2022). Due to the lack of a licensed vaccine or antiviral medication for treating or preventing HMPV infection, HMPV has been extremely common around the world and continues to cause a substantial medical burden in the community (Ma et al., 2023). In this virus, the sensitivity and specificity in their structure and of cell culture detection methods were found to be 68% and 99%, respectively, in comparison to real-time RT-PCR detection of HMPV. Cell culture is rarely used to diagnose HMPV infection these days; instead, molecular techniques like RT-PCR and/or real-time RT-PCR are more frequently employed (Matsuzaki et al., 2010).

Therapeutic and Preventive Strategies

Only symptomatic treatment is available for HMPV infection, as is the case with the majority of viral infections. Despite the development and evaluation of numerous treatment approaches by researchers worldwide, no antiviral medication specifically targeted for HMPV has yet to enter clinical trials.

Nucleoside Analogues

The antimetabolites known as nucleoside analogues (NA) imitate physiological nucleosides in order to be absorbed into freshly synthesised DNA and prevent additional DNA synthesis, which ends the chain. Numerous

NAs were evaluated as antiviral substances. One such NA that works well against pneumoviruses both in vitro and in vivo is ribavirin, which has also been utilised to treat HMPV infection cases (Chu et al., 2014). In addition to blocking viral RNA synthesis, ribavirin also affects the host immune system by causing CD4+ and CD8+ T cells to secrete more T helper (Th) 1 cytokines, such as TNFα, IFNγ, and IL2, and decreasing the secretion of Th2 cytokines, such as IL10, which further limits viral pathogenesis (Safdar et al., 2008). In order to treat HMPV infections, ribavirin has also been administered intravenously (IV) in conjunction with intravenous immunoglobulin (IVIg); nevertheless, the outcomes have been highly inconsistent. While a few other authors have reported that intravenous ribavirin/oral ribavirin combined with IVIg could successfully treat the infection in different categories of patients (Dokos et al., 2013), and found that the effect of, i.e., ribavirin combined with IVIg was not significant in treating the HMPV infection (Park et al., 2013).

Fusion Inhibitors

For a viral infection to begin, the HMPV F protein must fuse the viral envelope with the host cell membrane (Cox et al., 2012). Peptides that can stop this fusion process may reduce the virus's capacity to replicate within a host. A small number of peptides produced from the heptad repeat domains of the HMPV F protein were discovered by Deffrasnes et al., who then evaluated their efficacy in lowering the virus's morbidity and mortality. One of the peptides, HRA2, was quite effective in reducing levels of pro-inflammatory cytokines/chemokines, pulmonary inflammation, airway obstruction, and lung virus load in treated BALB/c mice (Deffrasnes et al., 2008). HRA2 peptide, when expressed in Nicotiana tabacum, has been able to inhibit virus binding to HEp2 cells under in vitro conditions (Márquez-Escobar et al., 2015). Additional research has been conducted to assess the effectiveness of the production of different peptides produced in plant and their system in suppressing the harmful damage of the virus in animal models. Recently, a fusion inhibitor, JNJ-5371867, has been reported for RSV, which is another pneumovirus closely related to HMPV (Roymans et al., 2017).

Sulfated Sialyl Lipid, NMSO3

It has been demonstrated that the sulfated sialyl lipid NMSO3 exhibits vigorous antiviral activity against HMPV (Wyde et al., 2004). Spetch et al., evaluated how NMSO3 medication affected HMPV infection. The inflammation of lung cells and the viral load in the lungs were both considerably decreased in BALB/c mice treated with a single dose of NMSO3 at 50 mg kg−1 body weight at the time of infection. Under NMSO3 medication, there was also a considerable decrease in the clinical disease and the amount of pro-inflammatory cytokines/chemokines affected in a part of the lungs. It was hypothesised that NMSO3 possesses anti-inflammatory properties in the recipient host in addition to its antiviral properties, which include preventing the entry and multiplication of viruses in host cells (Spetch et al., 2008).

Interfering RNAs

This type of small interfering RNAs (siRNAs) or short hairpin RNAs (shRNAs) has long been utilised in RNA interference to silence target genes specifically. The effectiveness of siRNAs targeted at different types of viral genes encoding nucleoprotein (N) and phosphoprotein (P) as a treatment strategy for HMPV. The most conserved region of HMPV nucleocapsid mRNA was the target of the 2′-O-methyl modified siRNA (Darniot et al., 2012), which demonstrated that it could partially inhibit viral replication. They also verified that the siRNA had no off-target effects and that cytokines had no role in this inhibitory effect (Deffrasnes et al., 2008).

Monoclonal Antibodies

Infected patients may be protected or have their disease severity reduced by monoclonal antibodies that target and preserve various parts of the epitopes of the virus's immunogenic proteins. Palivizumab is a monoclonal antibody that is effective in preventing RSV infection in high-risk individuals. The HMPV fusion protein is strongly immunogenic and invariant between virus types and subtypes (Cseke et al., 2007). In nasal aspirates and lungs of infected HMPV permissive mice, monoclonal antibodies that are present in humans, 54G10, are directly preserved by the different types of structural epitopes of the HMPV fusion protein, and have recently been shown to be strongly neutralising and effective in reducing the viral titer. 54G10's therapeutic and prophylactic effectiveness was greater than palivizumab when it came to the viral titer in lung homogenates and equal to that of palivizumab when it came to the viral titer in nasal aspirates (Schuster et al., 2015). Replication and transcription of HMPV in immortalised cells that are isolates of bronchial epithelial cells was recently examined and found to exhibit that, consistent with other filoviruses and rhabdoviruses, the development of inclusion bodies in the cytoplasm is essential to the replication and transcription of the HMPV genome (Munoz et al., 2017).

Future Directions

Human metapneumovirus appears to be a significant health concern, especially for the most vulnerable, such as small children, the elderly, and people with compromised immune systems. The highest goals need to be focused on demanding the preventive vaccines that offer long-term protection to the children and guard against multiple types of genotypes of viruses, especially for the likes of small children, the elderly, and immunocompromised individuals. The absence of specific antiviral medicines currently available means that future research will likely focus on developing effective antiviral drugs, improved diagnostic tools, and treatments that also consider the body's immune response. Higher attention has been paid to mRNA vaccine platforms as well as nanoparticle-based formulations at an early stage to counter the genetic diversity seen in HMPV strains. In summary, a multidisciplinary framework based on genetics, in the field of immunology, epidemiology, and various clinical research, is necessary to improve our knowledge and clinical practices of HMPV and minimise its impact. The burden of the disease should decrease worldwide. Precision medicine approaches enabled by applying clinical outcomes together with HMPV genotype information to create predictive models for disease severity. HMPV has different severities in children and can cause different symptoms. To better understand the role of host genetic determinants and co-infections with other respiratory viruses on the pathogenesis of the disease, further research is also needed.

Conclusion

Human metapneumovirus is still a severe respiratory infection, particularly among young children, older adults, and immunocompromised individuals. The genetic diversity, with two major genotypes (A and B) and their subclades (A1, A2, B1, B2), determines the virulence of the disease, its infectivity, and its capacity for immune escape. Epidemics and patient outcomes are reliant on the identification of such factors as monitoring, evolution, and the creation of supporting vaccines. Technological developments have dramatically improved our capacity for the identification and tracking of HMPV genotypes in molecular diagnostics such as real-time PCR and next-generation sequencing. It belongs to the Paramyxoviridae family. The structure of HMPV contains two subtypes. Genotype B is related to longer infections that are less severe in symptoms, and genotype A has been linked to increased inflammatory reactions in the human body and respiratory infection. Our ability to detect and track HMPV genotypes has been significantly enhanced by advances in molecular diagnostics processes, such as real-time PCR and next-generation sequencing, which are used as important molecular tools. Using these molecular techniques in the diagnosis of HMPV is very helpful for humans. These tools have strengthened epidemiological surveillance through the generation of valuable data on regional distribution, seasonality, and genotype-specific pathogenicity. Despite these advances, there are as yet no licensed vaccines or antiviral therapies for HMPV, and therefore, symptomatic therapy remains the sole major approach. Future research would mainly have to concentrate on genotype-specific vaccines and antiviral interventions in an attempt to slow down the global spread of HMPV. Valuable information concerning immune evasion mechanisms and disease pathogenesis can also be gained by studying the host immune system and viral pathogenesis. Furthermore, the advancements in different areas of immunology and bioinformatics, reinforcing public health controls, can make way for more effective medicinal treatments. For better patient care, development of preventive strategies, and improved diagnostic accuracy, a well-established knowledge of HMPV genotypes and their clinical significance is vital. In order to reduce the impact of HMPV among vulnerable populations and enhance global respiratory health, further research will be critical.

References

Arnold, J. C., Singh, K. K., Milder, E., Spector, S. A., Sawyer, M. H., & Gavali, S. (2009). Human metapneumovirus associated with central nervous system infection in children. *Pediatric Infectious Disease Journal, 28*(12), 1057–1060. https://doi.org/10.1097/INF.0b013e3181acd221.

Biacchesi, S., Skiadopoulos, M. H., Boivin, G., Grimley, K. A., Richardson, C. D., & Collins, P. L. (2007). Genetic engineering of human metapneumovirus to generate live attenuated vaccine candidates. *Journal of Virology, 81*(24), 1696–1702. https://doi.org/10.1128/JVI.00710-07.

Biacchesi, S., Skiadopoulos, M. H., Tran, K. C., Murphy, B. R., Collins, P. L., & Buchholz, U. J. (2004). Recovery of human metapneumovirus from cDNA: Optimization of growth in vitro and expression of additional genes. *Virology, 321*(2), 247–259. https://doi.org/10.1016/j.virol.2003.12.025.

Centers for Disease Control and Prevention (CDC). (2024). *About human metapneumovirus guidelines*. https://www.cdc.gov/human-metapneumovirus/about/index.html.

Chan, P. C., Wang, C. Y., Wu, P. S., Chang, P. Y., Yang, T. T., & Chiang, Y. P. (2007). Detection of human metapneumovirus in hospitalized children with acute respiratory tract infection using real-time RT-PCR in a hospital in northern Taiwan. *Journal of the Formosan Medical Association, 106*(1), 16–24. https://doi.org/10.1016/S0929-6646(09)60211-4.

Chang, A., Masante, C., Buchholz, U. J., & Dutch, R. E. (2012). Human metapneumovirus (HMPV) binding and infection are mediated by interactions between the HMPV fusion protein and heparan sulfate. *Journal of Virology, 86*(6), 3230–3243. https://doi.org/10.1128/JVI.06706-11.

Chu, H. Y., Renaud, C., Ficken, E., Thomson, B., Kuypers, J., & Englund, J. A. (2014). Respiratory tract infections due to human metapneumovirus in immunocompromised children. *Journal of Pediatric Infectious Diseases Society, 3*(4), 286–293. https://doi.org/10.1093/jpids/piu100.

Collins, P. L., Fearns, R., & Graham, B. S. (2013). Respiratory syncytial virus: Virology, reverse genetics, and pathogenesis of disease. *Current Topics in Microbiology and Immunology, 372*, 3–38. https://doi.org/10.1007/978-3-642-38919-1_1.

Cong, S., Wang, C., Wei, T., Xie, Z., Huang, Y., Tan, J., et al., (2022). Human metapneumovirus in hospitalized children with acute respiratory tract infections in Beijing, China. *Infectious Genetics and Evolution, 106*, 105386. https://doi.org/10.1016/j.meegid.2022.105386.

Cox, R. G., Livesay, S. B., Johnson, M., Ohi, M. D., & Williams, J. V. (2012). The human metapneumovirus fusion protein mediates entry via an interaction with RGD-binding integrins. *Journal of Virology, 86*(22), 12148–12160. https://doi.org/10.1128/JVI.01133-12.

Cseke, G., Wright, D. W., Tollefson, S. J., Johnson, J. E., Crowe, J. E., Jr, & Williams, J. V. (2007). Human metapneumovirus fusion protein vaccines that are immunogenic and protective in cotton rats. *Journal of Virology, 81*(2), 698–707. https://doi.org/10.1128/JVI.00844-06.

Cummings, R. D. (2019). Stuck on sugars – How carbohydrates regulate cell adhesion, recognition, and signaling. *Glycoconjugate Journal, 36*(5), 241–257. https://doi.org/10.1007/s10719-019-09893-5.

Darniot, M., Schildgen, V., Schildgen, O., Sproat, B., Kleines, M., Ditt, V., et al., (2012). RNA interference in vitro and in vivo using Dsi RNA targeting the nucleocapsid N mRNA of human metapneumovirus. *Antiviral Research, 93*, 364–373. https://doi.org/10.1016/j.antiviral.2012.01.004.

Deffrasnes, C., Hamelin, M. E., Prince, G. A., & Boivin, G. (2008). Identification and evaluation of highly effective fusion inhibitor for human metapneumovirus. *Antimicrobial Agents and Chemotherapy, 52*(1), 279–287. https://doi.org/10.1128/AAC.00793-07.

Deffrasnes, C., Hamelin, M. E., Prince, G. A., & Boivin, G. (2008). Identification and evaluation of highly effective fusion inhibitor for human metapneumovirus. *Antimicrobial Agents and Chemotherapy, 52*(1), 279–287. https://doi.org/10.1128/AAC.00793-07.

Dick, G., Akslen-Hoel, L. K., Grøndahl, F., Kjos, I., & Prydz, K. (2012). Proteoglycan synthesis and Golgi organization in polarized epithelial cells. *Journal of Histochemistry & Cytochemistry, 60*(11), 926–935. https://doi.org/10.1369/0022155412459853.

Dokos, C., Masjosthusmann, K., Rellensmann, G., Werner, C., Schuler, L. S., & Muller, K. M. (2013). Fatal human metapneumovirus infection following allogeneic hematopoietic stem cell transplantation. *Transplant Infectious Disease, 15*(1), 97–101. https://doi.org/10.1111/tid.12074.

Dokos, C., Masjosthusmann, K., Rellensmann, G., Werner, C., Schuler-Luttmann, S., Müller, K. M., et al., (2013). Fatal human metapneumovirus infection following allogeneic hematopoietic stem cell transplantation. *Transplant Infectious Disease, 15*, E97–E101. https://doi.org/10.1111/tid.12074.

Falsey, A. R., Erdman, D., Anderson, L. J., & Walsh, E. E. (2003). Human metapneumovirus infections in young and elderly adults. *Journal of Infectious Diseases, 187*(5), 785–790. https://doi.org/10.1086/367901.

Falsey, A. R., Erdman, D., Anderson, L. J., & Walsh, E. E. (2003). Human metapneumovirus infections in young and elderly adults. *Journal of Infectious Diseases, 187*(5), 785–790. https://doi.org/10.1086/367901.

Feuillet, F., Lina, B., Rosa-Calatrava, M., & Boivin, G. (2012). Ten years of human metapneumovirus research. *Journal of Clinical Virology, 53*(2), 97–105. https://doi.org/10.1016/j.jcv.2011.10.002.

Hamelin, M. E., Côté, S., Laforge, J., Lampron, N., Bourbeau, J., & Weiss, K. (2005). Human metapneumovirus infection in adults with community-acquired pneumonia and exacerbation of chronic obstructive pulmonary disease. *Clinical Infectious Diseases, 41*(4), 498–502. https://doi.org/10.1086/431981.

Ishiguro, N., Akutsu, Y., Azuma, K., Yonekawa, M., Sato, D., Ishizaka, A., et al., (2021). Evaluation of a novel immunochromatographic assay using monoclonal antibodies against the matrix protein of human metapneumovirus. *Clinical Laboratory, 67*(10), 1. https://doi.org/10.7754/Clin.Lab.2021.210232.

Jia, N., Byrd-Leotis, L., Matsumoto, Y., Gao, C., Wein, A. N., Lobby, J. L., Kohlmeier, J. E., Steinhauer, D. A., & Cummings, R. D. (2020). The human lung glycome reveals novel glycan ligands for influenza A virus. *Scientific Reports, 10*(1), 5320. https://doi.org/10.1038/s41598-020-62194-w.

Kahn, J. S. (2006). Epidemiology of human metapneumovirus. *Clinical Microbiology Reviews, 19*(3), 546–557. https://doi.org/10.1128/CMR.00014-06.

Kim, J. I., Park, S., Lee, I., Park, K. S., Kwak, E. J., Moon, K. M., et al., (2016). Genome-wide analysis of human metapneumovirus evolution. *PLoS ONE, 11*(4), e0152962. https://doi.org/10.1371/journal.pone.0152962.

Liu, S., Wang, C., Wang, H., Zhang, Y., Li, J., & Zhao, Y. (2018). Association of genetic polymorphisms in Toll-like receptors with HMPV susceptibility. *BMC Infectious Diseases, 17*(1), 345. https://doi.org/10.1186/s12879-017-2472-0.

Luytjes, W., Krystal, M., Enami, M., Parvin, J. D., & Palese, P. (1989). Amplification, expression, and packaging of a foreign gene by influenza virus. *Cell, 59*(6), 1107–1113. https://doi.org/10.1016/0092-8674(89)90766-6.

Ma, S., Zhu, F., Xu, Y., Wen, H., Rao, M., Zhang, P., et al., (2023). Development of a novel multi-epitope mRNA vaccine candidate to combat HMPV virus. *Human Vaccines & Immunotherapeutics, 19*(3), 2293300. https://doi.org/10.1080/21645515.2023.2293300.

Márquez-Escobar, V. A., Tirado-Mendoza, R., Noyola, D. E., Gutiérrez-Ortega, A., & Alpuche-Solís, A. G. (2015). HRA2pl peptide: A fusion inhibitor for human metapneumovirus produced in tobacco plants by transient transformation. *Planta*. https://doi.org/10.1007/s00425-015-2277-5.

Matsuda, S., Nakamura, M., Hirano, E., Kiyota, N., Omura, T., & Suzuki, Y. (2013). Characteristics of human metapneumovirus infection prevailing in hospital wards housing patients with severe disabilities. *Japanese Journal of Infectious Diseases, 66*(3), 195–200. https://doi.org/10.7883/yoken.66.195.

Matsuzaki, Y., Mizuta, K., Takashita, E., Okamoto, M., Itagaki, T., & Katsushima, F. (2010). Comparison of virus isolation using the Vero E6 cell line with RT RT-PCR assay for detection of hMPV. *BMC Infectious Diseases, 10*, 170. https://doi.org/10.1186/1471-2334-10-170.

Melero, J. A., Mas, V., & McLellan, J. S. (2017). Structural, antigenic, and immunogenic features of respiratory syncytial virus glycoproteins relevant for vaccine development. *Vaccine, 35*(3), 461–468. https://doi.org/10.1016/j.vaccine.2016.11.112.

Munoz, N. C., Branttie, J., Slaughter, K. B., & Dutch, R. E. (2017). Human metapneumovirus induces formation of inclusion bodies for efficient genome replication and transcription. *Journal of Virology, 91*(24), e01282-17. https://doi.org/10.1128/JVI.01282-17.

Muñoz, N. C., Branttie, J., Slaughter, K. B., & Dutch, R. E. (2017). Human metapneumovirus induces formation of inclusion bodies for efficient genome replication and transcription. *Journal of Virology, 91*(24), e01282-17. https://doi.org/10.1128/JVI.01282-17.

Nao, N., Saikusa, M., Sato, K., Sekizuka, T., Usuku, S., Tanaka, N., et al., (2020). Recent molecular evolution of human metapneumovirus (HMPV): Subdivision of HMPV

A2b strains. *Microorganisms, 8*(9), 1280. https://doi.org/10.3390/microorganisms 8091280.

Panda, S., Mohakud, N. K., Pena, L., & Kumar, S. (2014). Human metapneumovirus: Review of an important respiratory pathogen. *International Journal of Infectious Diseases, 25*, 45–52. https://doi.org/10.1016/j.ijid.2014.03.1391.

Park, S., Baek, S., Lee, S., Choi, S., Kim, Y. S., Woo, J. H., et al., (2013). Efficacy of oral ribavirin in hematologic disease patients with paramyxovirus infection: Analytic strategy using propensity scores. *Antimicrobial Agents and Chemotherapy, 57*(3), 983–989. https://doi.org/10.1128/AAC.01961-12.

Perotin, J. M., Dury, S., Renois, F., Deslee, G., Wolak, A., & Duval, V. (2013). Detection of multiple viral and bacterial infections in acute exacerbation of chronic obstructive pulmonary disease: A pilot prospective study. *Journal of Medical Virology, 85*(5), 866–873. https://doi.org/10.1002/jmv.23495.

Pilger, D. A., Cantarelli, V. V., Amentea, S. L., & Leistner-Segal, S. (2011). Detection of human bocavirus and human metapneumovirus by real-time PCR from patients with respiratory symptoms in Southern Brazil. *Memórias do Instituto Oswaldo Cruz, 106*(1), 56–60. https://doi.org/10.1590/s0074-02762011000100009.

Piyaratna, R., Tollefson, S. J., & Williams, J. V. (2011). Genomic analysis of four human metapneumovirus prototypes. *Virus Research, 160*(1–2), 200–205. https://doi.org/ 10.1016/j.virusres.2011.06.006.

Principi, N., & Esposito, S. (2014). Paediatric human metapneumovirus infection: Epidemiology, prevention and therapy. *Journal of Clinical Virology, 59*(2), 141–147. https://doi.org/10.1016/j.jcv.2014.01.003.

Roymans, D., Alnajjar, S. S., Battles, M. B., Sitthicharoenchai, P., Furmanova-Hollenstein, P., Rigaux, P., et al., (2017). Therapeutic efficacy of a respiratory syncytial virus fusion inhibitor. *Nature Communications, 8*, 167–181. https://doi.org/10.1038/ s41467-017-00170-x.

Safdar, A. (2008). Immune modulatory activity of ribavirin for serious human metapneumovirus disease: Early i.v. therapy may improve outcomes in immunosuppressed SCT recipients. *Bone Marrow Transplantation, 41*(6), 707–708. https://doi.org/10.1038/bmt.2008.80.

Schmidt, A. C., Schaap-Nutt, A., Bartlett, E. J., Schomacker, H., Boonyaratanakornkit, J., & Collins, P. L. (2009). Progress in human metapneumovirus vaccine development. *Expert Review of Vaccines, 8*(4), 435–447. https://doi.org/10.1586/erv.09.15.

Schuster, J. E., Cox, R. G., Hastings, A. K., Boyd, K. L., Wadia, J., Chen, Z., et al., (2015). A broadly neutralizing human monoclonal antibody exhibits in vivo efficacy against both human metapneumovirus and respiratory syncytial virus. *Journal of Infectious Diseases, 211*, 216–225. https://doi.org/10.1093/infdis/jiu307.

Spetch, L., Bowlin, T. L., & Casola, A. (2008). Effect of NMSO3 treatment in a murine model of human metapneumovirus infection. *Journal of General Virology, 89*, 2709–2712. https://doi.org/10.1099/vir.0.2008/003301-0.

Uche, I. K., & Guerrero-Plata, A. (2018). Interferon-mediated response to human metapneumovirus infection. *Viruses, 10*(9), 499. https://doi.org/10.3390/v10090499.

Uddin, S., & Thomas, M. (2023, July 17). *Human Metapneumovirus*. In StatPearls. StatPearls Publishing. https://www.ncbi.nlm.nih.gov/books/NBK560910/.

Van den Hoogen, B. G., de Jong, J. C., Groen, J., Kuiken, T., de Groot, R., Fouchier, R. A. M., & Osterhaus, A. D. M. E. (2001). A newly discovered human pneumovirus isolated from young children with respiratory tract disease. *Nature Medicine, 7*(6), 719–724. https://doi.org/10.1038/89098.

Van den Hoogen, B. G., de Jong, J. C., Groen, J., Kuiken, T., de Groot, R., Fouchier, R. A. M., & Osterhaus, A. D. M. E. (2001). A newly discovered human pneumovirus isolated from young children with respiratory tract disease. *Nature Medicine, 7*(6), 719–724. https://doi.org/10.1038/89098.

Van den Hoogen, B. G., van Doornum, G. J., Fockens, J. C., Cornelissen, J. J., Beyer, W. E., & de Groot, R. (2003). Prevalence and clinical symptoms of human metapneumovirus infection in hospitalized patients. *Journal of Infectious Diseases, 188*(10), 1571–1577. https://doi.org/10.1086/379200.

Vinci, A., Lee, P. J., & Krilov, L. R. (2018). Human metapneumovirus infection. *Pediatrics in Review, 39*(12), 623–624. https://doi.org/10.1542/pir.2018-0003.

Walther, T., Karamanska, R., Chan, R. W. Y., Chan, M. C. W., Jia, N., Air, G., Hopton, C., Wong, M. P., Dell, A., Malik Peiris, J. S., Haslam, S. M., & Nicholls, J. M. (2013). Glycomic analysis of human respiratory tract tissues and correlation with influenza virus infection. *PLoS Pathogens, 9*(3), e1003223. https://doi.org/10.1371/journal.ppat.1003223.

Williams, J. V., et al., (2006). Differential virulence between HMPV subgroups. *Journal of Infectious Diseases, 193*(5), 579–586. https://doi.org/10.1086/500239.

Williams, J. V., Harris, P. A., Tollefson, S. J., et al., (2023). The burden of HMPV disease in hospitalized children. *Journal of the Pediatric Infectious Diseases Society, 12*(1), 11–18. https://doi.org/10.1093/jpids/piac057.

Williams, J. V., Martino, R., Rabella, N., Otegui, M., Parody, R., & Heck, J. M. (2005). A prospective study comparing human metapneumovirus with other respiratory viruses in adults with hematologic malignancies and respiratory tract infections. *Journal of Infectious Diseases, 192*(6), 1061–1065. https://doi.org/10.1086/432732.

Wyde, P. R., Moylett, E. H., Chetty, S. N., Jewell, A., Bowlin, T. L., & Piedra, P. A. (2004). Comparison of the inhibition of human metapneumovirus and respiratory syncytial virus by NMSO3 in tissue culture assays. *Antiviral Research, 63*, 51–59. https://doi.org/10.1016/j.antiviral.2004.02.006.

Zhang, Y., Wang, Z., Zhang, J., Wu, J., Zhang, Y., Wang, H., & Li, J. (2014). Toll-like receptor 3 polymorphisms and susceptibility to respiratory infections. *Journal of Clinical Immunology, 34*(4), 460–467. https://doi.org/10.1007/s10875-014-0011-0.

Chapter 11

Emerging Technologies for Human Metapneumovirus Research

Sahil Dhiman[1]
Deepshi Arora[1]
Deepak Singla[1]
and Ganga Reddy Velma[2,*]
[1]Guru Gobind Singh College of Pharmacy, Haryana, India
[2]Department of Pharmacology and Toxicology, R. K. Coit, College of Pharmacy, University of Arizona, Tucson, USA

Abstract

A big reason behind the occurrence of ARTIs (acute respiratory tract infections) is mostly the HMPV (human metapneumovirus), which can be dangerous for people with impaired immune systems, children and the elderly. Seroprevalence studies have shown that 90 to 100% of children have contracted HMPV by the time they are 5 to 10 years old. 5–10% of paediatric hospitalisations are due to the acute lower respiratory tract infections caused by HMPV. Children who were less than six months old with HMPV infection had a three times higher chance of being admitted to the hospital than children aged between six months and five years. Despite the widespread impact of HMPV, there are currently no approved antiviral or vaccines available for its treatment. This chapter includes the innovative diagnostic tools for improvement in the detection and sensitivity, like RT-RPA, RT-PCR, isothermal amplification techniques and RISPR/Cas12a-based assays. Antivirals like probenecid and remdesivir, monoclonal antibodies, RNA-based vaccinations and

* Corresponding Author's Email: vgreddy@pharmacy.arizona.edu

In: Human Metapneumovirus
Editors: Anjali Sharma, Vishnu Mittal, Devkant Sharma et al.
ISBN: 979-8-90134-063-9

peptide fusion inhibitors are some examples of promising treatment approaches. Next-generation and nanopore sequencing can be utilised to get important information about HMPV evolution, genetic diversity and epidemiological trends. Researchers working on the development of vaccines for HMPV with the help of live-attenuated viruses and recombinant technology are supposed to be successful in future against HMPV. Artificial intelligence can also be very helpful in the development of vaccines for this virus and in accelerating drug discovery. Together, these developments provide a route to better HMPV surveillance, prevention, as well as treatment and fill important gaps in respiratory virus management.

Keywords: emerging technologies, human metapneumovirus, research, respiratory tract, treatment

List of Abbreviations

HMPV	Human Metapneumovirus
ARTIs	Acute Respiratory Tract Infections
RT-RPA	Reverse Transcription Recombinase Polymerase Amplification
RT-PCR	Reverse Transcription Polymerase Chain Reaction
crRNA	CRISPR RNA
Cas12a	CRISPR-associated protein 12a
FQ	Fluorophore-Quencher
TEM	Transmission Electron Microscopy
Cryo-EM	Cryo-Electron Microscopy
PPI	Protein–Protein Interaction
qPCR	Quantitative Polymerase Chain Reaction
VSTs	Virus-Specific T Cells
mAb	Monoclonal Antibody.

Introduction

The infection of the respiratory system, which is caused by human metapneumovirus (HMPV), is a main reason for illness and deaths in elderly people, children and people with weak immune systems. It was initially discovered in 2001 and became a main cause of acute respiratory tract infections (ARTIs) globally (Akingbola et al., 2025). It is less lethal than COVID-19, but it is the reason behind the 1% mortality due to acute lower respiratory infection in children under the age of 5 years (Kumar, Subramaniam, & Kumar, 2025). According to data available on clinical research, there is no vaccine or antiviral available for the treatment of HMPV. New treatments based on RNA are in the development stage, even though small molecule inhibitors, fusion proteins and monoclonal antibodies are used to hinder the virus entry, its replication, and to modulate the immune system (Tewari, Bhardwaj, Ghosh, & Farhana, 2025). As there is currently no antiviral or vaccine treatment available for HMPV, preventive measures like physical distance and cleanliness play a crucial role. However, vaccine development with the help of AI and the development of portable diagnostic equipment will advance the treatment in future (Akingbola et al., 2025). The goal of current research is to understand the reproduction and evasion techniques of HMPV, which will help in the development of treatments.

HMPV Detection

RT-RPA Method

RT-RPA is a method that can quickly detect HMPV. This method eliminates the need for heat cycling, as this is an isothermal nucleic acid amplification method. In this method, RNA is collected from clinical respiratory samples using reverse transcriptase enzyme and is first transformed into complementary DNA. Recombinase polymerase amplification (RPA) uses recombinase proteins, primers, and DNA polymerase to make quick amplification of the target in 20-30 minutes, which is then utilised for the amplification of complementary DNA at a constant temperature, which is between 37 and 42°C. Because it takes very little time for reaction and also works at very low temperature, RT-RPA is an effective method for diagnosis of HMPV (Du et al., 2024).

CRISPR/Cas12a Method

Amplified target sequences, which are specific to HMPV, are detected by CRISPR/Cas12a technology. HMPV-related target DNA sequences are detected by Cas12a enzyme when it is guided by CRISPR RNA (crRNA). When single-stranded DNA goes through cleavage, this activity is demonstrated by Cas12a, and this engagement leads to the activation. The real-time detection is done by fluorescence emission, which is a result of cleavage of fluorophore-quencher (FQ) reporter probe, and this cleavage is done after Cas12a is activated. The fluorophore-quencher (FQ) reporter probe is a very important component of the reaction mixture. For application in the field, Lateral flow assays (LFA) can be used, in which cleaved reporter molecules provide a visible test line for simple result interpretation. Due to its specificity, sensitivity and quickness, this technique is very useful for HMPV detection (Du et al., 2024).

RT-PCR

In HMPV detection by the RT-PCR method, extraction and then purification of nucleic acid are necessary steps, which generate accurate as well as repeatable results. The extraction of RNA from respiratory samples is done automatically by platforms such as the NucliSENS easyMAG, MagNaPure Compact and QIAamp Viral RNA Mini Kit. Those primers that target conserved regions of the material, specifically the N gene, help in the improvement of sensitivity and reliability of the methods. RT-PCR reactions can be one or two-step, but two-step reactions show repeatability but have a higher chance of contamination. This detection technique includes probe hybridisation, gel-based electrophoresis and automated fluorescence capillary electrophoresis. Although the manufacturing cost is very high, great specificity is offered by real-time PCR using molecular beacon or TaqMan probes. Molecular beacon probes re-bind with every cycle, and TaqMan probes cleave at the time of amplification, which enhances fluorescence proportionately. Output, number of targets, and experience level all influence the format selection of the real-time PCR. In experiments that are based on fluorescence, ensuring probe specificity is very important in preventing the overlapping of spectra. Timely improvements in the method keep improving the detection of HMPV by precision and effectiveness (Jeong, Park, Song, & Kim, 2020).

Reverse Transcriptase-Mediated Isothermal Amplification Fluorescence Assay

To detect HMPV, a number of stages are required by reverse transcriptase-mediated isothermal amplification fluorescence test. Extraction of RNA starts with the collection and then processing of respiratory samples, such as nose and throat swabs and bronchoalveolar lavage, with the help of kits such as the NucliSENS easyMAG system or the QIAamp Viral RNA Mini Kit. The RNA extracted from the clinical respiratory sample is reverse transcribed and amplified isothermally in a single-step reaction technique like Recombinase Polymerase Amplification (RPA) or Loop-Mediated Isothermal Amplification (LAMP). This is all done by maintaining the temperature between 60 and 65°C. Specificity and sensitivity are guaranteed by targeting conserved HMPV genomic areas, like the M, F or N genes, with certain primers. Fluorescence-based detection is done by utilising fluorophore-quencher probe systems like TaqMan and dyes as EvaGreen or SYBR Green I. Real-time fluorescence signals are tracked by a qPCR system or a portable fluorescence reader. An increase in the intensity of fluorescence indicates the presence of HMPV RNA. With the help of positive and negative controls, the fluorescence signals are contrasted and the results are interpreted.

Electron Microscopy

Structural understanding of the HMPV has enhanced significantly due to the advancements in imaging techniques, particularly electron microscopy (EM). Modern cryo-electron microscopy (cryo-EM) and transmission electron microscopy (TEM) allow high-resolution visualisation of F and G proteins of HMPV. With the help of these tools, it is easy to reveal fine ultrastructural details of the virus components, which aids in the differentiation between different types of pneumoviruses. Cryo-EM has eased the conformational elucidation of the perfusion of the F protein, which is very critical for the development of vaccines. These types of advancements back the targeted delivery of antivirals by clarifying the interaction of virus and host at the molecular level (Satapathy et al., 2025). In 2020 cryo-EM was used in order to determine the high-resolution structure of HMPV polymerase-phosphoprotein (L–P) complex by Pan et al., Cryo-EM enabled visualisation (at a resolution of 3.7 Å) of the complex, revealing in-depth interactions between the catalytic L protein and its cofactor P. Overall architecture of the RNA-dependent RNA polymerase was captured by this technique in its functional state. How the P protein stabilises the conformation of the L protein was uncovered by cryo-EM conformation, supporting its replicative and transcriptional roles. More than 1 million particle images were selected and processed carefully using cryoSPARC and RELION software in order to get structural insights. This cryo-EM structure advances our understanding of replication mechanisms of HMPV because it is the first near-atomic model of a pneumovirus polymerase complex (Pan et al., 2020).

Treatment

Monoclonal Antibodies

The fusion (F) protein of HMPV is essential for viral entry and membrane fusion. This F protein is targeted by a potent monoclonal antibody (mAb 100) and inhibits the HMPV. Treatment of HMPV in a mouse model by mAb 100 caused a reduction in lung viral titers, showing effective antiviral potential when given both prophylactically and therapeutically. Viral fusion and replication are blocked by this antibody by binding to an epitope on the F protein, which causes the neutralisation of the HMPV. When the treated mice were compared with the controls, histopathological analysis of lung tissues showed a reduction in the inflammation and improvement in the health of treated mice (Fausther-Bovendo et al., 2022).

RNA-Based Therapies

A new vaccine, rather a new multi-epitope mRNA vaccine, is introduced to fight against HMPV. Our immune system is capable of identifying the HMPV-specific protein parts. Some examples of the epitopes from the virus protein are matrix, M2, small hydrophobic, glycoprotein and fusion proteins. Several epitopes from the protein of the virus are first identified and then combined. It has been shown using in-silico methods (like molecular docking) that these epitopes are encoded into a single mRNA and the vaccine stably attaches to the immunological receptors in order to trigger cellular and humoral responses (Ma et al., 2024).

Peptide-Based Fusion Inhibitors

The first step in the occurrence of infection is always the entry of the virus into the host. The F protein of HMPV is the main reason for the entry and multiplication of the virus into the host. That is why. This protein is always considered when developing any antiviral strategy. Heptad repeat A region, which is represented by the peptide HRA2, demonstrates strong antiviral activity. An in vitro test is done which shows the replication of HMPV is stopped by HRA2 in cell cultures. In an in vivo investigation, mice treated with HRA2 were completely protected from the clinical signs and mortality shown by HMPV. When compared with controls, these treated animals showed less inflammation and the lung virus was undetectable. These results imply that HRA2 and related peptides may be effective antiviral medicines for hMPV infections (Van Den Bergh, Bailly, Guillon, von Itzstein, & Dirr, 2022).

Drugs

Recent computational studies have investigated the use of some antiviral drugs, which are approved by the FDA with the help of ADMET profiling, dynamics simulations and molecular docking against HMPV. Remdesivir, with a binding energy of -9.5 kcal/mol, and Peramivir, with -9.2 kcal/mol, showed good binding affinities to the F protein of HMPV, making them candidates that can be used against HMPV. In the case of Remdesivir, the drug-protein interactions were found to be stable as demonstrated by molecular dynamics simulations, with a lowest root mean square deviation of 0.20 nm. Pharmacophore analysis highlighted the hydrogen bonding and hydrophobic interactions that are very necessary for antiviral activity. Minimum toxicity as well as high bioavailability (85% ± 3 for Remdesivir) were confirmed by ADMET profiling, which means Remdesivir is a safe treatment choice. These findings speed up the development of new antiviral drugs by providing a ground for research on clinically approved antivirals against HMPV. A computational study reduced the cost of drug screening by reducing the lengthy lab studies. Antiviral activity of these candidates can be confirmed by in vitro and in vivo studies in future. By combining computational and experimental methods, targeted therapies can be advanced in treating HMPV (Dubey, Kumar, Tufail, & Dwivedi, 2025).

Antiviral property of probenecid was assessed by Bergeron et al., for HMPV both in vivo and in vitro. For in vitro studies, LLC-MK2 cells, which were infected by the HMPV strain CAN83, were used, and the cells were exposed to concentrations of probenecid. According the results, virus replication was reduced significantly at concentrations of 0.5 μm and above. For the in vivo study, probenecid was given to BALB/c mice at doses of 2 mg/kg or 200 mg/kg 24 hours prior to infection or therapeutically 24 hours post-infection. Then the mice were given 10^6 PFU of HMPV strain CAN83 by intranasal route. Lung tissues, which were obtained on day 5 after infection, showed decreased viral titers in a dose-dependent manner and a 4-log drop was seen in the case of 200 mg/kg. These results confirm the potential of probenecid for treatment and prevention of HMPV (Bergeron, Crabtree, Nagy, Martin, & Tripp, 2024).

Genome Sequencing and Evolution Analyses

In order to fully understand the molecular epidemiology of HMPV, Wei et al., in 2023 studied whole genome sequencing and evolution of the virus. Quantitative PCR was used by researchers to identify HMPV-positive samples. The samples were taken from nasopharyngeal aspirates from hospitalised children under the age of 14 who were suffering from acute respiratory tract infections (ARTIs). The scientists were able to amplify and sequence 27 genomes of HMPV using 14 pairs of overlapping primers. When the samples of the genetic materials were studied, except the G gene of the virus, most of the genetic material was found to be the same in all samples. 111 nucleotides were the extra section that makes the G gene different from others (Wei et al., 2023).

In 2021, Tulloch et al., started developing a method and achieved success in sequencing the full genome. This was done to support other studies that were ongoing on its evolution. In order to detect all subtypes of the genomes, they targeted conserved regions. For amplifying the whole genome, PCR was done. Qubit Fluorimeter was then used for the measurement then purified, and prepared for sequencing. The Illumina iSeq 100 platform was used for sequencing, producing high-depth reads that were quality-filtered and put together using de novo and reference-guided assembly techniques. Sequence correctness was validated by the confirmation of genetic diversity and subtype classification by phylogenetic analysis. With the improvement in genomic investigation of HMPV, this method aids in epidemiological research (Tulloch, Kok, Carter, Dwyer, & Eden, 2021).

Ponana et al., examined the prevalence, evolution and genetic diversity of HMPV in Spain between 2014 and 2021. This study shows that the prevalence was 2.5 % according to their analysis of laboratory-confirmed HMPV cases, with February-March as the seasonal maximum. The prevalence of HMPV subtypes A and B alternated before the COVID-19 pandemic. But HMPV occurrence was disturbed after SARS-CoV-2, and no such cases were seen until summer and winter of 2021. The prevalence of the A2c_111dup variant of HMPV increased during this time. 70% of the fusion protein was subject to negative selection, and G and SH proteins were the most variable proteins according to genetic analysis. Annually, the mutation rate in the HMPV genome was calculated to be 6.95×10^{-4} substitutions/site. This shows how COVID-19 affected HMPV epidemiology and stressed on the value of ongoing virological investigation to find and track new variants (Piñana et al., 2023).

To get the HMPV whole genome sequence from the clinical samples directly, Groen et al., used MinION nanopore sequencing technology in 2021. The researchers made overlapping primers that can target conserved regions of the genome to amply the RNA of HMPV from patient samples. Then the amplified RNA went through MinION sequencing, which enabled long-read, real-time sequencing of the HMPV genome. This method was equally sensitive for all four HMPV sublineages (A1, A2, B1, B2), including the highly variable G gene and created complete HMPV genomes with good coverage. This proved to be a useful tool for research in HMPV epidemiology, to study the genetics and evolution of HMPV (Groen et al., 2021).

Vaccines

Tian et al., in 2023 made a novel influenza virus vaccine that can express the epitopes of the HMPV fusion protein. This was done in order to produce immunity against HMPV. A recombinant influenza virus named rFLU-HMPV/F-NS was created by scientists by using reverse genetics, which added partial HMPV-F sequences to the influenza A/Puerto Rico/8/34 (PR8) virus non-structural (NS) segment. This virus showed proliferation in pathogen-free chicken embryos while retaining morphological characteristics similar to those of the wild-type influenza virus. BALB/c mice were given the vaccine and immunised through rFLU-HMPV/F-NS. This was done through the intranasal route. After this immunisation, when the mice were exposed to the virus, the vaccinated mice were seen developing a strong immune response. Tissue damage in the lungs was very little and the virus load was significantly reduced (Chongyu et al., 2023).

Omics Technology

Intractome Analysis

A study was done in 2020 by Rouka and colleagues to know the way by which HMPV interact with host cells. They used computer-based omics tools for this study. They study the interaction at the molecular level with the help of a database available for protein-protein interactions. The findings of the study showed that the main targets for the virus were pathways related to cell death, the immune system and cell signalling. By using the findings of this research, we can easily make ways to fight HMPV (Rouka et al., 2020).

Transcriptomics

How lung cells respond to HMPV was studied in 2008 by Bao and his team. They used microarray technology to study the changes in the activity of genes. They found that there were many changes in the genes when they interacted with the virus. Especially those genes that were altered were involved in cell death, the immune system, and inflammatory mechanisms. These type of studies helps us to know the process of infection by a virus at the genetic level, as there were also some findings that during infection, some genes related to inflammation, like RANTES and IL-8, were turned on more than usual (Bao et al., 2008).

Quantitative Proteomics

In 2017, Ren and his team used quantitative differential proteomics to determine the changes in proteins when the M2-2 protein present in HMPV induces changes inside the nucleus of host cells. By analysing with some advanced techniques like mass spectroscopy, it was found that levels of some nuclear proteins were altered by M2-2. Changes in gene regulations, RNA processing and cell functioning were some of the findings that M2-2 did. This shows that in order to develop and replicate itself, HMPV disturbs the host cell system (Ren et al., 2017).

AI and Computational Approaches

Exploring Chemical Space to Identify Partial Binders against hMPV Nucleocapsid Protein

Verma et al., investigated the chemical space in order to find binders for the HMPV nucleocapsid (N) protein, which is an important part for RNA replication and encapsulation. They studied compounds of natural origin as well as their derivatives from the ZINC database by using structure-based virtual screening, and then, by using 250-nanosecond molecular dynamics simulations, they evaluated binding stability. RMSD, RMSF, and radius of gyration revealed that M1 (ZINC85629735) and M3 (ZINC85569125) had favourable structural stability and strong docking affinities of -9.6 and -10.7 kcal/mol, respectively, among the compounds identified. The binding potential of these compounds was further validated by using MMGBSA calculations, and the energy value comes out to be -81.94 kcal/mol (M1) and -99.63 kcal/mol (M3) (Verma, Panchal, & Yadav, 2025).

Repurposing Metal-Based Therapeutics for Human Metapneumovirus (HMPV)

In 2025, Dubey screened a large number of metal-based drugs to find out ways by which these drugs interact with the virus. The use of metal-based drugs in combating HMPV was studied by Dubey and his colleagues. They used computer-based techniques to find a way to eliminate viruses with metal-based drugs. This study opens new ways to think about how to treat HMPV infections. Some of the results by molecular docking showed that the interactions were very strong and stable, which is necessary for selecting a candidate. Compounds based on platinum and gold demonstrated antiviral potential because they formed stable contact with the F and N proteins of HMPV. These results imply that metal-based drugs can be a potential candidate for the antiviral activity against HMPV (Dubey, Kumar, Tufail, & Dwivedi, 2025).

Vaccine

AI greatly aid the development of antiviral vaccines for HMPV, which can target the F protein of the virus. The structural confirmation of the F protein has been studied and optimised with the help of deep learning models like Rosetta and Alpha Fold, which guarantee that its highly immunogenic perfusion state. With the help of AI, protein engineering makes it possible to identify stable mutations that stop refolding prematurely into the less useful form post-fusion. Antigenicity and thermostability of vaccine candidates have been improved by the scientists through the use of molecular dynamics simulations and computational modelling. AI-assisted epitope mapping also made it possible to select conserved regions, which guarantees broad immune coverage against a number of strains of HMPV. This technique shortens the time for experiments, which results in the early development of vaccines for HMPV. The use of codons in mRNA sequences is maximised by AI-guided design, improving translational efficiency and expression of host cell protein. These developments help in the production of vaccines that are stable and highly immunogenic, exhibiting outstanding neutralising antibody responses. (Bakkers et al., 2024).

Future

Future immunologic methodologies to HMPV are likely to give emphasis to vaccine development and targeted immunotherapy. One promising strategy for immunocompromised patients, such as those undergoing transplantation of hematopoietic stem cells, is the adoptive transfer of virus-specific T cells. The identification of antigens which are immunodominant, including the matrix (M), nucleocapsid (N) and fusion (F) proteins, is greatly opening ways for the development of immunotherapies and targeted vaccines. Experimental models based on animals also play a vital role in understanding host immune responses and vaccine design. Research inspired by SARS-CoV-2 vaccine development also increases the feasibility for the development of vaccines for HMPV, as there is no approved one yet. A detailed study of the immunologic profile of HMPV can uncover immune markers as well as pathways to develop therapy. Collectively, the aim of all these approaches is to enhance protection against hMPV and reduce the severity of disease in populations (Hsieh et al., 2022; Adedokun et al., 2021).

Conclusion

This chapter systematically explores the advancements made in diagnostic, preventive, and therapeutic strategies against HMPV, which becomes a major cause of ARTs, in populations with weak immune systems. Technologies such as RT-PCR, RT-RPA and CRISPR/Cas12a have considerably improved the sensitivity, speed and point-of-care detection of HMPV. In treatment, computational approaches accelerate molecular targeting and drug repurposing, while peptide fusion inhibitors, RNA-based vaccines and monoclonal antibodies show promising antiviral efficacy. Subtype variability and evolutionary insights are revealed by genome sequencing done with the help of next-generation platforms, aiding in the surveillance of epidemiology. Vaccine development with the help of AI-guided design, chimeric viruses and recombinant platforms has opened new possibilities for long-term protection. Deep understanding of host-pathogen interactions is provided by omics technologies like interactome, proteomics and transcriptomic analysis. Altogether, the combination of all these and more tools holds potential for prevention, early detection and treatment of HMPV, thereby addressing the gaps to be filled in the management of respiratory viruses.

References

Adedokun, K. A., Kamorudeen, R. T., & Bello, I. O. (2021). Authorization of the first COVID-19 emergency vaccines: The matters arising. *EXCLI journal*, *20*, 655.

Akingbola, A., Adegbesan, A. A., TundeAlao, S., Adewole, O., Ayikoru, C., Benson, A. E., Shekoni, M., & Chuku, J. (2025). Human metapneumovirus: An emerging respiratory pathogen and the urgent need for improved diagnostics, surveillance, and vaccine development. *Infectious Diseases, 1*(7), 1–7.

Bakkers, M., Ritschel, T., Tiemessen, M., Dijkman, J., Zuffianò, A., Yu, X., Overveld, D., Le, L., Voorzaat, R., Haaren, M., de Man, M., Sem, T., Fits, L., Zahn, R., Juraszek, J., & Langedijk, J. (2024). Efficacious human metapneumovirus vaccine based on AI-guided engineering of a closed prefusion trimer. *Nature Communications, 15,* Article 50659.

Bao, X., Sinha, M., Liu, T., Hong, C., Luxon, B. A., Garofalo, R. P., & Casola, A. (2008). Identification of human metapneumovirus-induced gene networks in airway epithelial cells by microarray analysis. *Virology, 374*(1), 114–127.

Bergeron, H. C., Crabtree, J., Nagy, T., Martin, D. E., & Tripp, R. A. (2024). Probenecid inhibits human metapneumovirus (HMPV) replication in vitro and in BALB/c mice. *Viruses, 16*(7), 1087.

Chongyu, T., Guanglin, L., Fang, S., Zhuoya, D., Hao, Y., Cong, L., Xinyu, L., et al., (2023). A chimeric influenza virus vaccine expressing fusion protein epitopes induces protection from human metapneumovirus challenge in mice. *Frontiers in Microbiology, 13,* 1012873.

Dubey, A., Kumar, M., Tufail, A., & Dwivedi, V. D. (2025). Exploring FDA-approved antiviral drugs for human metapneumovirus treatment: Integrative computational insights. *bioRxiv,* 2025-01.

Dubey, A., Kumar, M., Tufail, A., & Dwivedi, V. D. (2025). Repurposing metal-based therapeutics for human metapneumovirus (HMPV): An integrative computational approach. *bioRxiv,* 2025-01.

Du, Y., Liu, X., Gao, H., Liu, X., Huang, M., Chai, Q., Xing, Z., Zhang, T., & Ma, D. (2024). Rapid and one-tube detection of human metapneumovirus using the RT-RPA and CRISPR/Cas12a. *Journal of Virological Methods, 329,* 115001.

Fausther-Bovendo, H., Hamelin, M.-E., Carbonneau, J., Venable, M.-C., Checkmahomed, L., Lavoie, P.-O., Ouellet, M.-È., Boivin, G., D'Aoust, M.-A., & Kobinger, G. P. (2022). A candidate therapeutic monoclonal antibody inhibits both HRSV and HMPV replication in mice. *Biomedicines, 10*(10), 2516.

Groen, K., van Nieuwkoop, S., Bestebroer, T. M., Fraaij, P. L., Fouchier, R. A. M., & van den Hoogen, B. G. (2021). Whole genome sequencing of human metapneumoviruses from clinical specimens using MinION nanopore technology. *Virus Research, 302,* 198490.

Hsieh, C. L., Rush, S. A., Palomo, C., Chou, C. W., Pickens, W., Más, V., & McLellan, J. S. (2022). Structure-based design of prefusion-stabilised human metapneumovirus fusion proteins. *Nature communications*, *13*(1), 1299.

Jeong, S., Park, M. J., Song, W., & Kim, H. S. (2020). Advances in laboratory assays for detecting human metapneumovirus. *Annals of Translational Medicine, 8*(9), 608.

Kumar, S., Subramaniam, G., & Kumar, K. J. S. (2025). Human metapneumovirus (HMPV) outbreak: An urgent call for enhanced surveillance and public health action. *Journal of Medical Virology, 97*(2), e70199.

Ma, S., Zhu, F., Xu, Y., Wen, H., Rao, M., Zhang, P., Peng, W., et al., (2024). Development of a novel multi-epitope mRNA vaccine candidate to combat the HMPV virus. *Human Vaccines & Immunotherapeutics, 20*(1), 2293300.

Pan, J., Qian, X., Lattmann, S., El Sahili, A., Yeo, T. H., Jia, H., ... & Lescar, J. (2020). Structure of the human metapneumovirus polymerase phosphoprotein complex. *Nature*, *577*(7789), 275–279.

Piñana, M., González-Sánchez, A., Andrés, C., Abanto, M., Vila, J., Esperalba, J., Moral, N., et al., (2023). The emergence, impact, and evolution of human metapneumovirus variants from 2014 to 2021 in Spain. *Journal of Infection, 87*(2), 103–110.

Ren, Y., Choi, E., Zhang, K., Chen, Y., Ye, S., Deng, X., Zhang, K., & Bao, X. (2017). Detection of nuclear protein profile changes by human metapneumovirus M2-2 protein using quantitative differential proteomics. *Vaccines, 5*(4), 45.

Rouka, E., Hatzoglou, C., Gourgoulianis, K. I., & Zarogiannis, S. G. (2020). Interactome networks between the human respiratory syncytial virus (HRSV), the human metapneumovirus (HMPV), and their host: In silico investigation and comparative functional enrichment analysis. *Microbial Pathogenesis, 141*, 104000.

Satapathy, T., Satapathy, A., Satapathy, A., Yadav, N., Chandrakar, M., & Chandrakar, K. (2025). Recent outbreaks of Human Metapneumovirus (HMPV): Prevention, Diagnosis and Therapeutic insights. *Journal of Drug Delivery & Therapeutics*, *15*(2).

Tewari, S., Bhardwaj, S. K., Ghosh, A., & Farhana, K. (2025). Therapeutic intervention against human metapneumovirus (HMPV) associated symptoms. *Journal of Advances in Microbiology Research, 6*(1), 1–5.

Tulloch, R. L., Kok, J., Carter, I., Dwyer, D. E., & Eden, J.-S. (2021). An amplicon-based approach for the whole-genome sequencing of human metapneumovirus. *Viruses, 13*(3), 499.

Van Den Bergh, A., Bailly, B., Guillon, P., von Itzstein, M., & Dirr, L. (2022). Antiviral strategies against human metapneumovirus: Targeting the fusion protein. *Antiviral Research, 207,* 105405.

Verma, M., Panchal, N. S., & Yadav, P. K. (2025). Exploring chemical space to identify partial binders against hMPV nucleocapsid protein. *Journal of Cellular Biochemistry, 126*(1), e30618.

Wei, T., Wang, C., Ma, F., Guo, J., Chen, A., Huang, Y., Xie, Z., & Zheng, L. (2023). Whole genome sequencing and evolution analyses of human metapneumovirus. *Virus Genes, 59*(4), 524–531.

Chapter 12

Global Initiatives for Controlling Human Metapneumovirus (HMPV)

Himanshu Sharma[1]
Akashdeep Singh[1]
Vishnu Mittal[2]
Pooja Mittal[3]
and Vinit N. Deshmukh[4,*]
[1]Chitkara College of Pharmacy, Chitkara University, Rajpura, Punjab, India
[2]Adesh College of Pharmacy, Kurukshetra
[3]GITAM School of Pharmacy, GITAM (Deemed to be) University, Rudraram, Patancheru, Sangareddy District, Hyderabad, India
[4]Department of Molecular Biology & Genetics, Krishna Vishwa Vidyapeeth (Deemed to be University), Malkapur, Karad (Dist - Satara), Maharashtra, India

Abstract

The Paramyxoviridae family includes the important respiratory pathogen known as human Metapneumovirus (HMPV), which was identified in 2001 and causes a significant amount of morbidity and mortality worldwide. HMPV has no particular therapies or vaccinations, and it is still underdiagnosed despite its clinical consequences. By investigating its virological traits, epidemiology, clinical manifestations, pathogenesis, diagnostic techniques, and management strategies, this viewpoint seeks to present a thorough understanding of HMPV as a newly developing respiratory pathogen. By analysing peer-reviewed papers from 2001 to 2025, this review summarises the present body of knowledge on HMPV

* Corresponding Author's Email: vinitdeshmukh1825@gmail.com

In: Human Metapneumovirus
Editors: Anjali Sharma, Vishnu Mittal, Devkant Sharma et al.
ISBN: 979-8-90134-063-9

and looks at its virological traits, epidemiology, clinical symptoms, pathogenesis, and therapeutic strategies. Lower respiratory tract infections affect an estimated 14.2 million children under five each year, leading to 643,000 hospital admissions and 16,100 in-hospital fatalities. HMPV is the cause of 5–10% of child respiratory hospitalisations worldwide. Improvements in diagnostics, especially in molecular methods, have improved the capacity for detection. Even while therapeutic research is focused on antiviral drugs, monoclonal antibodies, and vaccine candidates employing modern platforms like nanoparticle and mRNA technology, the majority of current therapy is supportive care. To combat HMPV, new therapeutic strategies, quicker vaccine development, and expanded worldwide surveillance are required. Understanding immune evasion mechanisms, long-term immunity, and the effects of the environment on transmission are among the top research goals. To convert scientific findings into practical treatments that lessen the public health burden of HMPV, cooperation between academics, business, public health organisations, and regulatory agencies is crucial.

Keywords: human metapneumovirus (HMPV), vaccines, surveillance, random reverse transcription-polymerase chain reaction

List of Abbreviations

HMPV	Human Metapneumovirus
RSV	Respiratory Syncytial Virus
ARI	Acute Respiratory Infection
RT-PCR	Reverse Transcription Polymerase Chain Reaction
RADTs	Rapid Antigen Detection Tests
CTLs	Cytotoxic T Lymphocytes
NK cells	Natural Killer Cells
PD-1	Programmed Cell Death Protein 1
PD-L1	Programmed Death-Ligand 1
COPD	Chronic Obstructive Pulmonary Disease
BAL	Bronchoalveolar Lavage
mAbs	Monoclonal Antibodies
IVIg	Intravenous Immunoglobulin
RNAi	RNA Interference
ELISA	Enzyme-Linked Immunosorbent Assay
DFA	Direct Fluorescent Antibody

NGS	Next-Generation Sequencing
PM2.5	Particulate Matter less than 2.5 micrometers.

Overview of Human Metapneumovirus (HMPV)

The human metapneumovirus (HMPV) is a common cause of respiratory tract infections in children, adults, the elderly, and people with compromised immune systems (Haas et al., 2013). Recent research, however, indicates that hMPV, particularly in susceptible groups, may have detrimental and sometimes lethal consequences when paired with influenza and respiratory syncytial virus (RSV). Furthermore, an estimated 101,400 people die each year as a result of RSV. Recent estimates of the worldwide burden of respiratory illnesses have brought attention to their substantial impact (Porwal et al., 2025).

The growing importance of hMPV in the public health discourse has been highlighted by the World Health Organisation's most recent outbreak warnings, particularly the 2024 pandemic in China. A deeper understanding of the epidemiology, transmission dynamics, and therapeutic implications of hMPV is essential due to its substantial contribution to ARI-related morbidity and death(Maurya, 2025). The two genera that make up the Pneumoviridae family are Orthopneumovirus, which comprises RSV, and Metapneumovirus, which contains hMPV. Although it mostly affects small children and the elderly, the hMPV may cause respiratory tract infections in persons of all ages. Asthma symptoms may worsen during the illness, and both traditional and non-classical acute respiratory infections are included in the burden of hMPV. The epidemiology, pathophysiology, clinical symptoms in hospital and community settings, distinct transmission patterns, and difficulties in identifying and treating hMPV were all investigated in this study. In order to better contextualise its effects and support further research and public health initiatives, it also made analogies to other respiratory viruses.

Discovery and Classification

Using electron microscopy and random reverse transcription-polymerase chain reaction (RT-PCR) on archival nasopharyngeal samples from 28 infants with respiratory problems, Dutch researchers discovered HMPV in

2001(Carelli, 2019). Despite the absence of hemadsorption, this new virus showed cytotoxic effects on tertiary monkey kidney epithelial cells. Up to 88% of the avian metapneumovirus's genome and serotype C are the same (van Boheemen, 2014). Nevertheless, the recently identified virus spreads more readily in monkeys than in birds. There were HMPV-2 neutralising antibodies in the serum from the 1950s. Together, these findings demonstrate that HMPV has existed for a considerable amount of time without being recognized (Brynes, 2024).

Epidemiology

Serological testing has shown that the human metapneumovirus has been present in the Netherlands since 1958, but it wasn't until 2001 that it was discovered to cause clinical symptoms in infants (de Graaf et al., 2008). HMPV infections may happen on any continent, although they are more common in the northern hemisphere in late winter and early spring, despite the fact that they are recorded throughout the year. Whether the four main subgroups, A1, A2, B1, and B2, cause diseases of different severity is unknown. Additionally, no strain is more prevalent than any other. With an average age of 22 months, HMPV is more common in the pediatric population, particularly in children under the age of two. According to seroprevalence studies, 90–100% of children had acquired HMPV by the time they were 5–10 years old (Yousafzai et al., 2018) . Five to ten per cent of all child hospitalisations are related to acute lower respiratory tract infections caused by HMPV. Compared to children aged 6 months to 5 years, children under 6 months who had an HMPV infection had a threefold higher chance of being admitted to the hospital. Re-infection may also result from different virus genotypes or from an inadequate response to the first infection. Adults often only have mild flu-like symptoms, but those who are elderly, have compromised immune systems, or have chronic lung conditions may experience more challenges (Huang et al., 2025).

Virology of HMPV

Structure and Genome

Nine proteins, nucleoprotein (N), phosphoprotein (P), matrix protein (M), fusion protein (F), matrix-2 proteins (M2-1 and M2-2), small hydrophobic (SH) protein, glycoprotein (G), and large (L) polymerase protein are encoded by eight genes that make up the approximately 13,000-nucleotide genome (van den Hoogen, 2004). Similar to other paramyxoviruses, the viral replication complex is made up of three proteins: N, L, and P. HMPV and avian metapneumovirus share a genome with RSV; however, they differ in their gene ordering and do not include the non-structural proteins NS1 and NS2. HMPV resembles a paramyxovirus in morphology because to its short protein spike projections 2 and size range of 150–600 nm (Aftab et al., 2017).

Pathogenesis and Immunity

Antibodies that neutralise HMPV are developed by both humans and animals. Neutralising antibodies in mice peak four to six weeks after infection and appear five to seven days later. A single HMPV infection in mouse models 40 and 80 prevents re-infection, and in small animal models 93–96, antibodies could be enough to provide protection. Nevertheless, despite the formation of serum antibodies, viral replication was found when macaques were challenged weeks after the first HMPV infection, and no protection was shown when they were challenged 8 months later. According to these findings, re-infection is possible since both humans and primates gradually lose their antibody levels. Antibodies provide some protection, as shown by a prospective human investigation that found older adults who later developed HMPV had lower baseline levels of HMPV antibodies than those who did not.

In mice, cytotoxic T lymphocytes (CTLs) aid in the removal of HMPV infection. As soon as the infection starts, monocytes, lymphocytes start to penetrate the perivascular and peribronchial regions of the lung (Parks, 2024). The development of total bronchoalveolar lavage cells starts on day 1 and peaks on day 7, after which they gradually decrease to levels that are close to normal by days 21–80. It's unknown what natural killer (NK) cells do. Another research used anti-CD49 to restrict NK cells and observed lower viral replication, while another study used the more specific antibody anti-NK1.1

to limit NK cells and found no impact. T cells may exacerbate conditions linked to HMPV even though they are essential for preventing illness. Reduced pulmonary inflammation, narrower airways, and much reduced weight loss were the results of either CD4+ + or CD8 + T cell depletion (Jones et al., 2002). Modified signalling, decreased cytokine production, decreased motility, and a diminished ability to activate CD4+ + T cells are possible outcomes of HMPV infection.

By upregulating programmed cell death-1 (PD-1), a T-cell surface receptor that suppresses the immunological response and compromises the function of CD8+ + T cells, HMPV circumvents the adaptive immune response. CD8+ + T-cell exhaustion, which has been linked to malignancies and persistent infections, is comparable to this disease. Lung CD8+ + T-cell effector capabilities were significantly reduced, and PD-1 expression rose after re-infection with subsequent HMPV infection. According to our findings, the PD-1/PD-L1 pathway may be linked to re-infection and contributes significantly to immune response evasion during both initial and recurrent HMPV infections (Rogers, 2018).

Clinical Manifestations

Frequent symptoms include rhinorrhea, wheezing, coughing, and fever. Hospitalisation, and further oxygen therapy are required in severe cases of respiratory distress (Cheng et al., 2006). Older persons frequently suffer from severe morbidity, although infections in healthy adults are usually moderate or subclinical. Although the symptoms are similar to those in children, adults may have worsening of heart failure or COPD (Janssen et al., 2011). HMPV's clinical significance in this population is highlighted by community-acquired pneumonia linked to the virus. Immunocompromised people: HMPV infections are frequently severe and protracted in immunocompromised patients, including as organ transplant recipients and chemotherapy patients (Ivanova et al., 2015). Secondary bacterial infections, respiratory failure, and elevated mortality are among the complications. For these high-risk populations, early identification and intervention are essential.

Global Epidemiology of HMPV

HMPV has been found in populations all around the world since its discovery, with late winter and early spring marking seasonal maxima. Geographical variations exist in prevalence rates; research indicates that HMPV is responsible for 5–15% of respiratory illnesses (Porwal et al., 2025; Satapathy et al., 2025). Its widespread nature is highlighted by serological data, which show almost universal exposure by the age of five. The effects of epidemics on hospitalised and long-term care patients with compromised immune systems are highlighted (Watson & Wilkinson, 2021). Immunosuppression, congenital cardiac abnormalities, chronic lung illness, and preterm birth are risk factors for severe disease. Co-infection of HMPV with other respiratory viruses, like rhinovirus, increases the severity of the illness and makes diagnosis more difficult (Georgakopoulou, 2024). The goal of international monitoring programs is to clarify viral epidemiological patterns and guide public health measures. Recent studies indicate that seasonality and HMPV transmission are significantly influenced by environmental factors. In temperate regions, HMPV has elevated activity during the colder months, similar to that of many respiratory viruses (Xu et al., 2021). Low ambient temperatures and decreased humidity, for example, can make viruses more stable and spread more easily while weakening the host's mucosal defences and making them more vulnerable to infection (Moriyama et al., 2020). Person-to-person transmission is further facilitated by indoor crowding in the winter.

Through changing seasonal patterns, shifting geographic distributions that affect respiratory health and air quality, climate change may have an impact on HMPV dynamics (Mirsaeidi et al., 2016). For instance, elevated levels of urban air pollution, especially fine particulate matter (PM2.5), might worsen respiratory disorders and make people more vulnerable to viral infections, such as HMPV. The conventional epidemiological calendar of HMPV may be altered by warmer winters in some areas, either prolonging the seasons of transmission or altering the peak times (Lianou et al., 2025).

Diagnostic Strategies

A combination of test confirmation and clinical suspicion is necessary for an accurate diagnosis of HMPV. RT-PCR, the gold standard for HMPV detection with excellent sensitivity and specificity, is one of the common diagnostic modalities (Duong & Ginocchio, 2016). The simultaneous identification of co-infecting respiratory viruses is made possible by multiplex PCR assays, which facilitate thorough diagnostic evaluation. (a) Antigen detection (Kim et al., 2009). Rapid antigen detection tests (RADTs) are less sensitive than molecular procedures, but they offer point-of-care results. The goal of recent developments in immunoassay design has been to increase diagnostic precision. (c) Serology: Although serological assays can identify immune responses and prior exposure, they are not very useful for acute diagnosis (O'Kennedy & Murphy, 2017). New diagnostic tools, like as biosensors and next-generation sequencing, have the potential to improve HMPV surveillance and detection.

RT-PCR and Molecular Tools

For the diagnosis of HMPV, real-time reverse transcription polymerase chain reaction is considered the gold standard (Jeong et al., 2020). All four HMPV lineages can be detected, and the circulating HMPV lineages can be identified using a one-step real-time RT-PCR assay in Pune, India. Conserved regions of the nucleoprotein gene were used to design a probe and real-time primers. This molecular method finds HMPV RNA in respiratory secretions like nasopharyngeal swabs or bronchoalveolar lavage specimens (BAL) (Rishmawi, 2007).

Antigen-Based Tests

The implementation of appropriate infection control measures, which reduce nosocomial transmission, is made possible by rapid testing for HMPV infection diagnosis (Brendish, 2019). These tests also aid in the assessment of timely antiviral medicine treatment. HMPV-specific monoclonal antibodies have been used in rapid antigen tests for HMPV detection. A direct fluorescent-antibody test (DFA) for HMPV was developed by Diagnostic Hybrids (Bartels; Trinity Biotech) (Greene[1] et al., 2016).

Cell Culture and Serology

A major cause of acute respiratory tract infections is the human metapneumovirus (HMPV), a member of the Paramyxoviridae family. HMPV is still difficult to isolate and grow in vitro, and little is known about its cellular tropism and replication kinetics (Kinder, 2020). Furthermore, a thorough characterisation of HMPV's stability under various environmental conditions is required. On the other hand, LLC-MK2 and Vero cells showed the most permissiveness among cell lines originating from non-human primates. Notably, LLC-MK2 cells continue to be the favoured substrate for effective HMPV proliferation because of their resistance to trypsin treatment (Kinder, 2020). Additionally, inoculating monolayer-cultured cells with HMPV significantly increased its infectivity. Serological tests like enzyme-linked immunosorbent tests (ELISA) are very important for seroepidemiological studies and for finding out about human metapneumovirus (HMPV) infections that happened in the past (Kroll & Weinberg, 2011). Serological techniques are not the best for early diagnosis and acute patients (Hodinka, 2016).

Current Therapeutic Approaches

Antiviral medications, antibodies, fusion inhibitors, and RNA interference (RNAi) are the mainstays of HMPV treatment strategies (Bergeron et al., 2024). To determine the effectiveness of treatment for this respiratory virus, these methods are presently being used in a number of in vitro and in vivo models. Antiviral research has looked at ribavirin, which has been demonstrated to reduce viral replication & pulmonary inflammation in BALB/c mice and to interact with HMPV in vitro (Hamelin et al., 2005). Even though there are a few case studies on its application in people, more clinical research is required to ascertain its effectiveness.

Monoclonal and polyclonal antibodies (mAbs), two antibody-based therapeutic modalities, have also shown promise. Intravenous immunoglobulin (IVIg) demonstrated neutralising action in vitro, but mAbs 234 and 338 were effective in reducing lung virus titers in hamsters and mice, respectively. mAb MPE8 showed efficacy against respiratory syncytial virus and HMPV in preclinical studies (Schuster et al., 2015). In order to effectively control HMPV infections and reduce the burden of respiratory diseases, these advancements in therapy development are essential.(Alotaibi et al., 2025).

Potential for Vaccination and Diagnostic Development

With several vaccine platforms now being researched, a successful vaccination would be a major step toward reducing hMPV (Abdaal et al., 2024). Conventional formalin-inactivated vaccine strategies have shown increased disease severity when challenged, which has been troublesome. Better safety profiles have been shown by innovative methods that use inactivation based on nano-emulsion. In animal models, live attenuated vaccines produced by temperature-sensitive mutations or gene deletion have demonstrated promising outcomes (Luongo et al., 2012).

Numerous contenders focus on the F protein's prefusion conformation, taking advantage of advancements in immunogenicity a tactic that worked well in RSV vaccination studies (Nasrollahzadeh et al., 2020). Using a variety of delivery methods, such as subunit vaccines, a class of vaccinations that include certain viral pathogens rather than the full viral pathogen that target the F protein, have shown promise (Liljeqvist & Ståhl, 1999). Another intriguing strategy is the use of virus-like particles. These particles avoid the dangers of live virus vaccines while successfully simulating viral structure. Because of the genetic variety of hMPV, cross-protection is essential. To increase prophylactic coverage, some researchers look into multivalent strategies that combine the hMPV and RSV antigens (Capone et al., 2013; Quan et al., 2020). HMPV surveillance has been improved with the use of better diagnostic techniques. Hospital-acquired infections are decreased when quick, precise testing directs isolation and patient triage procedures. Furthermore, since health authorities monitor which germs are most prevalent in certain epidemics and adjust their activities appropriately, these devices provide real-time epidemiological evaluations.

Using Accomplished Panels to Strengthen Surveillance Systems

hMPV and other respiratory pathogens can be detected simultaneously thanks to sophisticated multiplex PCR panels and NGS technologies (van Zyl, 2022). Health officials may monitor patterns of pathogen prevalence in local epidemics thanks to these tools, which also provide real-time epidemiological assessments. The timely implementation of control measures & quick identification of outbreak patterns are made possible by the integration of laboratory networks & data-sharing platforms (Gao et al., 2020). This scientific plan, which includes keeping antiviral medications on hand and keeping track of how many beds are available in acute care units, assists with better resource allocation. One benefit of teaching these skills in countries that used to be bad at diagnosing diseases is that they will be better at spotting outbreaks and providing people the care they need right away, especially for populations who are more likely to become sick. Clinical results is made possible by efficient communication between hospitals, clinics, and public health organisations (Buehler et al., 2016).

With this unified approach, healthcare institutions can quickly identify abnormalities, including increases in hMPV-positive testing, and take immediate corrective action. In the end, effective hMPV management depends on resources and policies that are supportive. Using RSV and influenza modelling, governments should give hMPV vaccine development top priority when allocating funds (Sachdeva & Ahmed). Increasing diagnostic capacity guarantees fair access to quick, precise testing, particularly in underserved areas. Long-term public health initiatives can support hygiene and other preventative measures. Its substantial impact on morbidity in children and the elderly is recognised by integrating hMPV preparedness into larger pandemic frameworks. Clinical standards of care will be further improved by guiding principles for immunomodulatory usage, antibiotic stewardship, and infection control.

Public Health Implications and Future Directions

Enhanced surveillance systems and global collaborative efforts are essential to improve hMPV detection and response strategies (Kumar et al., 2025). With Surveillance and Monitoring, integration with respiratory virus surveillance involves coordinating hMPV monitoring with influenza and RSV programs, and Global Health Policies need for better diagnostic accessibility in developing regions. Also, the Public Awareness Campaigns educate healthcare professionals and the public about hMPV (Akingbola et al., 2025). Due to the lack of a vaccine or antiviral treatment for hMPV, the cost of treatment continues to fall on the global healthcare system. All of the anti-hMPV techniques that have been studied so far are included in this review. Peptidomimetics and small-molecule inhibitors that target specific F protein domains involved in receptor binding or the fusion process have shown promise in preventing viral infection in addition to monoclonal antibodies.

Conclusion

The human metapneumovirus is still a major cause of acute respiratory infections (ARIs) worldwide, especially in young children, the elderly, and people with weakened immune systems. Virus has a clear seasonal pattern and frequently co-occurs with influenza and RSV, making diagnosis more difficult and increasing the cost of healthcare. Although hMPV detection has increased due to advancements in diagnostic techniques, especially PCR-based molecular assays, quick point-of-care diagnostics are still required for efficient clinical management. Understanding viral development, transmission dynamics, and the influence of environmental factors on disease epidemics requires ongoing epidemiological observation. Currently no approved vaccine or particular hMPV antiviral treatment, despite its significant morbidity and financial impact. Nonetheless, therapeutic research and vaccine development are advancing, with live-attenuated vaccine candidates and monoclonal antibodies demonstrating promise in preclinical and early clinical trials.

References

Abdaal, K., Batool, A., Navid, M., Ahmed, S., Qazi, A., Safdar, W., Ali, H., Rashid, M., & Rafaqat, S. (2024). Advancements in vaccination strategies: from historical milestones to modern innovations in viral disease prevention and public health. *Res J Vet Pract*, *12*(1), 11-21.

Aftab, S., Tazeen, A., Ali, S., Broor, S., Ahmed, A., & Parveen, S. (2017). Human Metapneumovirus (hMPV) Proteins, their Therapeutics and Vaccine Potentials. *Indian Journal of Health Sciences and Care*, *4*(3), 126-140.

Akingbola, A., Adegbesan, A., TundeAlao, S., Adewole, O., Ayikoru, C., Benson, A. E., Shekoni, M., & Chuku, J. (2025). Human metapneumovirus: an emerging respiratory pathogen and the urgent need for improved diagnostics, surveillance, and vaccine development. *Infectious Diseases*, *57*(3), 304-310.

Alotaibi, B. S., Habib, M., Habib, A., Syed, F., Shah, N. N., & Tantry, B. A. (2025). Human Metapneumovirus: A Review of Epidemiology, Pathogenesis, Diagnosis, and Future Prospects. *Journal of Pure & Applied Microbiology*, *19*(2).

Bergeron, H. C., Crabtree, J., Nagy, T., Martin, D. E., & Tripp, R. A. (2024). Probenecid inhibits human metapneumovirus (HMPV) replication in vitro and in BALB/c mice. *Viruses*, *16*(7), 1087.

Brendish, N. (2019). *Molecular point-of-care testing for respiratory viruses* University of Southampton].

Brynes, A. (2024). *Human Metapneumovirus Small Hydrophobic Protein Degrades JAKs to Block Immune Signals* University of Pittsburgh].

Buehler, S. S., Madison, B., Snyder, S. R., Derzon, J. H., Cornish, N. E., Saubolle, M. A., Weissfeld, A. S., Weinstein, M. P., Liebow, E. B., & Wolk, D. M. (2016). Effectiveness of practices to increase timeliness of providing targeted therapy for inpatients with bloodstream infections: a laboratory medicine best practices systematic review and meta-analysis. *Clinical microbiology reviews*, *29*(1), 59-103.

Capone, S., D'Alise, A. M., Ammendola, V., Colloca, S., Cortese, R., Nicosia, A., & Folgori, A. (2013). Development of chimpanzee adenoviruses as vaccine vectors: challenges and successes emerging from clinical trials. *Expert Review of Vaccines*, *12*(4), 379-393.

Carelli, M. (2019). Development of a new duplex real-time polymerase chain reaction assay for detection and quantification of KIHPyV and WUHPyV in pediatric samples.

Cheng, M.-F., Chen, B.-C., Kao, C.-L., Kao, C.-H., Hsieh, K.-S., & Liu, Y.-C. (2006). Human metapneumovirus as a causative agent of lower respiratory tract infection in four patients: the first report of human metapneumovirus infection confirmed by RNA sequences in Taiwan. *Scandinavian journal of infectious diseases*, *38*(5), 392-396.

de Graaf, M., Osterhaus, A. D., Fouchier, R. A., & Holmes, E. C. (2008). Evolutionary dynamics of human and avian metapneumoviruses. *Journal of General Virology*, *89*(12), 2933-2942.

Duong, S., & Ginocchio, C. C. (2016). Molecular tests for the identification of viruses. *Manual of Commercial Methods in Clinical Microbiology: International Edition*, 97-120.

Gao, F., Tao, L., Huang, Y., & Shu, Z. (2020). Management and data sharing of COVID-19 pandemic information. *Biopreservation and biobanking*, *18*(6), 570-580.

Georgakopoulou, V. E. (2024). Insights from respiratory virus co-infections. *World Journal of Virology*, *13*(4), 98600.

Greene[1], W. H., Menegus, M. A., & Truant, A. L. (2016). Rapid Antigen Devices and Instruments for. *Manual of Commercial Methods in Clinical Microbiology*, 87.

Haas, L. E., Thijsen, S. F., Van Elden, L., & Heemstra, K. A. (2013). Human metapneumovirus in adults. *Viruses*, *5*(1), 87-110.

Hamelin, M.-E. v., Yim, K., Kuhn, K. H., Cragin, R. P., Boukhvalova, M., Blanco, J. C., Prince, G. A., & Boivin, G. (2005). Pathogenesis of human metapneumovirus lung infection in BALB/c mice and cotton rats. *Journal of virology*, *79*(14), 8894-8903.

Hodinka, R. L. (2016). Serologic tests in clinical virology. In *Lennette's Laboratory Diagnosis of Viral Infections* (pp. 133-150). CRC Press.

Huang, Y., Li, S., Ye, W., Wang, H., Su, J., Gao, L., Shi, R., Mou, X., Leng, S. X., & Xiao, C. (2025). Viral Infections in Elderly Individuals: A Comprehensive Overview of SARS-CoV-2 and Influenza Susceptibility, Pathogenesis, and Clinical Treatment Strategies. *Vaccines*, *13*(4), 431.

Ivanova, L., Tsaneva, D., Stoykova, Z., & Kostadinova, T. (2015). Viral diseases in transplant and immunocompromised patients. In *Immunopathology and Immunomodulation*. IntechOpen.

Janssen, D. J., Spruit, M. A., Uszko-Lencer, N. H., Schols, J. M., & Wouters, E. F. (2011). Symptoms, comorbidities, and health care in advanced chronic obstructive pulmonary disease or chronic heart failure. *Journal of palliative medicine*, *14*(6), 735-743.

Jeong, S., Park, M.-J., Song, W., & Kim, H.-S. (2020). Advances in laboratory assays for detecting human metapneumovirus. *Annals of Translational Medicine*, *8*(9), 608.

Jones, H. P., Tabor, L., Sun, X., Woolard, M. D., & Simecka, J. W. (2002). Depletion of CD8+ T cells exacerbates CD4+ Th cell-associated inflammatory lesions during murine mycoplasma respiratory disease. *The Journal of Immunology*, *168*(7), 3493-3501.

Kim, S. R., Ki, C.-S., & Lee, N. Y. (2009). Rapid detection and identification of 12 respiratory viruses using a dual priming oligonucleotide system-based multiplex PCR assay. *Journal of virological methods*, *156*(1-2), 111-116.

Kinder, J. T. (2020). Pneumovirus Infections: Understanding RSV and HMPV Entry, Replication, and Spread.

Kroll, J. L., & Weinberg, A. (2011). Human metapneumovirus. Seminars in respiratory and critical care medicine.

Kumar, S., Subramaniam, G., & Kumar, K. S. (2025). Human Metapneumovirus (HMPV) Outbreak: An Urgent Call for Enhanced Surveillance and Public Health Action. *Journal of Medical Virology*, *97*(2), e70199.

Lianou, A., Tsantes, A. G., Ioannou, P., Bikouli, E. D., Batsiou, A., Kokkinou, A., Tsante, K. A., Tsilidis, D., Lampridou, M., & Iacovidou, N. (2025). hMPV Outbreaks: Worldwide Implications of a Re-Emerging Respiratory Pathogen. *Microorganisms*.

Liljeqvist, S., & Ståhl, S. (1999). Production of recombinant subunit vaccines: protein immunogens, live delivery systems and nucleic acid vaccines. *Journal of biotechnology*, *73*(1), 1-33.

Luongo, C., Winter, C. C., Collins, P. L., & Buchholz, U. J. (2012). Increased genetic and phenotypic stability of a promising live-attenuated respiratory syncytial virus vaccine candidate by reverse genetics. *Journal of virology*, *86*(19), 10792-10804.

Maurya, L. (2025). Epidemiology, Etiological Causes and Preventive Measures of Human Metapneumovirus (HMPV): A Review.

Mirsaeidi, M., Motahari, H., Taghizadeh Khamesi, M., Sharifi, A., Campos, M., & Schraufnagel, D. E. (2016). Climate change and respiratory infections. *Annals of the American Thoracic Society*, *13*(8), 1223-1230.

Moriyama, M., Hugentobler, W. J., & Iwasaki, A. (2020). Seasonality of respiratory viral infections. *Annual review of virology*, *7*(1), 83-101.

Nasrollahzadeh, M., Sajjadi, M., Soufi, G. J., Iravani, S., & Varma, R. S. (2020). Nanomaterials and nanotechnology-associated innovations against viral infections with a focus on coronaviruses. *Nanomaterials*, *10*(6), 1072.

O'Kennedy, R., & Murphy, C. (2017). *Immunoassays: development, applications and future trends*. CRC Press.

Parks, O. B. (2024). *The role of age and complement in CD8+ T cell function during human metapneumovirus (HMPV) infection* University of Pittsburgh].

Porwal, S., Malviya, R., Sridhar, S. B., Shareef, J., & Wadhwa, T. (2025). Global impact of hMPV virus: Transmission, pathogenesis, diagnostic and treatment. *Diagnostic Microbiology and Infectious Disease*, 116809.

Quan, F.-S., Basak, S., Chu, K.-B., Kim, S. S., & Kang, S.-M. (2020). Progress in the development of virus-like particle vaccines against respiratory viruses. *Expert Review of Vaccines*, *19*(1), 11-24.

Rishmawi, N. H. (2007). *Molecular detection and characterization of human metapneumovius (HMPV) in hospitalized children residing in Southern Palestine* Birzeit University].

Rogers, M. C. (2018). Immune regulation and evasion of acute respiratory virus infection.

Sachdeva, A., & Ahmed, N. Human Metapneumovirus in India (HMPV): Unveiling the Silent Respiratory Threat and Forging a Path to Resilient Healthcare Solutions. *Public health*, *8*, 11.

Satapathy, T., Satapathy, A., Satapathy, A., Yadav, N., Chandrakar, M., & Chandrakar, K. (2025). Recent outbreaks of Human Metapneumovirus (HMPV): Prevention, Diagnosis and Therapeutic insights. *Journal of Drug Delivery & Therapeutics*, *15*(2).

Schuster, J. E., Cox, R. G., Hastings, A. K., Boyd, K. L., Wadia, J., Chen, Z., Burton, D. R., Williamson, R. A., & Williams, J. V. (2015). A broadly neutralizing human monoclonal antibody exhibits in vivo efficacy against both human metapneumovirus and respiratory syncytial virus. *The Journal of infectious diseases*, *211*(2), 216-225.

van Boheemen, S. (2014). Virus discovery and characterization using next-generation sequencing.

van den Hoogen, B. G. (2004). Human metapneumovirus. Discovery, characterisation and associated disease.

van Zyl, G. U. (2022). New technological developments in identification and monitoring of new and emerging infections. *Encyclopedia of Infection and Immunity*, 463.

Watson, A., & Wilkinson, T. M. (2021). Respiratory viral infections in the elderly. *Therapeutic advances in respiratory disease*, *15*, 1753466621995050.

Xu, B., Wang, J., Li, Z., Xu, C., Liao, Y., Hu, M., Yang, J., Lai, S., Wang, L., & Yang, W. (2021). Seasonal association between viral causes of hospitalised acute lower respiratory infections and meteorological factors in China: a retrospective study. *The Lancet Planetary Health*, *5*(3), e154-e163.

Yousafzai, M. T., Ibrahim, R., Thobani, R., Aziz, F., & Ali, A. (2018). Human metapneumovirus in hospitalized children less than 5 years of age in Pakistan. *Journal of Medical Virology*, *90*(6), 1027-1032.

Chapter 13

Exploring the Role of Artificial Intelligence in the Diagnosis, Prognosis, and Treatment of Human Metapneumovirus-Related Diseases

Biruk Demisse Ayalew[1,*]
Shree Rath[2]
Nourhan Saeed Bakry[3]
Zemichael Getu Alemayehu[4]
and Habib Omari Ramadhani[5]

[1]Infectious Disease Unit, Department of Internal Medicine, St. Paul's Hospital Millennium Medical College, Addis Ababa, Ethiopia
[2]All India Institute of Medical Sciences, Bhubaneswar, India
[3]Senior Research Associate, Children's Cancer Hospital, Egypt
[4]Addis Ababa University, College of Health Sciences, School of Medicine, Addis Ababa, Ethiopia
[5]Institute of Human Virology, University of Maryland School of Medicine, Baltimore, MD, USA

Abstract

Human metapneumovirus (HMPV) is a common respiratory infection, now witnessing a rising trend worldwide. The recent surge in cases noticed in certain countries has prompted focus on the disease, its manifestations and early cure. Poor management can ultimately lead to multiple complications like respiratory distress and multiorgan failure. This stresses the need for early identification of the disease and risk-

* Corresponding Author's Email: bdemisse21@gmail.com

In: Human Metapneumovirus
Editors: Anjali Sharma, Vishnu Mittal, Devkant Sharma et al.
ISBN: 979-8-90134-063-9

stratification of patients to aid in rapid recovery. Artificial intelligence (AI) models are crucial in aiding healthcare diagnostics. The predictive value of these models allows for the detection of early signs of any disease. AI models have been evolving particularly for viral infections, allowing for early identification even in prodromal stages or when patients have non-specific symptoms. Recent studies have explored the use of AI models in detecting HMPV, as well as manufacturing its vaccine. In this chapter, we aim to summarise key studies on these models, highlight their success and identify potential healthcare decisions that could be facilitated by AI models.

Keywords: Human Metapneumovirus (HMPV), artificial intelligence in healthcare, machine learning models, AI-driven diagnosis and prognosis, viral infection prediction, AI-guided vaccine development

List of Abbreviations

AI	Artificial Intelligence
ML	Machine Learning
DL	Deep Learning
CDS	Clinical Decision Support
CNN	Convolutional Neural Network
SAE	Stacked Auto Encoder
DBN	Deep Belief Network
RNN	Recurrent Neural Network
ICH	Intracranial Haemorrhage
DNA	Deoxyribonucleic Acid
NLP	Natural Language Processing
PCR	Polymerase Chain Reaction
CS	Clinical Symptoms
LT	Laboratory Tests
NIR	Near Infrared
hRSV	Human Respiratory Syncytial Virus
MPV	Metapneumovirus
Pre:F	Prefusion F protein
Post:F	Postfusion F protein
RSV	Respiratory Syncytial Virus
IFA/IFB	Influenza Virus Type A/Type B
MP	Mycoplasma Pneumonia

QID	Quasi: Quasi-identifier
LSDA	Large-Scale Data Analytics
XAI	Explainable Artificial Intelligence
LIME	Local Interpretable Model Agnostic Explanations
SHAP	Shapley Additive Explanations
CDSS	Clinical Decision Support Systems
SaMD	Software as a Medical Device
FDA	Food and Drug Administration
MDR	Medical Device Regulation
PMA	Pre-Market Approval
IEC	International Electrotechnical Commission
ISO	International Organization for Standardization
IMDRF	International Medical Device Regulators Forum
GDPR	General Data Protection Regulation
LMIC	Low and Middle Income Countries
BERT	Bidirectional Encoder Representations from Transformers
XLNet	Generalised Autoregressive Pretraining for Language Understanding
ALBERT	A Lite BERT
ELECTRA	Efficiently Learning an Encoder that Classifies Token Replacements Accurately
RobERTa	Robustly Optimised BERT Pretraining Approach
ReCaP	Residue Classification for Protein Design
CRISPR	Clustered Regularly Interspaced Short Palindromic Repeats.

AI and Machine Learning for Healthcare

Artificial intelligence (AI) is a broad concept that allows computers to think like humans (Gupta et al., 2021). The beginning of AI traces back to 1956 when a group of computer scientists described human intelligence as a set of principles that could be precisely analysed, described, and taught to machines, enabling the machines to simulate it. Early AI was characterised by classical reprogramming in which computational methods provided hardcoding for each rule that governs a particular scenario (Choi et al., 2020).

Over time, AI evolved into a more specialised term called machine learning (ML). In contrast to classical reprogramming, ML was designed to handle more complex tasks that are not based on precisely pre-set algorithms coded for the task. Instead, ML is allowed to learn based on a subset of input data, called training datasets (Choi et al., 2020). This learning process is facilitated by certain methods rather than being precisely reprogrammed (Gupta et al., 2021). Upon learning, ML can generate new algorithms based on the training dataset and apply this learning to new datasets: validation and test datasets (Choi et al., 2020). ML represents a shift from classical reprogramming to self-learning and adaptive data-driven models that can identify patterns and make decisions, representing a new paradigm in artificial intelligence. The learning methods utilised by ML include supervised, unsupervised, semi-supervised, and reinforcement learning, and the learning components include the input data, referred to as features, and the outcome, referred to as target or label. The supervised method involves training datasets on certain features in correlation to the target. After validation and testing, the model can utilise this correlation with the target in interpreting new datasets (James et al., 2021). In the unsupervised method, the model uses unlabeled data to look for patterns with the goal of exploration. Subsequently, each pattern is classified into a certain category (James et al., 2021).

In the semi-supervised method, the model combines the benefits of the specific guidance provided by the supervised model and the exploration provided by the unsupervised model. This approach utilised the supervised learning method in a small dataset of labelled data and the unsupervised learning method in the remaining unlabeled data to generate a training dataset. Then the model can be validated and tested on new datasets. The reinforcement learning model resembles the human learning experience, where the model learns by trial and error. After several trials, the model achieves the desired action and then the desired action is rewarded, hence reinforced for this action in the following trials (Choi et al., 2020; Gupta et al., 2021). Later, a subset of ML, namely deep learning (DL), was introduced. In contrast to ML models that require manual feature engineering, which is labour-intensive, knowledge-based, and unsuitable for high-throughput data, DL models can automatically learn features from raw data and, therefore, outperform ML models in high-throughput data (Angermueller et al., 2016). DL utilises multiple layers of ML models called neural networks. This name was inspired by their ability to process and organise information mimicking the human brain (Gupta et al., 2021).

Introduction into AI Models

AI models mainly involve rule-based systems, machine learning models, and deep learning models (Joshi et al., 2022). Rule-based systems (RBS) are foundational AI models that can operate based on preset rules; hence they can only handle situations that were previously explicitly programmed into their systems. They have been widely applied in Clinical Decision Support (CDS) tools, where they utilise guidelines and expert opinion as the rule for decision-making. For instance, utilising relevant guidelines, RBS can identify patients at risk of developing certain conditions based on their vital signs and laboratory results (Joshi et al., 2022). One advantage of RBS is its transparency since it operates based on evidence-based guidelines. However, RBS represents inflexible systems since they operate based on fixed rules and are not adaptable (Shortliffe & Sepúlveda, 2018). Additionally, these systems were associated with false-positive alerts (Joshi et al., 2022).

In contrast, ML methods are adaptable since they identify and learn new patterns from input datasets and adapt accordingly. The classical models that are used in ML include: linear regression, logistic regression, decision trees, and random forests, among others. The linear regression models set a linear relationship between one or more features, in the form of numeric variables, and a target outcome. Linear regression models are utilised mainly for predicting numerical outcomes. The logistic regression model establishes a relationship between certain features and outcome probabilities in a non-linear fashion. These models are utilized for predicting binary outcomes. The decision trees and random forests model work by recursive partitioning, where the dataset, represented as the first node, is split into the next level, two nodes, based on their homogeneity in a certain feature. The two new nodes are either terminal groups, which are homogenous regarding the feature, or decision groups that will be further split based on another feature. Decision trees and random forests are mainly used in classifications (Choi et al., n.d.; *Encyclopedia of Bioinformatics and Computational Biology*, 2018).

Deep learning algorithms operate by transforming input data into outcomes via multi-layered algorithms. Examples of algorithms utilised in DL are convolutional neural networks (CNNs), stacked auto-encoders (SAEs), deep belief networks (DBNs), recurrent neural networks (RNNs), and others (Dong et al., 2021; Litjens et al., 2017). Among them, the most successful model is CNNs, which is widely applied in medical imaging analysis. CNNs work by converting images into disease/outcome by self-learning high-throughput features. Therefore, it helps in processing complex datasets (Litjens et al., 2017) (Figure 1).

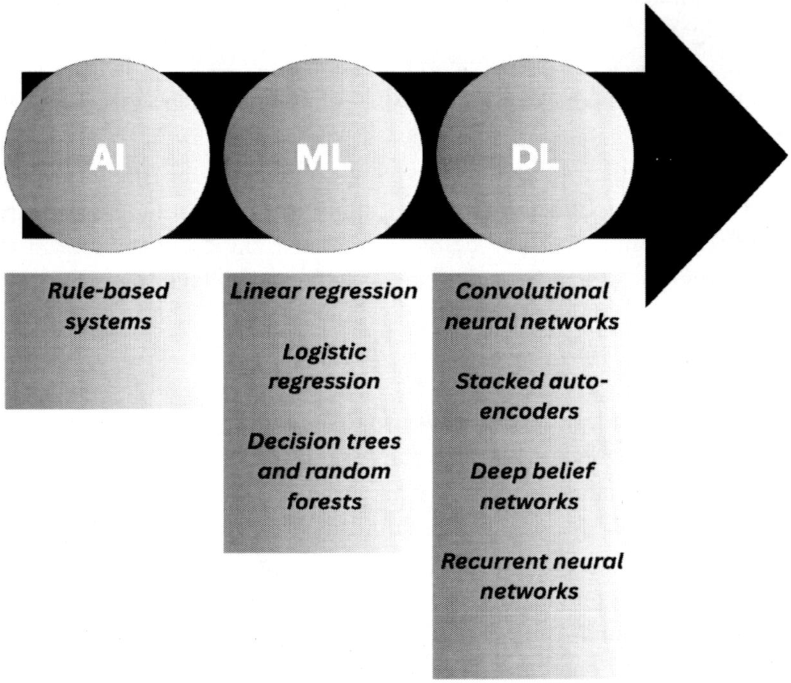

Figure 1. The evolution from artificial intelligence to machine learning and deep learning.

AI and Its Role in Healthcare Settings

Artificial intelligence has transformed the healthcare sector in several areas, including medical imaging, pathology, personalised medicine, medical operations, drug discovery, and clinical trials.

- Medical imaging

DL models have been trained to read X-rays, MRIs, CT scans, mammography, and ultrasound. DL models were able to identify interstitial lung disease, tumours, fractures, haemorrhages, and embolisms (Litjens et al., 2017). For example, DL models, trained on 37500 CT scans of intracranial haemorrhage (ICH), were able to diagnose more than 9000 new ICH cases and identify subtle ICH ones that were missed by radiologists. This suggests the utility of DL models in decreasing physicians' workload and improving diagnostic accuracy (Arbabshirani et al., 2018).

- Pathology

Digital microscopes are a very popular area for applying DL models in pathology. These models can segment cellular components, such as nuclei, cytoplasm, and mitochondria, detect large organs, such as colonic glands and neuronal membranes, and identify tumour-infiltrating lymphocytes. Additionally, they can classify and diagnose cancer. Also, ML models were able to detect biological processes such as mitosis (Litjens et al., 2017).

- Patient outcome prediction and disease progression forecasting

ML models have been utilised in outcome prediction. Several ML models have been developed to predict cardiovascular outcomes. For instance, ML models can utilise features, such as heart rate, to predict sudden cardiac death (Patel & Sengupta, 2020). Additionally, ML models have been utilised to predict surgical complications, i.e., following lung and gastrointestinal cancer surgeries, by monitoring patient-reported outcomes (Hassan et al., 2022). ML also contributed to the identification of distinct genomic subgroups by integrating genomic data of patients with myeloproliferative neoplasm and their clinical phenotypes. These genomic subgroups displayed distinct clinical phenotypes, including event-free survival and risk of leukemic transformation (Grinfeld et al., 2018). These applications highlight the potential of ML in predicting patients' prognosis, hence improving patient' care.

- Personalized medicine

The advent of big data in medicine has yielded large datasets that show that humans vary at the genomic level, and this variation might affect their treatment outcomes. And since the interpretation of these data is complex, it highlights the need for AI to analyse and interpret such data. In addition, utilising these interpretations, we can identify patients who are most likely to benefit from therapy. For instance, AI has been utilized to identify patterns in DNA sequencing results. Utilising such patterns to identify potential targets for therapy is pivotal in the application of personalised medicine (Schork, 2019).

- Medical operations

Reinforcement learning models, which use trial and error and reward successful actions to guide decisions, have been applied in the field of robotic surgeries. Robotic surgeries are a new and evolving field in surgery that aims at enhanced precision, smaller incisions, quick recovery and reduced surgeons' fatigue. Robotic surgeries mainly utilise reinforcement models to learn optimal surgical methods (Qian & Ren, 2023). Interestingly, a recent fully robotic double lung transplant surgery was conducted on a female patient to replace her diseased lungs with a donor's lungs. This surgery utilised small incisions, which led to less pain and quicker recovery when compared to conventional methods (*I Was Cut Open by a Robot — Now I Can Breathe Again*, n.d.). Additionally, a kidney transplant robotic-assisted surgery was conducted on a 60-year-old female patient. In this surgery, the physician utilised a small incision that led to fewer complications such as infection and hernia (Kehren, 2023). These examples highlight the potential of robotic surgeries to improve surgical outcomes (Jumper et al., 2021; Rajkomar et al., 2019).

AI and Machine Learning in Virology

Artificial intelligence is revolutionising the virology field and epidemiological studies. AI provides a good platform for understanding viral-host interactions, which aids in understanding the natural history of the disease (Zhang et al., 2024). Additionally, ML models have been utilised to aid in viral prevention and vaccine development (Olawade et al., 2024), control of outbreaks (Zhang et al., 2024), diagnosis (Mc Cord—De Iaco et al., 2023), mass screening (Huang et al., 2024) and antiviral therapy prediction (Zhang et al., 2024), as well as classifying novel viruses(Randhawa et al., 2020) (Figure 2). For example, by utilising a machine learning-based alignment-free approach along with digital signal processing and decision trees to analyse genomic sequences of over 5000 SARS-CoV-2 sequences, the authors were able to identify the taxonomic classification of SARS-CoV-2 with 100% accuracy and no need for biological data integration (Randhawa et al., 2020). The role of AI models in the diagnosis and therapy prediction of respiratory viruses, with a focus on respiratory syncytial viruses, is shown in Table 1.

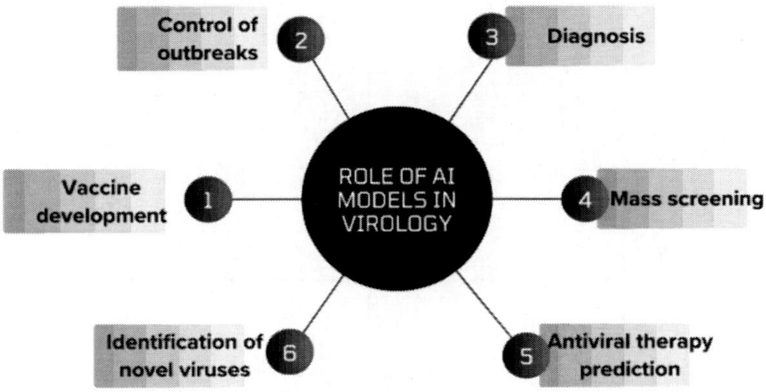

Figure 2. Role of AI models in virology.

AI and Machine Learning in HMPV

Study 1: Explainable AI for HMPV

This mainly served to assess the responsiveness and attitudes of the general population to the growing cases of HMPV (Apu et al., 2025). An XLNet model was used, which is a natural language processing (NLP) model known to perform better than other NLP models like BERT. Its autoregressive design, coupled with bidirectional context and the ability to create multiple representations of language, is a key feature that boosts the performance of the model. This study used data from the comments section of several YouTube videos to train the model. Results of the study concluded a higher performance of the XLNet model, superseding the performance of models like ELECTRA, BERT, RobERTa, ALBERT and DistilBERT. Overall accuracy of the model was good at 93.5%. The model was successful in predicting sentiments based on a few keywords. The study set an initial development on NLPs and their use in sentiment analysis systems in future.

Table 1. Shows the role of AI models in the diagnosis and therapy prediction of respiratory viruses with a focus on respiratory syncytial viruses

Study	Model used	Virus	Inputs	Outcome
Lopes et al., 2023	Artificial neural network techniques and genetic algorithms.	hRSV	Biological, structural, and physicochemical properties of flavonoids	Therapy prediction Recognising more than 83% hit rates.
Mc Cord—De Iaco et al., 2023	LightGBM model	hRSV and pertussis	PCR, clinical symptoms (CS), and/or laboratory tests (LT)	Diagnosis Recall rate for hRSV: 0.68 (CS + LT) and 0.72 (CS only) Recall rate for pertussis: 0.72 (CS + LT) and 0.74 (CS only)
Chang et al., 2023	Logistic regression, random forest, gradient boosting, and extreme gradient boosting models	Adenovirus (adv), influenza virus types A and B (IFA and B), parainfluenza virus (PIV), hRSV, mycoplasma pneumonia (MP)	PCR Clinical and laboratory data Age	Diagnosis AUROC of 0.84, 0.86, 0.77, 0.80,0.73, and 0.87 for hRSV, adv, IFA, IFB, PIV, and MP, respectively.
Huang et al., 2024	variable selection utilizing the Variable Importance in Projection	hRSV and Sendai virus	Near-infrared (NIR) spectroscopy spectral data	Diagnosis Enhance the specificity of NIR spectroscopy to diagnose hRSV and Sendai virus with a classification accuracy of 0.88 and 0.94, respectively.

Study 2: HMPV Vaccine Development by AI Models

Bakkers et al., (Bakkers et al., 2024) developed an efficacious HMPV vaccine aided by AI-guided engineering of the components. This study presented the development of an AI-guided HMPV vaccine candidate based on engineering a stabilised prefusion conformation of the HMPV fusion (F) protein. Central to this work was the AI-driven design strategy. The team developed a convolutional neural network, ReCaP (Residue Classification for Protein Design), trained on a vast dataset of protein structures from the Protein Data Bank. ReCaP analysed atomic microenvironments to predict stabilising substitutions, particularly at protomer interfaces. This approach identified mutations like V112R and D209E, which were overlooked by conventional methods. These substitutions significantly improved trimer stability and expression, as validated by biochemical assays, cryo-EM, and thermal shift analyses. The F protein was engineered for double cleavage, mimicking the natural processing of related pneumoviruses like RSV. This step resolved steric clashes caused by the extended F2 C-terminus, enabling trimer closure. The final construct, MPV-2c, exhibited a melting temperature of 71.8°C, surpassing previous Pre-F designs, and retained a closed conformation without requiring heterologous trimerization domains.

In animal studies, the AI-optimized Pre-F trimer induced high titers of cross-neutralizing antibodies in mice and near-complete protection against HMPV challenge in cotton rats. Notably, the vaccine candidate boosted pre-existing immunity in pre-exposed mice and demonstrated superior efficacy compared to postfusion F (Post-F) immunogens. Therefore, integrating AI with biophysical validation helped in developing a vaccine of higher efficacy than traditional techniques, holding promise for AI-driven vaccine development.

Integration of Existing Models and Extrapolation to HMPV

Comparison of Accuracy and Performance between HMPV and Other Similar Viral Infections

The building of diagnostic models for viral infections now heavily relies on machine learning (ML) techniques due to their potential to enhance accuracy compared to standard diagnostic procedures. With regard to HMPV, some studies have proven the effectiveness of such models. Take, for instance, the study dedicated to the detection of RSV. It demonstrates the power of model-based detection relying on the set of clinical symptoms. The model, based on a longitudinal analysis of symptom evolution, had a high sensitivity and specificity. It had a high success rate for identifying infected patients, successfully excluding 75.6% of non-infected patients, thus offering a suitable alternative to rapid antigen tests (Mc Cord-De Iaco et al., 2023).

The models predictive of viral infections did not perform uniformly, with both RSV and influenza having superior discrimination when compared to rhinovirus and adenovirus (Mai, 2014). As for the patients stratified in the high and low risk groups, the machine learning models did splendidly for RSV, hMPV, influenza, and parainfluenza, but the same models did not work well for adenovirus and rhinovirus. Models were able to ensure that almost all positive cases were detected, or sensitivity stayed high across the board, but specificity changed on a case-by-case basis, with influenza achieving 100% sensitivity at 46% specificity and striking a balance between identifying positive cases and limiting non-essential tests. The addition of structured clinical data to unstructured text-mining methods, especially those using MetaMap, enhanced the predictive performance of RSV models, which shows how beneficial applying natural language processing methods for disease detection can be (Mai & Krauthammer, 2017).

The models for HMPV and other similar respiratory infection candidates, such as RSV, appear to perform well. In the case of RSV mentioned in the analysis, those models that had symptom progression and the timing of symptom onset were more accurate. The proposed machine learning methods for RSV also appeared to be robust in correctly diagnosing true positives and true negatives while presenting very few false positives. This is important in the case of diagnosing viral infections. These viruses differ from one another in their nature as well as the data needed for accurate detection. For example, cough, wheezing, and nasal discharge are the major symptoms in the RSV models, while detection of HMPV may need more variables, like other diseases and atypical symptom expressions. The study on RSV also underscores the need for explanation and calibration of the model, which is another important feature that would be required for similar diagnostic devices for HMPV (Kawamoto et al., 2024). If there is no explainability, the models would be less trusted and hence not used. In addition, the problem of incorporating data from people without a medical background, the way it is done in RSV detection, may pose other challenges for HMPV detection, which would need careful design to avoid providing unreliable and invalid data.

Comparison of Predictive Model Performance for Different Viral Infections is shown in Table 2.

Table 2. Comparison of predictive model performance for different viral infections

Viral Infection	Discriminative Ability	Sensitivity	Specificity	Key Observations
RSV	High	High	Varies	Models effectively identify high- and low-risk patients, particularly with symptom progression data. Sensitivity improved within the first six days of illness.
Influenza	High	High	Moderate	Achieved perfect sensitivity but lower specificity. Good for early identification of influenza, reducing unnecessary testing.
hMPV	Moderate	High	Moderate	Performance is comparable to RSV models, with sensitivity guiding the detection process.
Parainfluenza	High	High	Varies	Similar performance to influenza and RSV in identifying at-risk patients.
Adenovirus	Low	High	Low	Models showed minimal predictive power. Low specificity and sensitivity, not as effective for detection.
Rhinovirus	Low	High	Low	Similar to adenovirus, low predictive value with low specificity and sensitivity.

Integration of Models

Given the successful prediction of RSV and influenza, the same method may be employed for hMPV detection. Machine learning hMPV models based on clinician-reported symptomatology seem feasible in hMPV detection. Structured clinical data integrated with symptom escalation patterns could be utilised. An RSV model that employed exclusion thresholds equal to those of rapid antigen tests had already successfully classified 75.6% of infected patients. Employing this approach on hMPV could improve its early detection and decrease unnecessary confirmatory tests (Kawamoto et al., 2024). Furthermore, combining clinical variables and natural language processing methods for hMPV detection, as done for RSV, could improve hMPV prediction, especially when dealing with unstructured admission notes (Mai & Krauthammer, 2017).

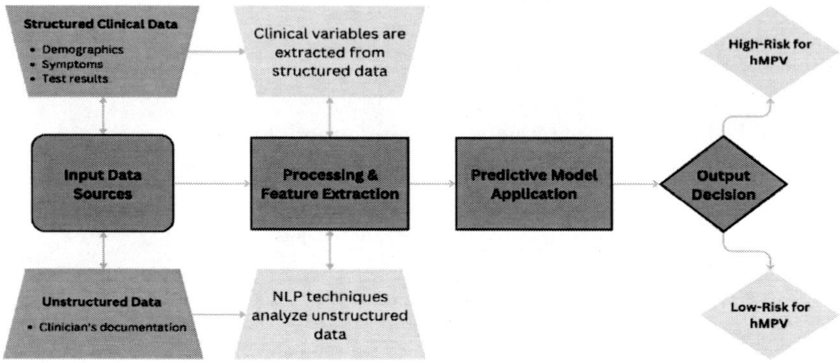

Figure 3. Integration of Predictive Models for hMPV Detection.

Just like with RSV models, hMPV models face similar limitations. A bigger problem emerges with generalizability because many models have been created and validated using data from one single institution, so they need external validation in other populations before they can be put to use (Kawamoto et al., 2024). The heterogeneity in clinicians' documentation and the small size of the dataset limited the ability of text-mining methods to make accurate predictions, and this may also be true for hMPV models (Mai & Krauthammer, 2017). Also, hMPV might have unique patterns of symptom evolution as compared to RSV, which would require a change in model training and calibration. These models tend to have high sensitivity, but the tradeoff is that they are often accompanied by false positives, which can lead to unnecessary testing or isolated measures being taken (Mai, 2014). These problems aside, incorporating near-real-time surveillance data and better tailoring model calibration by demographic groups is likely to enhance hMPV detection and improve the usefulness of these models for clinical decision support (Kawamoto et al., 2024). Integration of Predictive Models for hMPV Detection is shown in Figure 3.

Challenges of Integrating AI and Machine Learning in Healthcare

Ethical Concerns

The adoption of AI in healthcare faces major barriers because of ethical problems regarding accountability, privacy, and decision-making. The use of

AI has raised significant concerns regarding the lack of transparency and interpretability present with the so-called 'black box' form of AI. One of the many concerns is the shift of the burden of proof. Who is at fault when something is wrong? Physicians certainly do not design or maintain these algorithms, but at the same time, it seems unreasonable to shift blame to those who do not interact with patients. In addition, there are no industry-wide criteria that serve as the boundary with which AI could be incorporated into healthcare for it to remain ethical. Existing organisations like the Food and Drug Administration (FDA) and the National Health Service (NHS) are yet to come up with comprehensive safety measures and criteria regarding AI technology implementations in the healthcare industry and are still battling with the issues (Aung et al., 2021). It is safe to say that apart from establishing ethical guides, the use of AI technologies in interventions will have to deal with various legislation and legal systems that need focus.

Integrating AI into healthcare comes with its own issues, such as managing sensitive biomedical data. The issue arises from the challenge of maintaining privacy and even utility. Data sources in Large-Scale Data Analytics (LSDA) in precision medicine are vast as well as diverse. This requires strong encryption, automated access restrictions, and even forms of de-identification to ensure the confidentiality of patient data. Quasi-identifiers, for example, QIDs like genomic data, demographic data, and even imaging features, can have minimal invasive queries and differential privacy applied, which gives the opportunity for useful research to take place. Unfortunately, even when a data point in question does not uniquely identify an individual, the powerful automated data extraction may unintentionally leak private information due to multiple datasets being cross-referenced. Clinical notes identifying data can now easily be stripped by tools like Philtre to lessen these issues (Martínez-García & Hernández-Lemus, 2022). With the rapid integration of AI, new privacy concerns easily arise, and these issues will require robust privacy frameworks that can seamlessly change with the progression of data science as well as computational medicine.

Beyond privacy and security, ethical considerations around AI-driven decision-making for patient care must be considered. AI's increasing role in aiding decision-making, such as for treatment selection, disease forecasting, or resource allocation, raises additional issues of fairness and possible biases in the algorithms (Raparthi, 2020). The practices of informed consent need to adapt to guarantee that eligible patients understand the engagement of AI, its risks, and the possible advantages therein. The emphasis on Personalised Medicine—the application of an individual's genetics and clinical profile in tailoring treatment—also illustrates the urgency for data aggregation as well as the participation of the patient in the decision-making. Patients need to be given the freedom to determine the circumstances under which their data is disseminated or utilised, as this touches not only on their individual treatment preferences but also on the evaluation of public health issues (Martínez-García & Hernández-Lemus, 2022). Striking a compromise between innovation, privacy, and ethical accountability will inevitably call for concerted efforts from lawmakers, scholars, health practitioners, and patients themselves. In the end, the rational deployment of AI in medicine will depend on the existence of these policies, an open framework, and respectful relations between patients who stand to benefit from the advances of AI in medicine and the medical practitioners themselves.

Model Generalizability

In machine learning, generalizability is how well the model can function on completely new patient cohorts that are independent and whose data were not part of the model development process. Models that do not achieve this standard will have computation biases induced by data fabrication and processing instead of the expected relationship between outcomes and features. The result is even more exacerbated when one attempts to reproduce results or make predictions in real-world clinical situations (Yang et al, 2022). This issue is of particular importance in health care, where unaccounted backwards confounding differences, temporal change, observed clinical protocols, and deployment environments make centre generalizability challenging. One institution's data is heterogeneous in demographics, and the institution's collection and processing methods result in biases that are not general population-based. Therefore, attempting to validate models using the same dataset they were trained on is discouraged because they tend to perform dismally when put to the test on external patient cohorts. It is preferable to validate these models on multiple datasets; however, that is not always possible due to ethical, technical, and financial constraints in clinical data sharing. In order to improve the use of ML healthcare models in different hospital contexts, there is a need for model-customization techniques that are capable of transferring site-specific locally-trained models to new environments (Futoma et al, 2020).

Limited resource regions do tend to face the challenge of training the models from scratch, thereby increasing the necessity of adapting off-the-shelf models. These problems have been addressed by various techniques, including combined site training (which aggregates data from different institutions) and federated learning (where collaborative training takes place without direct data exchange). There is, however, a need for simultaneous data availability across institutions and a standard data sharing policy, which is quite hard because of the variation in data collection and technical infrastructure (Futoma et al, 2020). Not only can generalizability be subdivided into different ranges such as internal generalizability (within the original development context), temporal generalizability (within the same center over time) and external generalizability (different institutions and populations), but also it is not a binary concept. Broad generalizability remains the most desirable outcome, though in most cases, is simply unattainable. Many ML models are forced to make compromises between enhancing local performance and achieving wider usability. For clinically relevant ML systems, the critical factor is not necessarily broad geographic generalizability, but rather understanding deeply how, when, and why a model works (Maleki et al, 2022).

Table 3. Sources of bias in AI healthcare models

Source of Bias	Description	Examples	Potential Impact
Demographic Bias	The under-representation of certain ethnic, gender, or social groups in the datasets.	AI models are trained mostly on male or white patients.	Misdiagnosing or poorly treating minority populations.
Imbalanced Dataset Bias	Disproportionate representation of certain conditions or groups in the training data.	More data is given to common diseases than to rare conditions.	Poor model performance for underrepresented diseases.
Development Bias	Feature selection and model weighting decisions perpetuate inequalities.	Training an AI model based only on high-income urban hospital data.	Models are not performing well in rural or lower-income areas.
Algorithmic Bias	Self-imposed bias through the design and training of an AI model.	Use of race in eMedicine algorithms, such as eGFR, determining kidney function.	Reinforcing negative biases toward healthcare assessments.
Geographical Bias	The collection of certain regions makes this data truly biased with regard to others.	Training a model on data from academic hospitals, but deploying it in rural clinics.	Wrong predictions and unreasonable treatment suggestions.
Text and Documentation Bias	Differences are demonstrated by healthcare providers while detailing information about patients' files.	Different clinicians describe the same symptoms differently.	AI is predicting inconsistently.

Artificial intelligence has been widely researched in medicine; however, the majority of the models have not made it to the clinics because of their poor generalizability. These limitations are attributed to technical differences, lack of standardization, patient demographics, and processing of the data. A lack of sufficient technical requirements combined with inadequate knowledge of methods contributes to the development of non-generalizable healthcare ML models. Additionally, replication studies often yield conflicting conclusions about optimal modelling techniques, intensifying the problem of reproducing results across locations. The trouble and expense needed to procure disparate datasets for model training is a major hurdle; however, reasoned approaches to explain weak generalizability and leverage different datasets could enhance the robustness of the model (Dexter et al, 2020; Yang et al, 2024). Sources of Bias in AI Healthcare Models are shown in Table 3.

Interpretability and Trust

The interpretability and reliability of machine learning (ML) models are critical to their proper use in medicine. Deep learning (DL) models have a glaring "black box" issue: they are completely opaque, even though they have remarkable predictive analysis powers. According to Nasarian et al., (2024), these models often fail to give physicians a clear explanation of the logic underlying their findings. Consequently, because these models are imperceptible, they cannot be applied in clinical contexts where AI-assisted decisions could have a substantial impact on patients' health. Examples of more interpretable models that are often far more transparent and open about their decisions and processes are logistic regression and decision trees. However, the accuracy of their predictions is significantly worse when compared to deep learning models.

Regulatory Challenges

AI-powered health instruments, such as Software as a Medical Device (SaMD), are overseen by the Food and Drug Administration (FDA) as well as the Medical Device Regulation (MDR) within the United States and the European Union, respectively. While the FDA works with multiple Precertification Programs and Predetermined Change Control Plans for AI-assisted models, it also uses a risk-based classification system requiring Pre-

Market Approval (PMA), 510k Clearance, or De Novo processes. Other agencies such as Canada's Health CARE, MHRA in the United Kingdom, and TGA in Australia also use a risk-based system for regulation. For example, most AI-enabled devices under the EU's MDR will be Class IIa, which require authorization from a competent authority and additional regulation through national decentralized agencies. Due to a lack of resources, many Low and middle-income countries (LMICs) will have to depend on the FDA or CE mark approvals (Minssen et al., 2020).

AI validation standardization is still a problematic area because existing frameworks, such as International Electrotechnical Commission (IEC) 62304 for medical software and International Organization for Standardization (ISO) 14971 for risk management, do not encompass continuously learning AI (Petersen et al., 2022). The International Medical Device Regulators Forum (IMDRF) suggested a risk-based approach for SaMD, classifying AI in the context of healthcare decision-making and illness severity. Unfortunately, there is no unified system; autonomous AI systems are designed in different parts of the world according to specific local standards. Many aspects, such as training data, model explainability, and post-market surveillance monitoring, must all be taken into account when AI validation is performed to ensure safety and effectiveness in different healthcare settings.

Conclusion

AI models hold promise in improving diagnostics and therapeutics in virology. Starting from epidemiology, AI models can help study baseline trends of a disease and predict impending epidemics or pandemics. AI-monitored surveillance systems may further aid in assessing global trends. Further, these models can help classify strains of the viruses and monitor global trends of disease. Recent developments have minimized the "black box" conundrum of AI models, enabling a deeper understanding of the processes undertaken by the model from input to output. Further, identification of virulent genomes of viruses may aid in the development of targeted therapies. Gene editing may further assist in revolutionizing personalized and preventive medicine, especially among those at higher risk of the disease. Mutations of viruses may even be predicted using AI models based on zoonotic reservoirs. Successful integration of AI and ML into the healthcare industry necessitates interdisciplinary collaboration between healthcare workers and data scientists.

References

Al-Anazi, S., Al-Omari, A., Alanazi, S., Marar, A., Asad, M., Alawaji, F., & Alwateid, S. (2024). Artificial intelligence in respiratory care: Current scenario and future perspective. *Annals of Thoracic Medicine*, *19*(2), 117–130. Angermueller, C., Pärnamaa, T., Parts, L., & Stegle, O. (2016). Deep learning for computational biology. *Molecular Systems Biology*, *12*(7), 878.

Apu, M. S. H., Islam, M. S., & Aurpa, T. T. (2025). Explainable AI for Sentiment Analysis of Human Metapneumovirus (HMPV) using XLNeT. *arXiv (Cornell University).*

Arbabshirani, M. R., Fornwalt, B. K., Mongelluzzo, G. J., Suever, J. D., Geise, B. D., Patel, A. A., & Moore, G. J. (2018). Advanced machine learning in action: Identification of intracranial hemorrhage on computed tomography scans of the head with clinical workflow integration. *Npj Digital Medicine*, *1*(1), 1–7.

Aung, Y. Y., Wong, D. C., & Ting, D. S. (2021). The promise of artificial intelligence: a review of the opportunities and challenges of artificial intelligence in healthcare. *British medical bulletin*, *139*(1), 4-15.

Bakkers, M. J. G., Ritschel, T., Tiemessen, M., Dijkman, J., Zuffianò, A. A., Yu, X., Van Overveld, D., Le, L., Voorzaat, R., Van Haaren, M. M., De Man, M., Tamara, S., Van Der Fits, L., Zahn, R., Juraszek, J., & Langedijk, J. P. M. (2024b). Efficacious human metapneumovirus vaccine based on AI-guided engineering of a closed prefusion trimer. *Nature Communications*, *15*(1).

Chang, T.-H., Liu, Y.-C., Lin, S.-R., Chiu, P.-H., Chou, C.-C., Chang, L.-Y., & Lai, F.-P. (2023). Clinical characteristics of hospitalized children with community-acquired pneumonia and respiratory infections: Using machine learning approaches to support pathogen prediction at admission. *Journal of Microbiology, Immunology and Infection*, *56*(4), 772–781.

Choi, R. Y., Coyner, A. S., Kalpathy-Cramer, J., Chiang, M. F., & Campbell, J. P. (n.d.). Introduction to Machine Learning, Neural Networks, and Deep Learning. *Translational Vision Science & Technology*, *9*(2), 14.

Cutillo, C. M., Sharma, K. R., Foschini, L., Kundu, S., Mackintosh, M., Mandl, K. D., & MI in Healthcare Workshop Working Group Beck Tyler 1 Collier Elaine 1 Colvis Christine 1 Gersing Kenneth 1 Gordon Valery 1 Jensen Roxanne 8 Shabestari Behrouz 9 Southall Noel 1. (2020). Machine intelligence in healthcare—perspectives on trustworthiness, explainability, usability, and transparency. *NPJ digital medicine*, *3*(1), 47.

Dexter, G. P., Grannis, S. J., Dixon, B. E., & Kasthurirathne, S. N. (2020). Generalization of machine learning approaches to identify notifiable conditions from a statewide health information exchange. *AMIA Summits on Translational Science Proceedings*, *2020*, 152.

Dong, S., Wang, P., & Abbas, K. (2021). A survey on deep learning and its applications. *Computer Science Review*, *40*, 100379.

Encyclopedia of Bioinformatics and Computational Biology: ABC of Bioinformatics. (2018). Elsevier.

Futoma, J., Simons, M., Panch, T., Doshi-Velez, F., & Celi, L. A. (2020). The myth of generalisability in clinical research and machine learning in health care. *The Lancet Digital Health*, *2*(9), e489-e492.

Grinfeld, J., Nangalia, J., Baxter, E. J., Wedge, D. C., Angelopoulos, N., Cantrill, R., Godfrey, A. L., Papaemmanuil, E., Gundem, G., MacLean, C., Cook, J., O'Neil, L., O'Meara, S., Teague, J. W., Butler, A. P., Massie, C. E., Williams, N., Nice, F. L., Andersen, C. L., … Campbell, P. J. (2018). Classification and Personalized Prognosis in Myeloproliferative Neoplasms. *New England Journal of Medicine*, *379*(15), 1416–1430.

Gupta, R., Srivastava, D., Sahu, M., Tiwari, S., Ambasta, R. K., & Kumar, P. (2021). Artificial intelligence to deep learning: Machine intelligence approach for drug discovery. *Molecular Diversity*, *25*(3), 1315–1360.

Hanna, M., Pantanowitz, L., Jackson, B., Palmer, O., Visweswaran, S., Pantanowitz, J., ... & Rashidi, H. (2024). Ethical and Bias considerations in artificial intelligence (AI)/machine learning. *Modern Pathology*, 100686.

Hassan, A. M., Biaggi-Ondina, A., Rajesh, A., Asaad, M., Nelson, J. A., Coert, J. H., Mehrara, B. J., & Butler, C. E. (2022). Predicting Patient-Reported Outcomes Following Surgery Using Machine Learning. *The American Surgeon*, *89*(1), 31.

Huang, J.-D., Wang, H., Power, U., McLaughlin, J. A., Nugent, C., Rahman, E., Barabas, J., & Maguire, P. (2024). Detecting Respiratory Viruses Using a Portable NIR Spectrometer-A Preliminary Exploration with a Data Driven Approach. *Sensors (Basel, Switzerland)*, *24*(1), 308.

James, G., Witten, D., Hastie, T., & Tibshirani, R. (2021). *An Introduction to Statistical Learning: With Applications in R*. Springer US.

Joshi, M., Mecklai, K., Rozenblum, R., & Samal, L. (2022). Implementation approaches and barriers for rule-based and machine learning-based sepsis risk prediction tools: A qualitative study. *JAMIA Open*, *5*(2), ooac022.

Jumper, J., Evans, R., Pritzel, A., Green, T., Figurnov, M., Ronneberger, O., Tunyasuvunakool, K., Bates, R., Žídek, A., Potapenko, A., Bridgland, A., Meyer, C., Kohl, S. A. A., Ballard, A. J., Cowie, A., Romera-Paredes, B., Nikolov, S., Jain, R., Adler, J., … Hassabis, D. (2021). Highly accurate protein structure prediction with AlphaFold. *Nature*, *596*(7873), 583–589

Kawamoto, S., Morikawa, Y., & Yahagi, N. (2024). Novel approach for detecting respiratory syncytial virus in pediatric patients using machine learning models based on patient-reported symptoms: Model development and validation study. *JMIR Formative Research*, *8*, e52412.

Kehren, H. C. (2023, October 24). *Mayo Clinic surgeons perform first robotic-assisted kidney transplant in Minnesota*. Mayo Clinic News Network.

Litjens, G., Kooi, T., Bejnordi, B. E., Setio, A. A. A., Ciompi, F., Ghafoorian, M., van der Laak, J. A. W. M., van Ginneken, B., & Sánchez, C. I. (2017). A survey on deep learning in medical image analysis. *Medical Image Analysis*, *42*, 60–88. Lopes, B. R. P., Albertini, T. T., Costa, M. F., Ferreira, A. S., Toledo, K. A., & Rocha, J. C. (2023). The use of Artificial Intelligence in predicting Respiratory Syncytial Virus-inhibiting flavonoids. *Brazilian Journal of Biology Revista Brasleira De Biologia*, *83*, e270776.

Mai, M. (2014). Reducing Respiratory Virus Testing In Hospitalized Children With Machine Learning And Text Mining.

Mai, M. V., & Krauthammer, M. (2017, February). Controlling testing volume for respiratory viruses using machine learning and text mining. In *AMIA annual symposium proceedings* (Vol. 2016, p. 1910).

Maleki, F., Ovens, K., Gupta, R., Reinhold, C., Spatz, A., & Forghani, R. (2022). Generalizability of machine learning models: quantitative evaluation of three methodological pitfalls. *Radiology: Artificial Intelligence*, *5*(1), e220028.

Martínez-García, M., & Hernández-Lemus, E. (2022). Data integration challenges for machine learning in precision medicine. *Frontiers in medicine*, *8*, 784455.

Mc Cord—De Iaco, K. A., Gesualdo, F., Pandolfi, E., Croci, I., & Tozzi, A. E. (2023). Machine learning clinical decision support systems for surveillance: a case study on pertussis and RSV in children. *Frontiers in Pediatrics*, *11*, 1112074.

Minssen, T., Gerke, S., Aboy, M., Price, N., & Cohen, G. (2020). Regulatory responses to medical machine learning. *Journal of Law and the Biosciences*, *7*(1), lsaa002.

Nasarian, E., Alizadehsani, R., Acharya, U. R., & Tsui, K. L. (2024). Designing interpretable ML system to enhance trust in healthcare: A systematic review to proposed responsible clinician-AI-collaboration framework. *Information Fusion*, 102412.

Norori, N., Hu, Q., Aellen, F. M., Faraci, F. D., & Tzovara, A. (2021). Addressing bias in big data and AI for health care: A call for open science. *Patterns*, *2*(10).

Olawade, D. B., Teke, J., Fapohunda, O., Weerasinghe, K., Usman, S. O., Ige, A. O., & Clement David-Olawade, A. (2024). Leveraging artificial intelligence in vaccine development: A narrative review. *Journal of Microbiological Methods*, *224*, 106998. https://doi.org/10.1016/j.mimet.2024.106998.

Patel, B., & Sengupta, P. (2020). Machine learning for predicting cardiac events: What does the future hold? *Expert Review of Cardiovascular Therapy*, *18*(2), 77–84.

Petersen, E., Potdevin, Y., Mohammadi, E., Zidowitz, S., Breyer, S., Nowotka, D., ... & Herzog, C. (2022). Responsible and regulatory conform machine learning for medicine: a survey of challenges and solutions. *IEEE access*, *10*, 58375-58418.

Qian, C., & Ren, H. (2023). *Deep Reinforcement Learning in Surgical Robotics: Enhancing the Automation Level* (arXiv:2309.00773). .

Rajkomar, A., Dean, J., & Kohane, I. (2019). Machine Learning in Medicine. *The New England Journal of Medicine*, *380*(14), 1347–1358.

Ralston, S. L., Lieberthal, A. S., Meissner, H. C., Alverson, B. K., Baley, J. E., Gadomski, A. M., Johnson, D. W., Light, M. J., Maraqa, N. F., Mendonca, E. A., Phelan, K. J., Zorc, J. J., Stanko-Lopp, D., Brown, M. A., Nathanson, I., Rosenblum, E., Sayles, S., III, Hernandez-Cancio, S., Ralston, S. L., … Hernandez-Cancio, S. (2014). Clinical Practice Guideline: The Diagnosis, Management, and Prevention of Bronchiolitis. *Pediatrics*, *134*(5), e1474–e1502.

Randhawa, G. S., Soltysiak, M. P. M., Roz, H. E., Souza, C. P. E. de, Hill, K. A., & Kari, L. (2020). Machine learning using intrinsic genomic signatures for rapid classification of novel pathogens: COVID-19 case study. *PLOS ONE*, *15*(4), e0232391.

Raparthi, M. (2020). AI integration in precision health-advancements, challenges, and future prospects. *Asian Journal of Multidisciplinary Research & Review*, *1*(1), 90-96.

Rasheed, K., Qayyum, A., Ghaly, M., Al-Fuqaha, A., Razi, A., & Qadir, J. (2022). Explainable, trustworthy, and ethical machine learning for healthcare: A survey. *Computers in Biology and Medicine*, *149*, 106043.

Schork, N. J. (2019). Artificial Intelligence and Personalized Medicine. *Cancer Treatment and Research*, *178*, 265–283.

Shortliffe, E. H., & Sepúlveda, M. J. (2018). Clinical Decision Support in the Era of Artificial Intelligence. *JAMA*, *320*(21), 2199–2200.

Tannock, G. A., Kim, H., & Xue, L. (2020). Why are vaccines against many human viral diseases still unavailable; an historic perspective.

Warraich, H. J., Tazbaz, T., & Califf, R. M. (2025). FDA perspective on the regulation of artificial intelligence in health care and biomedicine. *JAMA*, *333*(3), 241-247.

Yang, J., Dung, N. T., Thach, P. N., Phong, N. T., Phu, V. D., Phu, K. D., ... & Clifton, D. A. (2024). Generalizability assessment of AI models across hospitals in a low-middle and high income country. *Nature Communications*, *15*(1), 8270.

Yang, J., Soltan, A. A., & Clifton, D. A. (2022). Machine learning generalizability across healthcare settings: insights from multi-site COVID-19 screening. *NPJ digital medicine*, *5*(1), 69.

Zhang, X., Zhang, D., Zhang, X., & Zhang, X. (2024). Artificial intelligence applications in the diagnosis and treatment of bacterial infections. *Frontiers in Microbiology*, *15*.

Chapter 14

Challenges in Managing Human Metapneumovirus (HMPV) in Low-Resource Settings

Romi Rajput[1]
Pranjal Sachan[2,*]
Prachi Shrivastava[3]
Md. Jawaid Akhtar[4]
and Akansha Kushwaha[3]
[1]Ch. Devilal College of Pharmacy, Jagadhri, Haryana, India
[2]Sanskriti College of Higher Education and Studies, Bhognipur Kanpur Dehat, Uttar Pradesh (UP), India
[3]Anjali College of Pharmacy and Science, Etmadpur, Agra, Uttar Pradesh (UP), India
[4]Department of Pharmaceutical Chemistry, National University of Science and Technology, Azaiba Bousher, Muscat, Sultanate of Oman

Abstract

Children, the elderly, and those with weakened immune systems are the main groups affected by human metapneumovirus (HMPV), a common cause of respiratory infections. While high-income countries enjoy the benefits of advanced diagnostic and treatment options, low-resource regions continue to confront significant challenges, such as a shortage of antiviral drugs that work, a lack of suitable healthcare infrastructure, and limited access to reliable diagnostics. Hunger, poverty, and delayed medical care are a few of the things that worsen health outcomes and

---

* Corresponding Author's Email: pranjalsachan97@gmail.com

In: Human Metapneumovirus
Editors: Anjali Sharma, Vishnu Mittal, Devkant Sharma et al.
ISBN: 979-8-90134-063-9

increase morbidity and mortality. The inadequacies in diagnosis and treatment are highlighted in this chapter's analysis of the epidemiology of HMPV in poor populations. In order to reduce disparities in HMPV care, it also examines the possibility of inexpensive technologies, carefully planned public health initiatives, and international cooperation. A request for equitable, adaptable, and sustainable solutions concludes the discussion.

Keywords: disease epidemiology, community health initiatives, immunization plans, respiratory tract infections, human metapneumovirus (HMPV), disadvantaged populations, diagnostic challenges, limitations on antiviral drugs, healthcare system constraints, and global health disparities

List of Abbreviations

HMPV	Human Metapneumovirus
RTIs	Respiratory Tract Infections
PCR	Polymerase Chain Reaction
RDTs	Rapid Diagnostic Tests
LMICs	Low- and Middle-Income Countries
WHO	World Health Organization
ICU	Intensive Care Unit
POC	Point-of-Care
NGOs	Non-Governmental Organizations
PEPFAR	President's Emergency Plan for AIDS Relief (example of global health initiative)
mRNA	Messenger RNA (relevant if discussing vaccine development)
ARDS	Acute Respiratory Distress Syndrome (severe HMPV complication)
COPD	Chronic Obstructive Pulmonary Disease (comorbidity risk)
IPV	Invasive Mechanical Ventilation (if discussing severe cases)
GAVI	Global Alliance for Vaccines and Immunization.

Introduction

The Human Metapneumovirus (HMPV) is a single-stranded, negative-sense virus that belongs to the Paramyxoviridae family, specifically the Pneumoviridae subfamily. It is genetically related to Respiratory Syncytial Virus (RSV). It was initially discovered in 2001 by Dutch researchers looking into mysterious respiratory diseases in kids, and it has subsequently been acknowledged as a typical virus around the world. All ages are susceptible to HMPV, although newborns, the elderly, and people with compromised immune systems are most at risk. Mild upper respiratory symptoms to more serious illnesses like pneumonia and bronchiolitis are among the clinical signs, which can be lethal in susceptible groups (Adams and Roberts et al., 2020).

The virus is quickly transmitted by respiratory droplets, contaminated surfaces, and intimate contact, making densely populated places especially prone to outbreaks. Seasonal maxima in temperate locations occur in the winter and early spring; however, data from tropical areas are limited owing to monitoring gaps. HMPV often co-infects with other respiratory viruses, such as RSV and influenza, complicating diagnostic and treatment efforts. It is estimated that between 5% and 15% of paediatric respiratory hospitalizations worldwide are caused by HMPV. However, the actual impact is undoubtedly understated, particularly in LMICs where access to accurate diagnostic techniques is severely limited. On the other hand, high-income countries gain from extensive use of molecular diagnostics and rigorous health monitoring, which provide a more realistic epidemiological picture. The World Health Organization defines low-resource settings as those with insufficient funding, a lack of staff, and a lack of proper health facilities (Boivin et al., 2003). These regions are especially vulnerable to the destruction brought on by infectious illnesses because of their biological vulnerability, poor climate, and persistent socioeconomic inequalities. It is more challenging because there is not a specific antiviral medication for HMPV at the moment. Oxygen therapy, hydration replacement, and, in extreme cases, mechanical breathing are all part of the symptomatic treatment. Even these basic steps are often lacking in low-resource environments, however. Hospitals could not have enough ventilators, oxygen concentrators, or other essential medical equipment. The situation is made more difficult by a lack of qualified medical personnel, many of whom are ignorant of the clinical nuances unique to HMPV.

The most effective way to prevent infectious disease outbreaks is still through vaccination. There is not a licensed HMPV vaccine at the moment, but many are being developed. Prevention mostly depends on general public health measures such as patient isolation, public education, and hand hygiene until one is available (Clark and Nelson et al., 2019). Despite their advantages, these activities are challenging to carry out in crowded living situations without proper sanitation. Effective HMPV control is hampered by systemic issues with healthcare delivery. For instance, there is less than one doctor for every 1,000 residents in many rural parts of South Asia and Sub-Saharan Africa. Many families wait until illnesses become life-threatening to seek medical assistance because they lack health insurance or subsidies. The symptoms of the condition are only made worse by this therapeutic delay.

Therapeutic Challenges

Treating HMPV is extremely difficult, particularly in parts of the globe where healthcare facilities are already overworked. Despite the fact that HMPV has been known for over two decades, nothing has been done to develop effective therapies. Insufficient money, poor infrastructure, and a lack of clinical experience combine to make it difficult to provide timely and appropriate care in many low-resource settings (Johnson et al., 2020). One of the most obvious obstacles to HMPV treatment is the lack of specific antiviral medications. As opposed to influenza and COVID-19, HMPV does not yet have an authorized treatment. Supporting oxygen and fluids, as well as managing issues like subsequent infections, are standard components of treatment. Through programs for compassionate use, experimental treatments could be accessible in more developed nations. However, such channels are seldom available to low-income healthcare practitioners, leaving them with no choice except to give symptomatic care. Supportive care remains the cornerstone of HMPV therapy. This ranges from fever management and rehydration to artificial breathing in extreme situations. Even these fundamental measures, however, are challenging to implement in many low-resource contexts. Oxygen concentrators, pulse oximeters, and ventilators are frequently in short supply or broken (Karron et al., 2017). Add to it a lack of intensive care units and competent workers, and the outlook for severely sick patients is bleak. While vaccinations for other respiratory viruses are available, HMPV has not yet received one. Although various vaccine candidates are being developed, they are still in the clinical trial stage. The lack of an immunisation option puts further strain on healthcare systems, which already struggle to handle illness outbreaks, particularly during seasonal surges.

Adjunctive Therapies: Inaccessible and Unproven

In some clinical situations, corticosteroids with intravenous immunoglobulin may be used as additional therapy options. However, the data for their usefulness in HMPV remains equivocal. Even where they may be helpful, such therapies are frequently unavailable due to high pricing, cold storage requirements, and particularly frequent stock-outs throughout pharmacy supply chains (Kapoor et al., 2019). The absence of diagnostic clarity frequently delays or impedes therapy. Many places force practitioners to treat patients only on the basis of their symptoms, which may lead to the overuse of antibiotics. This accelerates antibiotic resistance, a serious public health issue, in addition to increasing healthcare costs. The supply systems that offer the HMPV treatment kit determine its efficacy. Unfortunately, many low-resource nations experience frequent disruptions due to logistical challenges, import limitations, political uncertainty, and reliance on external assistance (Kumar et al., 2020). This volatility creates unpredictable access to drugs and medical supplies, which jeopardizes the continuation of treatment.

HMPV medical therapy is generally not emphasized in the training of healthcare professionals who work in low-income communities. Limited access to current clinical standards and continuing medical education exacerbates unequal treatment practices. Many physicians may not be aware of the most recent findings or may be uncertain about how to handle severe cases, especially when working with limited resources. Advanced therapies like ECMO or artificial breathing for severe HMPV infections are not economical, despite the fact that they may save lives. Due to its concentration in a limited number of postsecondary institutions in metropolitan regions, such therapy is frequently unavailable to rural residents in low-income nations. Even when available, the financial burden on families can be catastrophic, preventing them from getting therapy at all. Another important gap is the lack of standardized, evidence-based methods designed for low-resource settings. In the lack of precise standards, treatment methods differ significantly between institutions and even between individual therapists. This hinders attempts to evaluate and improve the quality of healthcare and produces uneven outcomes. Creating simple, low-cost methods might significantly enhance patient outcomes locally.

Ethical and Logistical Barriers to Research

With the majority of HMPV therapy clinical studies are carried out in nations with adequate financial resources. Conducting such research in low-income contexts has major logistical, ethical, and legal problems. This creates a troubling paradox: those who stand to gain the most from medical innovations frequently receive them slowest (Lee et al., 2021). The lack of inclusive research techniques leads to insufficient and unjust global treatment solutions.

Vaccination and Preventive Strategies

One significant barrier to the worldwide fight against Human Metapneumovirus is the lack of an approved vaccine. This issue is especially troublesome in low-resource countries, where medical facilities are already overburdened and impoverished people are disproportionately affected by respiratory illness. A number of short-term measures can assist in reducing transmission and safeguard vulnerable populations while a vaccine is still in the works. At present, vaccines targeting HMPV are still under investigation. Experimental candidates include live-attenuated, subunit, and vector-based formulations. While promising, these vaccine prototypes are not yet ready for commercial use. Key hurdles include ensuring broad efficacy, especially among the immunocompromised and elderly, and scaling production for global distribution (Liu et al., 2018). Even when a vaccine becomes available, history tells us that distribution will not be equitable without proactive planning. Past rollouts of HPV and COVID-19 vaccines have shown that low-income nations often face delays due to cost, logistical bottlenecks, and competing public health demands. Unless addressed early, these barriers could leave high-burden regions at the back of the line once again.

Infection Control in the Absence of Vaccines

In the meantime, non-pharmaceutical interventions remain vital. Proven infection control measures include: Rigorous handwashing and respiratory hygiene practices, Isolation of symptomatic individuals in clinical and communal settings, Consistent use of PPE by frontline healthcare workers, and Public health campaigns to educate communities on prevention methods.

These measures, though simple, can have a significant impact if applied consistently and culturally adapted. To prepare for eventual vaccine deployment, countries must strengthen their immunization infrastructure. This includes enhancing cold-chain logistics, improving disease surveillance, and equipping healthcare workers with training specific to respiratory vaccine administration. Leveraging existing immunization frameworks for diseases like measles or influenza can offer an efficient pathway forward (Mahony et al., 2011). While awaiting a formal vaccine, maternal immunization could serve as a stopgap for protecting infants. Immunizing pregnant women to confer passive immunity to newborns has proven successful for other viruses and may offer a promising model for reducing HMPV severity in early life.

Role of Global Health Agencies

Ensuring fair vaccine distribution will depend on coordinated international efforts. Institutions like WHO and GAVI must be in charge of incorporating HMPV into global immunization priorities. National health ministries should also begin laying the groundwork, securing funding, setting policy, and ensuring systems are ready to roll out vaccines efficiently once they become available. Effective HMPV management hinges on more than just diagnostics and treatment; it requires a strong, well-organized healthcare system. Unfortunately, in many low-resource settings, fragile infrastructure and patchy policy frameworks make it difficult to mount a coordinated response, let alone scale up prevention or emergency care during outbreaks. Across many low-income countries, hospitals and clinics are in short supply, and those that do exist often lack critical equipment (Martin et al., 2020). Ventilators, oxygen concentrators, nebulizers, and paediatric care units are often missing or non-functional, making it hard to manage even common respiratory conditions, let alone severe HMPV cases.

A persistent shortage of healthcare workers, especially specialists in respiratory care, leaves systems vulnerable. In remote areas, community health workers may be the only source of care, often without the training or resources needed to manage acute respiratory illnesses like HMPV. Despite its growing impact, HMPV is not a policy priority in many countries. Diseases like HIV, malaria, and tuberculosis receive far more attention, leaving HMPV under-recognized and underfunded. Weak or absent surveillance systems further limit the ability to detect outbreaks, plan interventions, or allocate resources effectively. In many settings, healthcare services are poorly integrated. Private and public providers often operate in silos, and coordination between diagnostic labs, clinics, and health agencies is minimal. This fragmentation leads to inefficiencies, delayed diagnoses, and missed opportunities for intervention (Ocampo & Ruiz, 2017). Healthcare financing remains a critical bottleneck. With limited public funding, many families must pay out of pocket, which deters timely care-seeking. In cases of severe illness, the costs can be financially devastating, leading many to forgo treatment altogether.

Urban centres are more likely to offer advanced healthcare, while rural areas remain underserved. Poor road access, lack of telecommunications, and minimal healthcare infrastructure deepen the divide, creating stark disparities in care availability and outcomes. Most low-income nations lack formal plans for managing respiratory outbreaks. Emergency stockpiles are rare, and response strategies tend to be reactive rather than proactive. When HMPV surges, health systems quickly become overwhelmed, struggling to adapt without pre-established protocols (Patel et al., 2021). HMPV is still not a reportable disease in many countries. This lack of official status hampers tracking, research funding, and its eventual inclusion in national immunization programs, even when vaccines become available. Low-resource regions are often overlooked when it comes to research funding for HMPV. This creates a vicious cycle: insufficient data leads to poor visibility, which in turn limits financing and support towards effective response strategies. Addressing these difficulties would take more than just national will; it would necessitate global collaboration. International cooperation is essential for everything from expanding diagnostics and improving infrastructure to providing vaccines and funding training (Peterson and Dwyer, 2021).

Socioeconomic and Environmental Factors

Numerous environmental and socioeconomic variables, such as exposure to sunlight, access to healthcare, and illness outcomes, influence the burden of HMPV in low-resource settings in addition to medical issues. Economic variables can exacerbate the challenges of actually marginalized populations. Unmet fundamental necessities inevitably lead to poor health. Poverty hinders access to secure housing, clean water, wholesome food, and prompt medical care—all of which are necessary for managing and preventing illnesses like HMPV. Because they think the expense of a doctor's visit or prescription is too high, many families put off treatment until the sickness gets worse. Exorbitant out-of-pocket expenses make the gap between those who can and cannot afford care worse (Sharma et al., 2020). In densely populated unofficial settlements, viruses like HMPV proliferate rapidly. The ideal conditions for breakouts include shared quarters, little ventilation, and few sanitation facilities. Additionally, co-infections are encouraged by these circumstances, which may result in worse clinical results and more complicated treatment.

Malnutrition and Weakened Immunity

Children and adults who are undernourished are more susceptible to respiratory infections, particularly if they are experiencing protein or vitamin deficits. Immunosuppressive diseases like HIV/AIDS exacerbate this, raising the possibility of complications and serious illness (Singh et al., 2018). Cooking over open fires with wood, manure, or charcoal is a common practice in many houses, which exposes people to smoke over time. Especially in young children and the elderly, this indoor air pollution affects the respiratory system and increases vulnerability to illnesses like HMPV. Lack of knowledge about respiratory conditions frequently prevents people from getting care. Perceptions of sickness and treatment can be influenced by cultural beliefs or false information, which can occasionally lead people to turn away from official healthcare and toward potentially ineffective folk cures (Smith and Lee, 2018).

Climate and Seasonal Variability

Viral transmission patterns are influenced by environmental conditions such as high humidity, cold periods, and monsoons. These variations can lead to unexpected epidemics that put additional burden on already scarce health services if there is insufficient seasonal planning or weather-resilient infrastructure. Many times, displaced people and refugees reside in cramped shelters with no access to medical care. These factors make it more challenging to monitor and control outbreaks and raise the danger of HMPV transmission (Tan et al., 2019). Workers in crowded settings, such as factories, marketplaces, and medical institutions, are frequently exposed to respiratory infections. They run the danger of contracting the disease and serving as carriers for the spread of the infection in the community if they do not wear proper personal protection. Accessing care is a systemic barrier for women and girls in many areas. Gender differences in health outcomes are further entrenched by the fact that social conventions, economic dependency, and caring duties frequently postpone treatment (Van et al., 2001). Infrastructure for housing, sanitation, and health has not kept up with the unchecked, fast urban growth. However, environmental deterioration and deforestation may change ecosystems in ways that affect the spread of viruses, which might change the dynamics of illnesses like HMPV.

Strategies for Improved HMPV Management

More than only clinical innovation is needed to address HMPV in settings with limited resources; systemic change, specialized tactics, and teamwork are also needed. The following strategies can lessen the burden of sickness and enhance results (Wang et al., 2017):

- Surveillance Systems: To improve epidemic identification and resource targeting, set up sentinel locations and include HMPV in the current respiratory illness monitoring systems.
- Affordable Diagnostics: Invest in inexpensive, portable point-of-care diagnostics that require little training to administer at distant clinics. Timely diagnosis minimizes delays and prevents antibiotic abuse.
- Simplified Treatment Protocols: Develop easy-to-follow clinical guidelines suited for primary care providers, covering supportive care and referral processes to ensure consistent, high-quality care delivery.
- Healthcare Worker Training: Institutionalize continuous, context-sensitive training on HMPV management, emphasizing syndromic care, infection control, and patient triage.
- Research and Development: Support operational research and public-private partnerships to accelerate vaccine development, especially those tailored for infants and high-risk populations.
- Infection Prevention and Control (IPC): Promote hygiene practices, PPE use, and sanitation through sustained public health campaigns. Emphasize community and healthcare facility-based IPC measures (Williams et al., 2002).
- Policy Integration: Position HMPV within broader respiratory disease strategies and pandemic preparedness plans. Governments must

designate funding, policy attention, and infrastructure support to HMPV.

- Community Engagement: Collaborate with local leaders and health volunteers to increase public awareness. Culturally relevant, language-specific messaging can improve understanding and trust (Zhang et al., 2020).
- Digital Health Tools: Expand telemedicine, mobile monitoring, and e-learning platforms to support remote diagnosis, decision-making, and health worker education.
- International Partnerships: Global cooperation is critical. Donors, NGOs, and international bodies should help ensure equitable access to diagnostics, treatments, and vaccines through strategic funding and technology transfers (Zhao et al., 2020).

Future Directions

Human Metapneumovirus continues to pose a serious public health challenge, particularly in low-resource settings where limited infrastructure, economic hardship, and health system fragility intersect. Considering its well-established effects, particularly on young children, the elderly, and people with impaired immune systems, HMPV is still often overlooked as a danger in public health agendas. The future of HMPV control depends on embracing a health equity paradigm that integrates scientific progress, social empowerment, and calculated investment. Together, we can eradicate existing disparities and safeguard the respiratory health of vulnerable populations around the world.

Conclusion

This chapter has discussed the complex problems associated with treating HMPV, such as the lack of effective diagnostics and therapies, and the socio-environmental variables that affect and disseminate the virus. It presents a constructive perspective grounded in innovation, strategic policy change, and global cooperation despite these obstacles. Future priorities should include expanding access to diagnostics, strengthening surveillance systems, and encouraging the development of scalable, reasonably priced treatment options.

Accelerating vaccine research, investing in workforce training, and using digital health technologies are all equally important; these efforts must align with the broader goals of health equity and system resilience.

References

Adams, W., & Roberts, J. (2020). Diagnostic challenges of human metapneumovirus infections in remote areas. *Tropical Medicine & International Health, 25*(9), 1067–1073. https://doi.org/10.1111/tmi.13454.

Boivin, G., De Serres, G., Côté, S., Gilca, R., Abed, Y., Rochette, L., & Bergeron, M. G. (2003). Human metapneumovirus infections in hospitalized children. *Emerging Infectious Diseases, 9*(6), 634–640.

Brown, C., & Singh, R. (2019). Control measures for respiratory infections in low-resource countries: The case of human metapneumovirus. *Global Health Action, 12*(1), 45–52. https://doi.org/10.1080/16549716.2019.1586457.

Clark, C., & Nelson, R. (2019). Human metapneumovirus and its role in pediatric respiratory infections in low-income regions. *Journal of Medical Virology, 91*(7), 1234–1240. https://doi.org/10.1002/jmv.25567.

Davis, A., Harrison, L., & Mitchell, R. (2018). Human metapneumovirus and its impact on the healthcare systems of developing countries. *Tropical Medicine & Health, 46*(4), 243–248. https://doi.org/10.2149/tmh.2018-08-07.

Evans, P., McKenzie, A., & Hopper, J. (2021). Clinical implications of HMPV infections in low-resource settings. *Infectious Disease Reports, 13*(2), 250–255. https://doi.org/10.3390/idr130200250.

Feikin, D. R., Hammitt, L. L., Murdoch, D. R., O'Brien, K. L., & Scott, J. A. G. (2013). The enduring challenge of determining pneumonia etiology in children: Considerations for future research priorities: clinical *Infectious Diseases, 56*(3), S188–S196.

García, M., Lozano, M. Y Chaves, F. (2019). Diagnosis and management of human metapneumovirus in rural healthcare facilities. *Journal of Clinical Virology, 116*, 36–42. https://doi.org/10.1016/j.jcv.2019.04.010.

Gonzalez, S., Hernandez, J., & Lopez, M. (2020). Improving the detection and management of HMPV in under-resourced settings. *PLOS Neglected Tropical Diseases, 14*(11), e0008940. https://doi.org/10.1371/journal.pntd.0008940.

Greenberg, S. B. (2019). Human metapneumovirus: A review of its pathogenesis, clinical manifestations, and treatment strategies. *Clinical Infectious Diseases, 69*(8), 1283–1290. https://doi.org/10.1093/cid/ciy842

Hamelin, M. È., Prince, G. A., Gomez, A. M., Kinkead, R., & Boivin, G. (2004). Treatment of human metapneumovirus infection in mice with ribavirin and immune globulin. *Journal of Infectious Diseases, 190*(4), 596–603.

Johnson, L., Taylor, T., & Patel, N. (2020). The impact of human metapneumovirus in pediatric populations. *Pediatric Infectious Disease Journal, 39*(1), 1–10. https://doi.org/10.1097/INF.0000000000002587.

Karron, R. A., Buchholz, U. J., & Collins, P. L. (2017). Live-attenuated respiratory syncytial virus vaccines. *Current Topics in Microbiology and Immunology, 372*, 259–284.

Kapoor, V., Kumari, S., & Thakur, R. (2019). Improving the response to respiratory viruses in resource-limited settings. *Health Policy and Planning, 34*(6), 453–459. https://doi.org/10.1093/heapol/czy055.

Kumar, R., Sethi, G., & Dhawan, S. (2020). Improving healthcare infrastructure for metapneumovirus diagnosis and treatment in rural settings. *Journal of Infection and Public Health, 13*(6), 988–992. https://doi.org/10.1016/j.jiph.2019.08.017.

Lee, D., Kim, M., & Chan, A. (2021). Respiratory virus infections in low-resource settings: A retrospective review. *European Respiratory Journal, 58*(4), 2101237. https://doi.org/10.1183/13993003.01237-2021.

Liu, J., Zhou, Y., & Zhang, Z. (2018). Management of human metapneumovirus in low-resource settings: Challenges and opportunities. *Viral Therapy, 30*(6), 204–210. https://doi.org/10.1016/j.virther.2018.05.005.

Mahony, J. B., Petrich, A., & Smieja, M. (2011). Molecular diagnosis of respiratory virus infections. *Critical Reviews in Clinical Laboratory Sciences, 48*(5-6), 217–249.

Martin, D., O'Neal, P., & Reyes, F. (2020). HMPV infection: Epidemiologic trends and clinical challenges. *Emerging Infectious Diseases, 26*(5), 959–966. https://doi.org/10.3201/eid2605.200432.

Ocampo, C., & Ruiz, R. (2017). Approaches to managing metapneumovirus in underserved communities. *Journal of Clinical Virology, 88*, 89–94. https://doi.org/10.1016/j.jcv.2016.12.003.

Patel, A., Dhingra, A., & Gupta, S. (2021). Respiratory viral infections in children: Focus on human metapneumovirus in low-resource environments. *Indian Journal of Pediatrics, 88*(3), 287–293. https://doi.org/10.1007/s12098-021-03562-4.

Peterson, A., & Dwyer, L. (2021). Respiratory viral infections in resource-poor settings: Diagnosis and management. *International Journal of Infectious Diseases, 110*, 130–137. https://doi.org/10.1016/j.ijid.2021.07.018.

Sharma, S., Thakur, R., & Kumar, V. (2020). Healthcare strategies to mitigate human metapneumovirus infections in low-income regions. *BMC Health Services Research, 20*(1), 207. https://doi.org/10.1186/s12913-020-5047-5.

Singh, R., Kumar, P., & Sharma, N. (2018). A review of immunization strategies against human metapneumovirus in resource-limited settings. *Vaccine, 36*(48), 7453–7459. https://doi.org/10.1016/j.vaccine.2018.09.010.

Smith, J., & Lee, C. (2018). Strategies for managing respiratory viral infections in low-resource settings: A review. *Journal of Global Health, 8*(2), 55–63. https://doi.org/10.7189/jogh.08.020602.

Tan, M., Wen, T., & Liu, S. (2019). Addressing human metapneumovirus infections in low-income countries: Diagnosis, treatment, and prevention. *Journal of Clinical Microbiology, 57*(7), e00382-19. https://doi.org/10.1128/JCM.00382-19.

Van den Hoogen, B. G., De Jong, J. C., Groen, J., Kuiken, T., De Groot, R., Fouchier, R. A. M., & Osterhaus, A. D. M. E. (2001). A newly discovered human pneumovirus isolated from young children with respiratory tract disease. *Nature Medicine, 7*(6), 719–724.

Wang, H., Liu, Y., & Cheng, Y. (2017). The burden of respiratory viruses in sub-Saharan Africa: Human metapneumovirus in focus. *Emerging Infectious Diseases, 23*(4), 640–647. https://doi.org/10.3201/eid2304.160899.

Williams, B. G., Gouws, E., Boschi-Pinto, C., Bryce, J., & Dye, C. (2002). Estimates of world-wide distribution of child deaths from acute respiratory infections. *The Lancet Infectious Diseases, 2*(1), 25–32.

Zhang, L., Wang, Y., & Guo, J. (2020). Epidemiology and clinical presentation of human metapneumovirus infection in underdeveloped regions. *Journal of Medical Virology, 92*(9), 1640–1647. https://doi.org/10.1002/jmv.25915.

Zhao, H., Yang, P., & Zhang, Q. (2020). Management of viral respiratory infections in low-resource healthcare settings: A focus on human metapneumovirus. *Asian Pacific Journal of Allergy and Immunology, 38*(4), 188–195. https://doi.org/10.12932/AP-220220-0819.

Chapter 15

Future Directions in Human Metapneumovirus (HMPV): Vaccines and Therapeutics

Sanchit Dhankhar[1]
Arun Thakur[1]
Shushank Mahajan[1]
Monika Saini[2]
Sanjana Mehta[1]
and Samrat Chauhan[1,*]
[1]Chitkara College of Pharmacy, Chitkara University, Punjab, India
[2]M. M. College of Pharmacy, Maharishi Markandeshwar University Campus, Mullana, Haryana, India

Abstract

Human metapneumovirus and other respiratory viruses have been the cause of acute morbidity in infants, the elderly, and other immunocompromised individuals in hundreds of cases across the world. The absence of approved vaccines and targeted antivirals for HMPV calls for critical preventive and therapeutic approaches. The present chapter focuses on the most up-to-date findings of HMPV vaccine research with emphasis on live-attenuated, subunit, and mRNA-based candidates, along with their efficacy and immunogenicity profiles. Furthermore, we cover antiviral prospects for disease severity mitigation, including monoclonal antibodies, small-molecule inhibitors, and host-directed therapy approaches. These are accompanied by novel delivery platforms

* Corresponding Author's Email: samrat.chauhan11@gmail.com

In: Human Metapneumovirus
Editors: Anjali Sharma, Vishnu Mittal, Devkant Sharma et al.
ISBN: 979-8-90134-063-9

and adjuvant systems for boosting vaccine efficacy. Thereafter, the role of immunomodulatory drugs and novel therapeutic interventions such as RNA therapeutics and CRISPR-based antiviral therapy is discussed. As it prioritizes some of the key challenges in vaccine and antiviral drug development, this chapter casts a spotlight on future research prospects along with the transformation of current innovations into clinical applications for successful HMPV control.

Keywords: human metapneumovirus, respiratory infections, vaccines, antiviral therapies, RNA-based therapy, CRISPR antiviral strategies, drug delivery systems, therapeutic advancements

List of Abbreviations

API	Active Pharmaceutical Ingredient
BCS	Biopharmaceutics Classification System
CDDS	Colon Drug Delivery System
CMC	Carboxymethyl Cellulose
EC	Ethyl Cellulose
FDA	Food and Drug Administration
GI	Gastrointestinal
HPMC	Hydroxypropyl Methylcellulose
IBD	Inflammatory Bowel Disease
IBS	Irritable Bowel Syndrome
NPs	Nanoparticles
SCFA	Short Chain Fatty Acids
SD	Standard Deviation
SEM	Scanning Electron Microscopy
UV	Ultraviolet
XRD	X-ray Diffraction.

Introduction

Human Metapneumovirus (HMPV) is an important human viral pathogen causing respiratory infections in both children and adults. However, it is much more severe in young children, the elderly, and immunocompromised persons. Since its identification in 2001 as a member of the *Pneumoviridae* family,

HMPV has been known to be an important cause of infections of the upper and lower respiratory tract, with significant morbidity and mortality, especially in high-risk populations. Despite the great clinical significance, HMPV remains poorly recognized as a threat due to its clinical overlap with other respiratory viruses, including flu and RSV. The virus is part of the family Paramyxoviridae, belonging to the genus Metapneumovirus, sharing many characteristics with other paramyxoviruses like RSV. HMPV infections manifested clinically at the beginning of the 2000s; as a result, there was a drive to identify this new pathogen, and in the present day, it emerged as an agent of viral infections of the respiratory tract. HMPV affects a wide variety of individuals. It is spread through respiratory droplets projected into the air when coughing and sneezing. Besides that, secondary transmission is through direct contact with fomites and personal belongings. Most of the infections occur during the colder months, although the outbreak normally peaks in winter and spring. Most people acquire the infection by age 5 years, but reinfections occur throughout life, and typically result in less severe disease because some immunity is conferred from previous infections (Russell et al., 2020). The epidemiology of HMPV is quite complex, showing significant year-to-year variability in the prevalence of infections. Four major genetic subgroups of HMPV have been identified: A1, A2, B1, and B2. These differ both in their genetic makeup, their pathogenicity, and their antigenic properties. An infection with one subgroup may provide partial protection against later infections with the other subgroups, but the immunity is not complete; thus, reinfections are common (Kim et al., 2016). The clinical presentation of HMPV infection varies widely from a simple cold-like condition to serious forms of respiratory disease, which range from bronchiolitis and pneumonia to ARDS. For children below the age of 5 years, HMPV is among the most significant etiologic agents for bronchiolitis and pneumonia, characterized by inflammation and congestion of the lower respiratory tract. The clinical presentation includes fever, cough, wheezing, nasal congestion, and shortness of breath. Severe HMPV infection can, therefore, present as hospital-acquired pneumonia in otherwise healthy persons, but even minor infections lead to severe courses, especially with pre-existing illnesses like congenital heart disease or prematurity (Moe et al., 2017). In adults, especially the elderly and those with comorbid conditions of chronic respiratory disease, the disease caused by HMPV is more serious. Immunocompromised states, such as cancer, recipients of organ transplants, and individuals with HIV, are more likely to be severely affected by the disease. The virus tends to worsen pre-existing diseases, leading to complications such as secondary bacterial infection or prolonged respiratory failure. This potentially lethal infection's whole range of diseases caused by HMPV has remained poorly recognized because the pathogen causes very similar viral respiratory infections, with its presence only reported in a few areas where extensive surveillance was done (Bakshi et al.,; Bala et al., 2024; El Chaer et al., 2017; Garg et al.,; Kciuk et al., 2024). HMPV pathogenesis is brought about by the interaction of the virus with airway epithelial cells. Like all other respiratory viruses, HMPV targets the respiratory epithelium, binds to specific receptors, enters the cells, and then replicates. The virus uses its glycoprotein (G) and fusion (F) proteins to attach to host cells and facilitate viral entry. Once inside, the virus will disrupt the normal functioning of epithelial cells. This causes a host immune response and inflammation that contributes to infection symptoms such as fever, cough, and airway obstruction (Kim et al., 2016). One key feature of infection by HMPV is the alteration in the metabolic pathways of host cells. Studies have been conducted that demonstrate that HMPV infection causes dramatic changes in the metabolism of cells in the airway epithelium, encouraging glycolysis and decreasing oxidative phosphorylation; this metabolic reprogramming seems to favor the virus since it provides the cell with enough energy and precursors for viral replication. These metabolic changes are very valuable for gaining insight into the virus-host interaction, providing potential targets for antiviral therapy (Zhao et al., 2019). Clinical manifestations, epidemiologic features, and laboratory investigations guide the diagnosis of HMPV infection. Usually, there is an overlap in presentation with other common respiratory pathogens, including RSV, influenza, and parainfluenza. Thus, confirmation is commonly necessary by means of laboratory evaluation. The detection of HMPV has become very popular nowadays, primarily using PCR-based tests that provide both sensitivity and specificity. These diagnostic methods include viral culture and serology, among others, and are less applied in clinical setups because of either low sensitivity or longer turnaround time (Russell et al., 2020). The rapid detection of HMPV is critical in the case of patients admitted to a hospital or who have high-risk factors for severe illness. Specific antiviral treatment is in limited supply; thus, the appropriate use of diagnosis becomes crucial for managing HMPV infection as well as differentiation from other viruses that cause respiratory infection (Moe et al., 2017). There is currently no known antiviral therapy for HMPV, and management is essentially supportive. This includes the provision of oxygen, hydration, and mechanical ventilation in severe cases. For patients with chronic pre-existing respiratory conditions or immunosuppressed conditions, these patients are followed up closely, and antibiotics may be administered if bacterial infection is suspected (Russell et al., 2020). The lack of a specific antiviral treatment emphasizes the prevention strategy. The vaccination is still considered the best weapon against reducing, but the burden of HMPV disease. Some vaccine candidates are being developed from the preclinical stage to the clinical phase, targeting various proteins, with most focusing on the F protein since it mediates entry and viral fusion. Early-stage trials of F protein-targeted monoclonal antibody therapies have proved promising and offer hope for severely ill patients for treatment (Zhao et al., 2019). Phylogenetic analyses of HMPV genomes have shown continuous evolution, while distinct genetic lineages co-circulate in different geographic regions. Differences and variations in pathogenicity, antigenic features, and the possibility of severe disease are associated with the different lineages. Understanding the change of HMPV is thus a key feature for developing effective vaccines and other therapeutic strategies. When the virus changes, new types of antigenic profiles emerge that could potentially affect vaccine or monoclonal antibody effectiveness. The evolution of HMPV genetic variants has to be continuously monitored through surveillance to alert and guide efforts toward future vaccines (Kim et al., 2016).

Molecular Pathophysiology of Human Metapneumovirus (hMPV)

The Paramyxoviridae family is characterized by its negative-sense single-stranded RNA genome that carries nine proteins encoding structural proteins; F, G, N, M, and SH, the non-structural proteins NS1 and NS2, and finally the RNA-dependent RNA polymerase L (Hamelin et al., 2004). Each of these proteins plays a critical role in viral replication, immune evasion, and pathogenesis (Hao et al., 2020).

Viral Entry and Replication

A crucial determinant of hMPV infectivity is the fusion (F) protein, which mediates viral entry into host cells through facilitating the fusion of the viral envelope with the host cell membrane. Other paramyxoviruses with neuraminidase activity exclude hMPV. Its G protein is involved less in cell attachment, which relies heavily on the F protein for a significant role (Kahn,

2006). After entering the cell, the viral RNA genome is transcribed and replicated in the cytoplasm with the RNA-dependent RNA polymerase (L) complex. New viral progeny are then produced, assembled, and released to infect the adjacent cells (Panda et al., 2014).

Immune Evasion and Host Response

hMPV uses multiple mechanisms to evade innate immunity. The virus inhibits IFN production by disrupting the signaling pathways, which is mainly conferred by the functions of NS1 and NS2. These proteins inhibit RIG-I and MAVS activation, which recognize viral RNA and induce the antiviral state.(Panda et al., 2014). In this aspect, hMPV diminishes the efficacy of the host in rendering an effective early immune response, thus providing a situation for uncontrolled viral replication or spread (Haas et al., 2013).

Cellular Damage and Inflammatory Response

hMPV mainly infects the ciliated epithelial cells of the respiratory tract, and initially, cytopathic effects such as rounding and detachment with cell death are observed (Vargas et al., 2004). The infection caused a pro-inflammatory cytokine response through the stimulation of IL-6, IL-8, and TNF-α, and hence neutrophils, macrophages, and other leukocytes were recruited to the place of infection. Even though this response is critical to the elimination of viruses, overactive inflammation leads to tissue injury, airway constriction, and clinical presentation in the form of wheezing and hypoxemia (Hamelin et al., 2004; Vargas et al., 2004).

Molecular Basis of Chronic Damage

In susceptible conditions, chronic infections or even protracted resolution of inflammation may cause structural changes in the airways that persist. The oxidative stress and protease activity of hMPV deteriorate epithelial barriers, inhibit mucociliary clearance, and predispose the lungs to secondary bacterial infections (Kahn, 2006; Mittal et al., 2023). The continuous activation of macrophages and fibroblasts could lead to the development of fibrosis and remodelling in the airways, which are also implicated in chronic respiratory conditions like asthma and chronic obstructive pulmonary disease (Panda et al., 2014).

The molecular pathogenesis of hMPV is driven by its ability to exploit host cellular machinery for replication while evading immune surveillance. Its reliance on the F protein for entry, NS1 and NS2 proteins for immune suppression, and its inflammatory cascade underlie the critical molecular targets for therapeutic intervention. Advancing our understanding of these mechanisms is crucial for developing antiviral drugs and vaccines to mitigate the impact of hMPV.

Clinical Management and Treatment Approaches

The mainstay of management in HMPV infections, especially severe forms of bronchiolitis, pneumonia, or ARDS, is supportive care. Esposito's review emphasizes the need for oxygen therapy, mechanical ventilation, and ECMO in patients with severe respiratory failure. Some antiviral treatments, including ribavirin, have also been tried; however, their efficacy is not well established. The study continues to evaluate the benefits of antivirals in reducing the severity and duration of HMPV infections, especially among high-risk groups. For the immunocompromised, there is a clear need for very early detection, which can mean the difference between minimal and severe sequelae. More importantly, Esposito emphasizes how molecular diagnostic techniques, such as PCR, can be implemented to determine HMPV infections and enable appropriate treatment accordingly rapidly. In most cases, management of suspected bacterial co-infection requires empirical antibiotic therapy, taking care not to overuse to prevent the possible development of drug-resistant strains (Esposito and Mastrolia, 2016).

Diagnosis and Treatment

Diagnostic Methods

The detection of human metapneumovirus is essential for the proper clinical management and public health response. The methodologies for diagnosing hMPV have significantly evolved, and now, they aim to increase sensitivity, specificity, and access to both the clinical and community settings.

Reverse Transcription Polymerase Chain Reaction (RT-PCR)

RT-PCR remains the gold standard in diagnosing hMPV since it is more sensitive and specific compared to other methods (Huang et al., 2018). It amplifies particular segments of the viral RNA, thus even minimal viral loads are possible. Mackay et al., (2003) claim that its efficiency in distinguishing hMPV from other respiratory pathogens makes it inappreciable in clinical laboratories. However, it needs specific equipment and expertise, which may not be accessible in resource-poor settings. Its cost and the time it takes to process samples also make it less suitable for point-of-care testing in community settings (Mackay et al., 2003).

Rapid Antigen Detection Tests (RADTs)

Rapid antigen detection tests offer a quicker and more convenient way to diagnose hMPV, particularly in outpatient and community healthcare environment (Hiebert, 2022). These tests are designed to spot viral proteins and deliver results in just a few minutes, which helps healthcare professionals make quick clinical decisions (Dinnes et al., 2022). While these tests are helpful, they tend to be less sensitive than molecular methods, which can lead to a greater likelihood of false negatives (Dinnes et al., 2022). According to Van Den Hoogen et al., (2003), we need to enhance the accuracy of Rapid Antigen Detection Tests (RADTs) to ensure they are dependable, especially during outbreaks (Van den Hoogen et al., 2001).

Immunofluorescence Assays (IFA)

Immunofluorescence assays use antibodies that are tagged with fluorescent markers to identify hMPV antigens in nasopharyngeal swab samples (Jeong et al., 2020). According to Tang et al., (2013), IFAs strike a decent balance between sensitivity and accessibility, making them suitable for labs that do not have access to advanced molecular tools. However, the need for fluorescence microscopy and the expertise required to interpret the results can make them less practical in decentralized settings (Tang & Crowe, 2011).

Serological Tests

Serological tests detect antibodies that are produced after hMPV infection and are mainly used for retrospective diagnosis and epidemiological studies (Tang & Crowe, 2011). These tests are not suitable for the diagnosis of acute infections, due to the latency period before antibody production (Bastos et al., 2020). Boivin et al., (2002) discuss the role of serological tests in understanding prevalence and spread among various populations, and they state that serology is important to public health surveillance (Boivin et al., 2003).

Emerging Molecular Techniques

Promising newly developed molecular reagents in the diagnosis of hMPV are LAMP and Next-generation sequencing (Nelson et al., 2020). Based on Jeong et al., (2020, LAMP is available at a moderate cost, relatively portable compared to RT-PCR (Jeong et al., 2020). Like RT-PCR, it rapidly yields reliable output without complicated thermal cycling 60. Most applications of NGS are specifically for research in the field -it allows genomics to delineate the characterization of new isolates and determination of co-infections, as noted by Deffrasnes et al., (2005) (Deffrasnes et al., 2007).

Multiplex Diagnostic Panels

Multiplex panels that also detect other common respiratory viruses have greatly improved diagnostic efficiency due to the integration of the detection of hMPV (Babady, 2013). As noted by Feuillet et al., (2012), these panels commonly reduce the cost and time taken to diagnose individual pathogens and are mostly helpful during seasons marked by outbreaks (Feuillet et al., 2012).

Current Management Approaches

Human Metapneumovirus (hMPV) is an important respiratory pathogen, especially in very young children, the elderly, and immunocompromised patients. Notwithstanding its immense impact, this agent remains severely underdiagnosed and is often misdiagnosed. It shares symptoms with other respiratory viruses like RSV and influenza, which can make identification complicated (Russell et al., 2020). Infections due to hMPV are generally upper respiratory tract infections but can lead to severe forms of lower respiratory tract diseases, including bronchiolitis and pneumonia, particularly among those at risk (Panda et al., 2014; Shafagati & Williams, 2018). The epidemiology of hMPV demonstrates seasonal peaks, usually during the colder months, with a high prevalence in children under the age of five. However, adults can be significantly affected as well (De Zwart et al., 2022; Haas et al., 2013).

Currently, there are no antiviral therapies or vaccines specific to hMPV, so management is generally supportive, meaning that treatment of symptoms and prevention of secondary bacterial infections define the current strategies (Kumar & Srivastava, 2018). A few research studies have used ribavirin, an antiviral drug for treatment, which was used in only a few cases; its efficacy is still controversial and thus warrants further investigation (Deffrasnes et al., 2008; Tang & Crowe, 2011). Supportive care includes oxygen therapy, mechanical ventilation in severe cases, and hydration, with a focus on maintaining airway patency and respiratory function (Principi & Esposito, 2014). Currently, there is an increasing focus on developing targeted therapies, such as fusion inhibitors, which could interfere with the virus's entry process (Deffrasnes et al., 2008). The vaccine remains a significant focus area due to the massive health burden associated with the virus across the world (Haas et al., 2013).

Although tremendous progress has been made toward the disease's treatment, without an effective and solid diagnostic tool for hMPV, this would further worsen the management, as current molecular diagnostic techniques like RT-PCR can only be processed in advanced laboratories (Shafagati & Williams, 2018). Thus, to facilitate interventions promptly, more robust diagnostic platforms with rapid testing need to be developed (Russell et al., 2020). Furthermore, detailed knowledge of hMPV's mechanisms of immune modulation and its mode of viral persistence will contribute significantly to vaccine design and development, along with designing new antiviral agents (Panda et al., 2014).

Prevention and Control

Although there is no specific vaccine for hMPV (Ren et al., 2015)Several approaches can be taken to reduce its transmission and severity. These include vaccination, antiviral treatment, infection control measures, and public health interventions.

Vaccination and Immunization

Residual development of a functional vaccine for hMPV thus constitutes one area that researchers are keenly focusing on in the area of respiratory viruses.

Though one vaccine targeting hMPV has not been licensed yet, the molecular biology of the virus, especially of the attachment protein, is of vital interest in developing potential vaccines. It allows the design of vaccines that can evoke immunity and block infection, since the attachment protein helps the virus gain entry into the host cells. Studies such as Liu L. help to find such targets in vaccines which might prevent binding of the virus to the host cells and eventually lighten the clinical burden (Liu, 2008).

As its relevance to respiratory viruses like hMPV, Carrico J. emphasizes vaccines as the only means of pre-exposure prevention against such infections as RSV that present strong similarities with hMPV. Vaccine intervention against RSV has already been proven to lower the attack rate of severe disease, especially in high-risk populations, which would be infants and the elderly. A similar strategy for hMPV may be very effective at preventing not only direct healthcare costs but also indirect productivity losses that occur with severe infections (Carrico et al., 2024).

Antiviral Treatments

Even though hMPV vaccines are under development, antiviral therapy is still one of the effective control strategies against the virus. Antiviral drugs that target the viral replication process or its attachment to host cells are being developed (Kausar et al., 2021). In this regard, Pacheco G. A. Bacterial and viral coinfections with RSV have been described, pointing to the urgency of antiviral therapy as soon as possible to decrease the severity of the infection and complications. For hMPV, early antiviral intervention would help decrease the duration and intensity of symptoms and reduce hospitalizations and healthcare costs (Pacheco et al., 2021).

Infection Control Measures

Infection control in health care settings is important to prevent the transmission of hMPV, especially in pediatric or geriatric units, where patients are most susceptible to respiratory infections. The importance of infection control practices like hand hygiene, isolation of infected patients, and the use of personal protective equipment (PPE) in controlling the clinical and economic burden of RSV among Spanish children. These are just as effective for hMPV. It should be noted that proper respiratory hygiene measures, including masks and tissues covering coughs and sneezes, can effectively cut down the incidence of hMPV transmission within community settings during seasonal peaks of respiratory infections (Martinón-Torres et al., 2022).

Public Health Interventions

Public health campaigns are the most important to raise awareness regarding hMPV and its prevention strategies (Alıravcı et al., 2023; Leung et al., 2022). The early diagnosis and treatment of hMPV infections is a way of reducing the healthcare burden and enhancing patient outcomes. Surveillance systems monitoring the incidence of hMPV can be helpful in informing public health responses and resource allocation. These systems also allow for the identification of at-risk groups, such that interventions, such as antivirals or potential vaccines, will be targeted toward those most likely to suffer from severe disease (Wang et al., 2021).

Community and Environmental Measures

This measure will control environmental spread in school settings, day care, and hospitals through proper cleaning and disinfection of any surface where the virus might find its home. As discussed by Ramocha L. M., given that children may face pulmonary sequelae following infection by hMPV, the risk of transmission at this initial phase must be halted as much as possible. Reducing the overall incidence of respiratory infections and especially vulnerable populations by implementing effective community-level strategies: community awareness of the presence of hMPV, promotion of vaccinations for other respiratory pathogens, including influenza and RSV (Ramocha, 2022).

Integrated Approach to Prevention

Shared clinical features of hMPV and other respiratory viruses, such as RSV, influenza, and parainfluenza, require a concerted approach for prevention and control. Preventing coinfections by hMPV and other respiratory pathogens will likely diminish the disease severity and improve the clinical outcome. The approach would involve concomitant vaccination with a range of multiple respiratory viruses as well as the use of broad-spectrum antiviral drugs (Pacheco et al., 2021). Even though the development of vaccines and antiviral treatments for hMPV remains an open challenge, the combination of infection control measures, public health strategies, and research into antiviral therapies will be important in controlling the spread of hMPV (Shah et al., 2012). Seroprevalence analysis, which deals with the knowledge of the patterns of transmission of hMPV and its prevalence in the population, is fundamental for proper planning in prevention (Lu et al., 2011).

Future Directions

Future research should focus on optimizing vaccine formulations to induce long-lasting, broad-spectrum protection across age groups and immunocompromised individuals. Innovative delivery platforms, such as nanoparticle and virus-like particle vaccines, along with next-generation adjuvants, could enhance immunogenicity. Antiviral development must address resistance, safety, and delivery concerns through robust clinical trials. Additionally, host-targeted therapies, RNA-based technologies, and CRISPR-driven antiviral strategies represent promising areas for intervention. A multidisciplinary approach—integrating virology, immunology, bioengineering, and regulatory science—will be essential to accelerate clinical translation, ensure global access, and mitigate the burden of HMPV infections worldwide.

Conclusion

Human metapneumovirus (HMPV) continues to pose a significant public health challenge, particularly among high-risk populations such as infants, the elderly, and immunocompromised individuals. Despite decades of research, the absence of licensed vaccines or targeted antiviral therapies limits effective clinical management of severe cases. Recent advances—including various vaccine platforms, monoclonal antibodies, and small-molecule antivirals—have shown promising preclinical and early clinical results. However, translating these findings into safe, effective, and accessible treatments requires overcoming key challenges related to immune durability, viral diversity, and production scalability.

References

Alıravcı, I. D., Çelik, T., Çelik-Ekinci, S., & Hamidi, A. A. (2023). Bibliometric Analysis of Human Metapneumovirus Studies. *Infectious Diseases & Clinical Microbiology*, *5*(4), 311.

Babady, N. E. (2013). The FilmArray® respiratory panel: an automated, broadly multiplexed molecular test for the rapid and accurate detection of respiratory pathogens. *Expert review of molecular diagnostics*, *13*(8), 779-788.

Bakshi, S., Yadav, A., Dhankhar, S., Chauhan, S., Mahajan, S., & Singla, D. Annona Muricata: Unveiling its Potential as a Complementary and Alternative Cancer Therapy.

Bala, R., Madaan, R., Chauhan, S., Gupta, M., Dubey, A. K., Zahoor, I., Brijesh, H., Calina, D., & Sharifi-Rad, J. (2024). Revitalizing allicin for cancer therapy: Advances in formulation strategies to enhance bioavailability, stability, and clinical efficacy. *Naunyn-Schmiedeberg's Archives of Pharmacology*, *397*(2), 703-724.

Bastos, M. L., Tavaziva, G., Abidi, S. K., Campbell, J. R., Haraoui, L.-P., Johnston, J. C., Lan, Z., Law, S., MacLean, E., & Trajman, A. (2020). Diagnostic accuracy of serological tests for covid-19: systematic review and meta-analysis. *bmj*, *370*.

Boivin, G., De Serres, G., Côté, S., Gilca, R., Abed, Y., Rochette, L., Bergeron, M. G., & Déry, P. (2003). Human metapneumovirus infections in hospitalized children. *Emerging Infectious Diseases*, *9*(6), 634.

Carrico, J., Hicks, K. A., Wilson, E., Panozzo, C. A., & Ghaswalla, P. (2024). The annual economic burden of respiratory syncytial virus in adults in the United States. *The Journal of Infectious Diseases*, *230*(2), e342-e352.

De Zwart, A., Riezebos-Brilman, A., Lunter, G., Vonk, J., Glanville, A. R., Gottlieb, J., Permpalung, N., Kerstjens, H., Alffenaar, J.-W., & Verschuuren, E. (2022). Respiratory syncytial virus, human metapneumovirus, and parainfluenza virus infections in lung transplant recipients: a systematic review of outcomes and treatment strategies. *Clinical Infectious Diseases*, *74*(12), 2252-2260.

Deffrasnes, C., Hamelin, M.-E., & Boivin, G. (2007). Human metapneumovirus. Seminars in respiratory and critical care medicine,

Deffrasnes, C. l., Hamelin, M.-E. v., Prince, G. A., & Boivin, G. (2008). Identification and evaluation of a highly effective fusion inhibitor for human metapneumovirus. *Antimicrobial agents and chemotherapy*, *52*(1), 279-287.

Dinnes, J., Sharma, P., Berhane, S., van Wyk, S. S., Nyaaba, N., Domen, J., Taylor, M., Cunningham, J., Davenport, C., & Dittrich, S. (2022). Rapid, point-of-care antigen tests for diagnosis of SARS-CoV-2 infection. *Cochrane database of systematic reviews*(7).

El Chaer, F., Shah, D. P., Kmeid, J., Ariza-Heredia, E. J., Hosing, C. M., Mulanovich, V. E., & Chemaly, R. F. (2017). Burden of human metapneumovirus infections in patients with cancer: risk factors and outcomes. *Cancer*, *123*(12), 2329-2337.

Esposito, S., & Mastrolia, M. V. (2016). Metapneumovirus infections and respiratory complications. Seminars in respiratory and critical care medicine,

Feuillet, F., Lina, B., Rosa-Calatrava, M., & Boivin, G. (2012). Ten years of human metapneumovirus research. *Journal of Clinical Virology*, *53*(2), 97-105.

Garg, N., Farhat, J., Dhankhar, S., Chauhan, S., Bala, R., Madaan, R., Sharma, H., Saini, M., Singh, T. G., & Aldahish, A. A. Vincristine in Cancer Therapy: Mechanisms, Efficacy, and Future Perspectives. *Current medicinal chemistry*.

Haas, L. E., Thijsen, S. F., Van Elden, L., & Heemstra, K. A. (2013). Human metapneumovirus in adults. *Viruses*, *5*(1), 87-110.

Hamelin, M.-È., Abed, Y., & Boivin, G. (2004). Human metapneumovirus: a new player among respiratory viruses. *Clinical Infectious Diseases*, *38*(7), 983-990.

Hao, W., Wang, L., & Li, S. (2020). Roles of the non-structural proteins of influenza A virus. *Pathogens*, *9*(10), 812.

Hiebert, R. (2022). *Clinical Evaluation of the ONETest, a Target-Capture Next Generation Sequencing Platform for the Identification of Respiratory Pathogens* University of Toronto (Canada)].

Huang, H.-S., Tsai, C.-L., Chang, J., Hsu, T.-C., Lin, S., & Lee, C.-C. (2018). Multiplex PCR system for the rapid diagnosis of respiratory virus infection: systematic review and meta-analysis. *Clinical Microbiology and Infection*, *24*(10), 1055-1063.

Jeong, S., Park, M.-J., Song, W., & Kim, H.-S. (2020). Advances in laboratory assays for detecting human metapneumovirus. *Annals of Translational Medicine*, *8*(9).

Kahn, J. S. (2006). Epidemiology of human metapneumovirus. *Clinical microbiology reviews*, *19*(3), 546-557.

Kausar, S., Said Khan, F., Ishaq Mujeeb Ur Rehman, M., Akram, M., Riaz, M., Rasool, G., Hamid Khan, A., Saleem, I., Shamim, S., & Malik, A. (2021). A review: Mechanism of action of antiviral drugs. *International journal of immunopathology and pharmacology*, *35*, 20587384211002621.

Kciuk, M., Garg, N., Dhankhar, S., Saini, M., Mujwar, S., Devi, S., Chauhan, S., Singh, T. G., Singh, R., Marciniak, B., Gielecińska, A., & Kontek, R. (2024). Exploring the Comprehensive Neuroprotective and Anticancer Potential of Afzelin. *Pharmaceuticals*, *17*(6), 701. https://www.mdpi.com/1424-8247/17/6/701

Kim, J. I., Park, S., Lee, I., Park, K. S., Kwak, E. J., Moon, K. M., Lee, C. K., Bae, J.-Y., Park, M.-S., & Song, K.-J. (2016). Genome-wide analysis of human metapneumovirus evolution. *PloS one*, *11*(4), e0152962.

Kumar, P., & Srivastava, M. (2018). Prophylactic and therapeutic approaches for human metapneumovirus. *Virusdisease*, *29*(4), 434-444.

Leung, M.-W., O'Donoghue, M., & Suen, L. K.-P. (2022). Personal and household hygiene measures for preventing upper respiratory tract infections among children: a cross-sectional survey of parental knowledge, attitudes, and practices. *International Journal of Environmental Research and Public Health*, *20*(1), 229.

Liu, L. (2008). Molecular biology of human metapneumovirus (HMPV) attachment protein.

Lu, G., Gonzalez, R., Guo, L., Wu, C., Wu, J., Vernet, G., Paranhos-Baccalà, G., Wang, J., & Hung, T. (2011). Large-scale seroprevalence analysis of human metapneumovirus and human respiratory syncytial virus infections in Beijing, China. *Virology journal*, *8*, 1-10.

Mackay, I. M., Jacob, K. C., Woolhouse, D., Waller, K., Syrmis, M. W., Whiley, D. M., Siebert, D. J., Nissen, M., & Sloots, T. P. (2003). Molecular assays for detection of human metapneumovirus. *Journal of clinical microbiology*, *41*(1), 100-105.

Martinón-Torres, F., Carmo, M., Platero, L., Drago, G., López-Belmonte, J., Bangert, M., Díez-Domingo, J., & Garcés-Sánchez, M. (2022). Clinical and economic burden of respiratory syncytial virus in Spanish children: the BARI study. *BMC Infectious Diseases*, *22*(1), 759.

Mittal, P., Dhankhar, S., Chauhan, S., Garg, N., Bhattacharya, T., Ali, M., Chaudhary, A. A., Rudayni, H. A., Al-Zharani, M., & Ahmad, W. (2023). A Review on Natural Antioxidants for Their Role in the Treatment of Parkinson's Disease. *Pharmaceuticals*, *16*(7), 908.

Moe, N., Krokstad, S., Stenseng, I. H., Christensen, A., Skanke, L. H., Risnes, K. R., Nordbø, S. A., & Døllner, H. (2017). Comparing human metapneumovirus and respiratory syncytial virus: viral co-detections, genotypes and risk factors for severe disease. *PloS one*, *12*(1), e0170200.

Nelson, P. P., Rath, B. A., Fragkou, P. C., Antalis, E., Tsiodras, S., & Skevaki, C. (2020). Current and future point-of-care tests for emerging and new respiratory viruses and future perspectives. *Frontiers in cellular and infection microbiology*, *10*, 181.

Pacheco, G. A., Gálvez, N. M., Soto, J. A., Andrade, C. A., & Kalergis, A. M. (2021). Bacterial and viral coinfections with the human respiratory syncytial virus. *Microorganisms*, *9*(6), 1293.

Panda, S., Mohakud, N. K., Pena, L., & Kumar, S. (2014). Human metapneumovirus: review of an important respiratory pathogen. *International journal of infectious diseases*, *25*, 45-52.

Principi, N., & Esposito, S. (2014). Paediatric human metapneumovirus infection: epidemiology, prevention and therapy. *Journal of Clinical Virology*, *59*(3), 141-147.

Ramocha, L. M. (2022). *Epidemiology and pulmonary sequelae in children with human metapneumovirus associated lower respiratory tract infection* School of Pathology, Faculty of Health Sciences, University of the Witwatersrand].

Ren, J., Phan, T., & Bao, X. (2015). Recent vaccine development for human metapneumovirus. *Journal of General Virology*, *96*(Pt_7), 1515-1520.

Russell, C. J., Penkert, R. R., Kim, S., & Hurwitz, J. L. (2020). Human metapneumovirus: a largely unrecognized threat to human health. *Pathogens*, *9*(2), 109.

Shafagati, N., & Williams, J. (2018). Human metapneumovirus-what we know now. *F1000Research*, *7*.

Shah, D. P., Ghantoji, S. S., Mulanovich, V. E., Ariza-Heredia, E. J., & Chemaly, R. F. (2012). Management of respiratory viral infections in hematopoietic cell transplant recipients. *American journal of blood research*, *2*(4), 203.

Tang, Y. W., & Crowe, J., James E. (2011). Respiratory syncytial virus and human metapneumovirus. *Manual of clinical microbiology*, 1357-1371.

Van den Hoogen, B. G., de Jong, J. C., Groen, J., Kuiken, T., de Groot, R., Fouchier, R. A., & Osterhaus, A. D. (2001). A newly discovered human pneumovirus isolated from young children with respiratory tract disease. *Nature medicine*, *7*(6), 719-724.

Vargas, S. O., Kozakewich, H. P., Perez-Atayde, A. R., & McAdam, A. J. (2004). Pathology of human metapneumovirus infection: insights into the pathogenesis of a newly identified respiratory virus. *Pediatric and Developmental Pathology*, *7*(5), 478-486.

Wang, X., Li, Y., Deloria-Knoll, M., Madhi, S. A., Cohen, C., Ali, A., Basnet, S., Bassat, Q., Brooks, W. A., & Chittaganpitch, M. (2021). Global burden of acute lower respiratory infection associated with human metapneumovirus in children under 5 years in 2018: a systematic review and modelling study. *The Lancet Global Health*, *9*(1), e33-e43.

Zhao, Y., Chahar, H. S., Komaravelli, N., Dossumbekova, A., & Casola, A. (2019). Human metapneumovirus infection of airway epithelial cells is associated with changes in core metabolic pathways. *Virology*, *531*, 183-191.

About the Editors

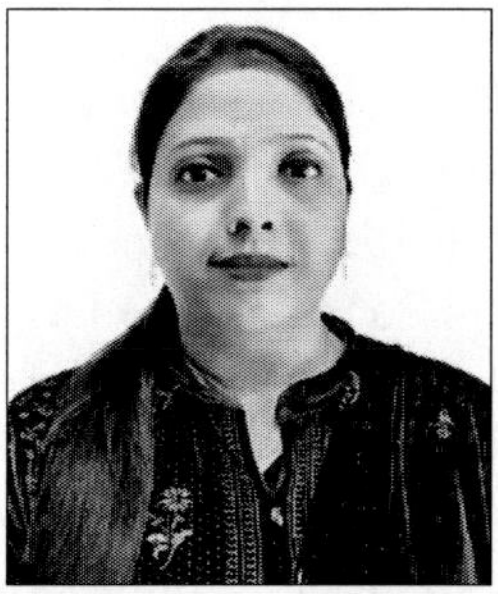

Dr. Anjali Sharma is presently working as an Associate Professor (Pharmaceutics) at Guru Gobind Singh College of Pharmacy, Yamuna Nagar, Haryana, India. She holds a B. Pharm. from Pt. B. D. Sharma University of Health Sciences, Rohtak, Haryana (India); an M. Pharm in Pharmaceutics from Uttarakhand Technical University, Dehradun, Uttarakhand, India (78.6%), and a PhD from Shobhit University, Gangoh, Uttar Pradesh, India. With over eleven years of teaching experience, including six years at the postgraduate level, she has mentored 10 M. Pharm (02 ongoing) and 03 PhD (ongoing) students. Her research focuses on nanotechnology-based drug delivery systems, enhancing drug efficacy and patient compliance. She has authored 50 research/review articles, 45 book chapters, four books, and holds 12 design patents and five copyrights. A committed educator and researcher, she is a Life Member of APTI and IPGA. Her excellence has been recognized through prestigious awards, including the Young Scientist Award (2021), Research Excellence Award (2023 & 2024), Global Faculty Award (2023), and Inspiring Academician Award (2024) by IPGA Uttarakhand State Branch. She has also been honored by the Bureau of Indian Standards (BIS) and other esteemed organizations for her contributions to science, education, and society.

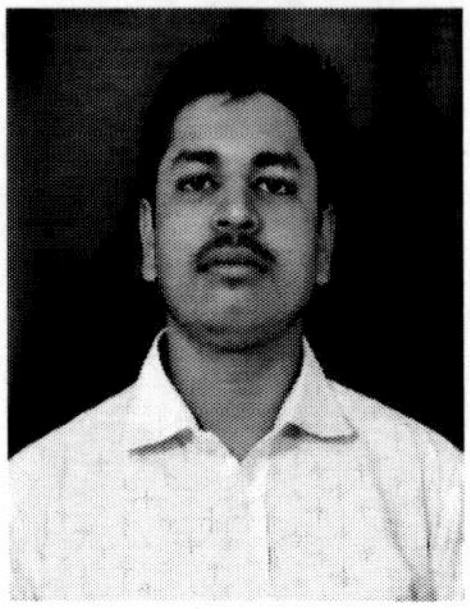

Mr. Vishnu Mittal is currently serving as an Assistant Professor at Adesh Institute of Pharmacy and Biomedical Sciences, Adesh University, Bathinda, Punjab, India. He holds both his Bachelor's and Master's degrees in Pharmacy (Pharmaceutics) from Pt. B. D. Sharma University of Health Sciences, Rohtak, has an impressive academic record. His primary research interests lie in the development of novel drug delivery systems aimed at enhancing drug efficacy and patient compliance. Mr. Mittal has authored over 20 research and review articles and contributed to around 20 book chapters, reflecting his scholarly dedication and innovative approach. Beyond his research, he actively engages in academic enrichment and professional development. He has participated in more than 25 conferences, workshops, and Faculty Development Programs (FDPs), sharing insights and collaborating with peers to stay abreast of emerging trends in the pharmaceutical domain. His achievements have earned him several recognitions, including the Indian Book of Records honor and awards for academic excellence and poster presentations.

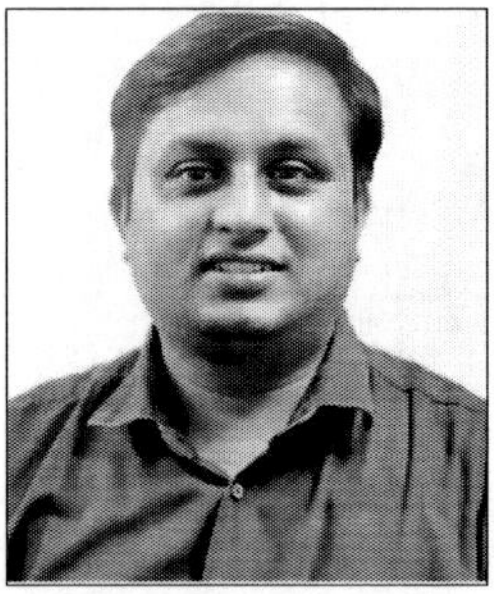

Dr. Devkant Sharma is currently an associate professor at Ch. Devi Lal College of Pharmacy, Jagadhri, Yamuna Nagar, Haryana (India). He holds a Bachelor of Pharmacy from Pt. B. D. Sharma University of Health Sciences,

Rohtak, Haryana (India); a Master of Pharmacy (Pharmaceutics) from Punjab Technical University, Jalandhar, Punjab (India), and a PhD in Pharmaceutical Sciences from Shobhit University, Gangoh (Uttar Pradesh, India). With over 12 years of teaching experience, Dr. Sharma has developed deep expertise in lipid-based drug delivery systems, which form the core of his research interests. He is presently supervising one M. Pharm. and two PhD scholars, contributing actively to academic mentorship and research development. Received the Pharma Excellence Award (2024) by IPGA Uttarakhand State Branch. Dr. Sharma has an impressive scholarly output, with 30 research and review articles, 40 book chapters, and three authored books to his credit. He also holds ten design patents and five copyrights, reflecting his commitment to innovation in pharmaceutical sciences.

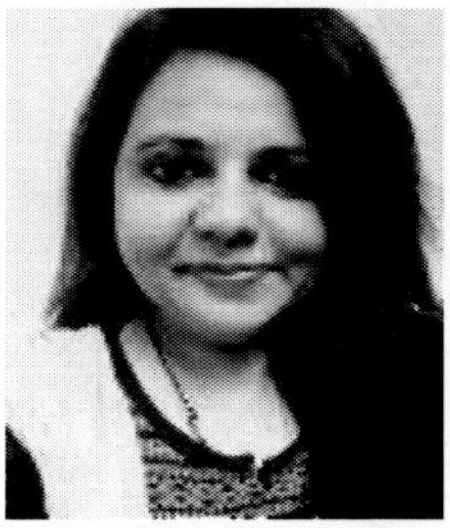

Professor (Dr.) Himani Bajaj is currently serving as Professor of Pharmaceutics at Adarsh Vijendra Institute of Pharmaceutical Sciences, Shobhit University, Gangoh, Saharanpur (U.P.), India. She holds a PhD in Pharmaceutical Sciences from Kumaun University, Bhimtal Campus, Nainital; an MPharm in Pharmaceutics from Hemwati Nandan Bahuguna Garhwal University, Srinagar (Uttarakhand); and a BPharm (Gold Medalist) from Sardar Bhagwan Singh Post Graduate Institute of Biomedical Sciences & Research, Dehradun. Her research expertise lies in the design and development of transdermal and novel drug delivery systems. Dr. Bajaj's academic and research excellence been widely recognized with numerous accolades, including the Best Researcher Award (2023), International Best Researcher Award (2024), Shodh Ratna Award (2023), and the Women Iconic Achievers Award (2025). She has also been honored with certificates and awards from the Smart Education Welfare Association, the Shoonya Foundation, and Aaron Education Welfare for her significant contributions to research and education.

List of Contributors

Abhishek Kumar Mishra
Medpharm, Durham, NC, USA

Akansha Kushwaha
Anjali College of Pharmacy and Science
Etmadpur, Agra, Uttar Pradesh (UP), India

Akash Jain
M. M. College of Pharmacy
M. M. (Deemed to be University)
Mullana, Ambala, Haryana

Akashdeep Singh
Chitkara College of Pharmacy
Chitkara University
Rajpura-140401, Punjab, India

Anand Singh Chouhan
ShriRam College of Pharmacy
Banmore, MP

Anjali Sharma
Guru Gobind Singh College of Pharmacy
Yamunanagar, Haryana-135001

Ankita Verma
ShriRam College of Pharmacy
Banmore, MP

Anu Chaudhary
Global Research Institute of Pharmacy
Nachraun, Radaur, Haryana

Anupama Ojha
Department of Biochemistry
Shri Gorakshnath Medical College Hospital and Research Center
Mahayogi Gorakhnath University
Gorakhpur, Sonbarsa-273007
Gorakhpur, India

Arun Thakur
Chitkara College of Pharmacy
Chitkara University
Punjab-140401, India

Biruk Demisse Ayalew
Infectious Disease Unit, Department of Internal Medicine
St. Paul's Hospital Millennium Medical College
Addis Ababa, Ethiopia

Deepak Singla
Guru Gobind Singh College of Pharmacy
135001, Haryana

Deepshi Arora
Guru Gobind Singh College of Pharmacy
135001, Haryana

Ganga Reddy Velma
Department of Pharmacology and Toxicology
R. K. Coit, College of Pharmacy
University of Arizona
Tucson, United States

Garima Maurya
Maharana Pratap College of Pharmaceutical Sciences
Kanpur UP

Gaurav Gupta
Centre for Medical and Bio-allied Health Sciences Research
Ajman University, Ajman, UAE
Centre for Research Impact & Outcome
Chitkara College of Pharmacy
Chitkara University, Punjab, India 140401

Habib Omari Ramadhani
Institute of Human Virology
University of Maryland School of Medicine

Himanshu Sharma
Chitkara College of Pharmacy
Chitkara University, Rajpura-140401
Punjab, India

Jasmine Chaudhary
M. M. College of Pharmacy
M. M. (Deemed to be University)
Mullana, Ambala, Haryana

Jeewon Rajesh
Department of Zoology
College of Science
King Saud University
P.O. Box 2455
Riyadh 11451, Saudi Arabia.

Kotthapalli Prashanth
Department of Microbiology
JSS Academy of Higher Education and Research
Mysuru, Karnataka, 570015, India

Md Jawaid Akhtar
Department of Pharmaceutical Chemistry
National University of Science and Technology
PO 620, PC 130, Azaiba Bousher, Musca
Sultanate of Oman

Mirunalini Gobinath
Department of Pharmacognosy and & Phytopharmacy
JSS College of Pharmacy
JSS Academy of Higher Education & Research
Ooty-643001, Tamil Nadu, India

Mohd Aftab Siddiqui
Faculty of Pharmacy
Integral University
Lucknow, U.P., India

Monika Saini
M. M. College of Pharmacy
Maharishi Markandeshwar University Campus
Mullana, Haryana 133207

Muskan
Guru Gobind Singh College of Pharmacy
Yamunanagar, Haryana-135001

Muskan Shingari
Guru Gobind Singh College of Pharmacy
Yamunanagar (135001), Haryana

Naina Mohamed Pakkir Maideen
Clinical Associate Professor of Pharmacology
College of Medicine
Mohammed Bin Rashid University of Medicine and Health Sciences
Dubai. UAE; Pharmacologist, Dubai Health, Dubai, UAE.

Neha Saini
Global Research Institute of Pharmacy
Nachraun, Radaur, Haryana

Nidhi Rani
Chitkara College of Pharmacy
Chitkara University, Punjab, India

Nikhil
M. M. College of Pharmacy
M. M. (Deemed to be University)
Mullana, Ambala, Haryana

Nourhan Saeed Bakry
Senior Research Associate
57357 Children's Cancer Hospital, Egypt.

Pallavi
Amity Institute of Pharmacy
Amity University
Rajasthan, Jaipur, India, 303002

Parthasarathi Behera
Department of Health Sciences
International Centre for Genetic Engineering and Biotechnology (ICGEB)
Aruna Asif Ali Marg, New Delhi – 110067, India

Pooja Mittal
GITAM School of Pharmacy
GITAM (Deemed to be) University
Rudraram, Patancheru, Sangareddy District
Hyderabad-502329

Prabhjot Kaur
Guru Gobind Singh College of Pharmacy
Yamunanagar, Haryana-135001

Prachi Shrivastava
Anjali College of Pharmacy and Science
Etmadpur, Agra, Uttar Pradesh (UP), India.

Pranjal Sachan
Sanskriti College of Higher Education and Studies
Bhognipur Kanpur Dehat
Uttar Pradesh (UP) 209111 India

Priya Sahani
Department of Biotechnology
Deen Dayal Upadhyaya Gorakhpur University
Gorakhpur 273009, Uttar Pradesh, India.

Priyanka Kriplani
Guru Gobind Singh College of Pharmacy
Yamunanagar, Haryana-135001

Rita Saini
Department of Pharmacy
Shree Dev Bhoomi Institute of Education, Science and Technology
Pondha, Dehradun, Uttarakhand, India

Romi Rajput
Ch. DeviLal College of Pharmacy
Jagadhri (135003), Haryana

Sahil Dhiman
Guru Gobind Singh College of Pharmacy
135001, Haryana

Samrat Chauhan
Chitkara College of Pharmacy
Chitkara University, Punjab-140401, India

Sanchit Dhankhar
Chitkara College of Pharmacy
Chitkara University, Punjab-140401, India

Sandeep Singh
Adesh Institute of Pharmacy & Biomedical Sciences
Adesh University, Bathinda, Punjab, India,151101

Sanjana Mehta
Chitkara College of Pharmacy
Chitkara University
Punjab-140401, India

Sarad Kumar Mishra
Department of Biotechnology
Deen Dayal Upadhyaya Gorakhpur University
Gorakhpur 273009, Uttar Pradesh, India.

Shefali Mehla
University Institute of Pharma Sciences
Chandigarh University

Shivanand Patil
Department of Pharmacy
Shree Dev Bhoomi Institute of Education, Science and Technology
Pondha, Dehradun, Uttarakhand, India

Shivani Sharma
Global Research Institute of Pharmacy
Nachraun, Radaur, Haryana

Shree Rath
All India Institute of Medical Sciences
Bhubaneswar, India.

Shushank Mahajan
Chitkara College of Pharmacy
Chitkara University, Punjab-140401, India

Soundarya R
Department of Pharmaceutics
JSS College of Pharmacy
JSS Academy of Higher Education & Research
Mysuru-643001, Karnataka, India

Sumana Kumar
Department of Microbiology
JSS Academy of Higher Education and Research
Mysuru, Karnataka, 570015, India

Tejaswini Reddy Jeeru
Department of Pharmaceutical Chemistry
JSS College of Pharmacy
JSS Academy of Higher Education & Research
Ooty-643001, Tamil Nadu, India

Thakur Gurjeet Singh
Chitkara College of Pharmacy
Chitkara University, Punjab, India

Vaishali Kamboj
M. M. College of Pharmacy
M. M. (Deemed to be University)
Mullana, Ambala, Haryana

Vinay Jain
ShriRam College of Pharmacy
Banmore, MP

Vinit N. Deshmukh
Department of Molecular Biology & Genetics
Krishna Vishwa Vidyapeeth (Deemed to be University)
Malkapur, Karad (Dist - Satara), Maharashtra, India-415539

Vishnu Mittal
Department of Pharmaceutics
Adesh Institute of Pharmacy and Biomedical Sciences
Adesh University, Bathinda, Punjab, India, Pin-151101

Yunes M. M. A. Alsayadi
University Institute of Pharma Sciences
Chandigarh University

Zemichael Getu Alemayehu
Addis Ababa University
College of Health Sciences, School of Medicine
Addis Ababa, Ethiopia

Index

A

B

C

D

E

N

O

P

Q

R

S

T

U

V

W

X